PUBLIC HEALTH
Nursing
Practicing Population-Based Care

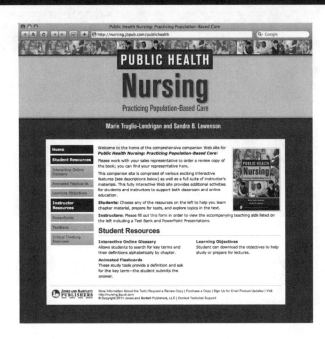

A companion Web site where students and instructors will find complete, current material to support the text!

For Instructors

PowerPoint Slides

Download our slides and use them in your course!

TestBank

Test your student's knowledge of key information with this downloadable TestBank! Use our questions exactly as they appear, or modify them to meet your needs.

Critical Thinking Exercises

Challenge students by using these exercises to further their understanding of topics covered chapter by chapter.

For Students

Animated Flash Cards

These study tools provide a definition and ask for the key term—the student submits the answer.

Interactive Glossary

Allows students to search for key terms and their definitions alphabetically by chapter.

Learning Objectives

Students can download the objectives to help study or prepare for lectures.

PUBLIC HEALTH
Nursing
Practicing Population-Based Care

Edited by

Marie Truglio-Londrigan, PhD, RN
Professor of Nursing
Mercy College
School of Health and Natural Sciences
Dobbs Ferry, New York

Sandra B. Lewenson, EdD, RN, FAAN
Professor
Lienhard School of Nursing
Pace University
Pleasantville, New York

JONES AND BARTLETT PUBLISHERS
Sudbury, Massachusetts
BOSTON   TORONTO   LONDON   SINGAPORE

World Headquarters

Jones and Bartlett Publishers	Jones and Bartlett Publishers	Jones and Bartlett Publishers
40 Tall Pine Drive	Canada	International
Sudbury, MA 01776	6339 Ormindale Way	Barb House, Barb Mews
978-443-5000	Mississauga, Ontario L5V 1J2	London W6 7PA
info@jbpub.com	Canada	United Kingdom
www.jbpub.com		

Jones and Bartlett's books and products are available through most bookstores and online booksellers. To contact Jones and Bartlett Publishers directly, call 800-832-0034, fax 978-443-8000, or visit our website, www.jbpub.com.

Substantial discounts on bulk quantities of Jones and Bartlett's publications are available to corporations, professional associations, and other qualified organizations. For details and specific discount information, contact the special sales department at Jones and Bartlett via the above contact information or send an email to specialsales@jbpub.com.

The authors, editor, and publisher have made every effort to provide accurate information. However, they are not responsible for errors, omissions, or for any outcomes related to the use of the contents of this book and take no responsibility for the use of the products and procedures described. Treatments and side effects described in this book may not be applicable to all people; likewise, some people may require a dose or experience a side effect that is not described herein. Drugs and medical devices are discussed that may have limited availability controlled by the Food and Drug Administration (FDA) for use only in a research study or clinical trial. Research, clinical practice, and government regulations often change the accepted standard in this field. When consideration is being given to use of any drug in the clinical setting, the health care provider or reader is responsible for determining FDA status of the drug, reading the package insert, and reviewing prescribing information for the most up-to-date recommendations on dose, precautions, and contraindications, and determining the appropriate usage for the product. This is especially important in the case of drugs that are new or seldom used.

Production Credits

Publisher: Kevin Sullivan
Acquisitions Editor: Amy Sibley
Associate Editor: Patricia Donnelly
Editorial Assistant: Rachel Shuster
Associate Production Editor: Lisa Cerrone
Marketing Manager: Rebecca Wasley
V.P., Manufacturing and Inventory
  Control: Therese Connell
Composition: Shepherd, Incorporated

Cover Design: Scott Moden
Cover Images: All courtesy of the Visiting Nurse
  Service of New York.
Printing and Binding: Malloy, Inc.
Cover Printing: Malloy, Inc.
Chapter opener photographic credits appear on
  page 393, which constitutes a continuation of the
  copyright page.

Library of Congress Cataloging-in-Publication Data

Public health nursing : practicing population-based care / [edited by] Marie Truglio-Londrigan, Sandra B. Lewenson.
    p. ; cm.
  Includes bibliographical references and index.
  ISBN-13: 978-0-7637-6654-2 (pbk.)
  ISBN-10: 0-7637-6654-2 (pbk.)
  1. Public health nursing—United States. 2. Evidence-based nursing—United States. I. Truglio-Londrigan, Marie. II. Lewenson, Sandra.
  [DNLM: 1. Public Health Nursing—United States. 2. Evidence-Based Nursing—United States. 3. Models, Organizational—United States. WY 108 P97625 2011]
  RT97.P8325 2011
  610.73'4—dc22
                                                                                            2009043593

6048

Printed in the United States of America
14 13 12 11 10   10 9 8 7 6 5 4 3 2 1

CONTENTS

FOREWORD

An honored nursing specialty, public health nursing is threaded through nursing history from its beginnings to the modern present. This book presents a fresh examination of the influences that shaped public health nursing and offers strategies to merge national issues and health agendas into public health nursing's agenda and activities.

Practicing Population-Based Care aptly describes the authors' intent for the reader, whether in global or local settings. Practical applications such as case vignettes, actual education and practice interventions, case findings, and advocacy case management represent the practice of population-based care of public health nursing. The strength of public health nursing within an interdisciplinary approach is foundational in all chapters.

Unique to the book, the editors created an innovative Public Health Nursing Assessment Tool (PHNAT), which incorporates nursing process and well-known documents, *Healthy People 2010* and the *Minnesota Department of Health Population-Based Public Health Nursing Practice Intervention Wheel*. Using a kaleidoscope approach, the focus shifts from simultaneous individual, family, or community assessments and provides the nurse with the ability to address priority needs in care. PHNAT may be expanded by the user and is designed for practice and education settings.

The voices of public health nurses like Lillian Wald and Florence Nightingale resonate with current and emerging health challenges such as SARS, Ebola, and the H1N1 pandemic. The authors present new ways that public health nurses are incorporating the latest knowledge and evidence-based practices to address health concerns in both the classroom and the practice arena. This text is comprehensive and contemporary while also being rich in history presented in an interesting, inviting manner.

In addition, the writers embrace new concepts concerning discrimination, social epidemiology, and technology. Broadening nursing's traditional epidemiological approach, social epidemiology is fully presented in usable, thought-provoking methods that include the little-discussed health effects of discrimination. Public health nurses share their experiences using new technologies in their practice. The authors discuss the potential that technology can have on the quality and outcomes in nurses' everyday practice.

All nurses are, indeed, public health nurses. To be effective, they must have knowledge, skills, and attitudes that incorporate the essence of public health nursing. As a timely and thought-provoking publication, this text will provide those foundations for both the new and seasoned public health nurse.

Cathleen M. Shultz, PhD, RN, CNE, FAAN
Dean and Professor of Nursing
College of Nursing
Harding University
Searcy, Arkansas

PREFACE

That morning's experience was a baptism of fire. . . . On my way from the sick-room to my comfortable student quarters my mind was intent on my own responsibility. To my inexperience it seemed certain that conditions such as these were allowed because people did not *know,* and for me there was a challenge to know and to tell. (Wald, 1915, p. 8)

The public's health involves all nurses in all settings. Whether nurses work in the emergency room, the operating room, a medical–surgical unit, an ambulatory care clinic, home care, or in schools, the idea of public health should permeate their educational and work experiences. The question of how to provide public health nursing using a population focus has been a dilemma throughout history and has created challenges to the way public health nursing is taught and practiced in the United States. Nursing leader Virginia Henderson saw an important connection between public health nursing and nursing of the individual when she said, "I think it is impossible to nurse an aggregate effectively until you have effectively nursed individuals and acquired considerable judgment as to what helps clients or patients prevent disease, cope with it, or die with dignity when death is inevitable" (Abrams, 2007, p. 384). To care for populations, as this is what public health nursing is about, nurses need to place the individual, family, and population within the context of community and the myriad environmental, social, economic, political, ethnic, and gender factors that influence health. Public health nurses share the unique ability to be able to see the relevancy of health-promoting programs while caring for the individual, family, and population.

GETTING STARTED

Raising Questions

Truglio-Londrigan and Lewenson, both public health nurse educators, conceived of this text as a way of exploring what it means to practice population-based public health nursing. The questions they raised about public health nursing at curriculum meetings, in the classroom, and in clinical settings led to the writing of this book. For example, they asked, "How do you provide clinical experiences in public health? Do students only need 'carry the bag' type experiences usually found in voluntary visiting nurses service associations, or should they also have surveillance-type activities found in publicly funded health departments? Or, should they have both?" Often, they argued that students could learn public health nursing by offering blood pressure screenings at social service type agencies, such as the Henry Street Settlement in New York City or at a recycling bottling plant near a homeless shelter, or even in a local shopping center. Other questions emerged that expanded their thinking, such as "How can evidence-based practice and technology be integrated into the work of public health nurses and how can we use history to explain how public health nursing has been defined over the past hundred years?" Questions about diversity and cultural competence became relevant as the authors further explored the ways to convey the concepts of public health to students, faculty, and other healthcare professionals. How can we speak to diversity and relate this to students and nurses engaged in the practice of public health nursing? And, finally, they wanted to understand what so many nurses have already asked, "What is public health nursing?"

These questions compelled Truglio-Londrigan and Lewenson to explore the books that were already published in public health and community health nursing. Although many excellent texts exist, there still seemed to be confusion about the differences between public health and community, and these differences led them to seek greater clarity.

Public Health Nursing: Practicing Population-Based Care offers a variety of different perspectives on community and public health nursing from other texts already being used. For example, the authors address the relevance of historical evidence in coming to know the meaning of the terms used to describe public health nursing, disaster nursing, and global perspectives; they explore the use of technology in public health; they provide the meaning of social epidemiology as well as the traditional content on epidemiology; and they offer an innovatively designed assessment tool that uses *Healthy People 2010: A Systematic Approach to Health Improvement,* as its framework. Another highlight of this text is the focus on the 17 intervention strategies identified in the *Population-Based Public Health Nursing Practice Intervention Wheel* developed by the Minnesota Department of Health in the mid 1990s. In addition, they examine how these interventions may be applied throughout the three levels of practice: individual/family, community, and systems levels (Minnesota Department of Health, 2001; Keller, Strohschein, & Briske, 2008). *Public Health Nursing: Practicing Population-Based Care* aims to add greater clarity to the body of public health nursing literature and serve as a useful tool for educators, students, and practitioners of public health nursing.

Audience for Text

This text can be used by nursing students in both baccalaureate and graduate degree programs. In addition, all nurses, whether practicing in public health, community health, or home care settings, would benefit from this book because it offers a way to understand how care of the individual, family, and population relates to larger systems and the care of communities. Nurses in the ever-expanding long-term care settings and acute care settings in the community will also find this book useful in their practice.

ORGANIZATION AND PEDAGOGICAL FEATURES OF TEXT

Each chapter begins with a quote and a photograph from nursing history that resonates with the content of the chapter. Objectives and key terms for each chapter offer direction to the reader as to what can be expected. Those chapters that address public health intervention strategies contain case studies. The use of history as evidence is threaded throughout the chapters where it illuminates the didactic content and case studies. To aid the reader further, a glossary defining the various key terms used in the text can be found at the end of the text. Although the authors wrote several chapters, they turned to experts to write many of the chapters throughout the text. These contributing authors represent a cadre of outstanding nursing professionals who were willing to rethink the way they practice and share their thoughts with the reader. Another unique feature of this book is that each contributor's "voice" can be heard in their own chapter. This means that consistency of style and pedagogy was purposely avoided by the authors so they could showcase a diversity of ideas in how to approach public health nursing.

The first chapter, "What Is Public Health and Public Health Nursing?" explores the ideas of health promotion and disease prevention and refers the reader to the evolutionary nature of nursing activities in primary, secondary, and tertiary prevention. Nursing care, Truglio-Londrigan and Lewenson point out, especially public health nursing, is not a linear process. Henderson's question raised earlier speaks to this nonlinear approach and encourages us to think about providing care for disease while simultaneously promoting health. This first chapter includes definitions of public health and public health nursing, the three core functions of public health, and the ten essential public health services, an explanation of Health People 2010. Truglio-Londrigan and Lewenson use these various documents and meanings of public health to help explain the work of public health nurses.

The reader finds an unusual approach to public health nursing history in Chapter 2, "Public Health Nursing in the United States: A History." Lewenson approaches this chapter from the standpoint of how changing definitions show the social, political, and economic influences that altered the work of nurses in the home setting. The author turns to past nursing leaders in public health nursing and examines how they defined public health nursing. Instead of writing a traditional history of public health nursing, Lewenson uses the past to explain the tensions that exist between and among the various titles nurses have used to delineate care provided in the community. District nurse, health visitor, public health nurse, community health nurse, and home care nurse are among the names used. These changing definitions and titles show the evolutionary nature of public health nursing and the response of these nurses to the social, political, and economic environment. The use of historical evidence also offers insight into the questions Truglio-Londrigan and Lewenson asked, including "What is public health nursing?," "How is public health nursing different from community health nursing or home care nursing?," and "How do we educate students into the role of public health nursing when the names and contextual meanings change over time?"

Chapter 3, "Assessment: Using the Public Health Nursing Assessment Tool," presents the innovative public health nursing assessment tool (PHNAT) designed by Lewenson and Truglio-Londrigan. The PHNAT engages nurses, nursing students, and public health nurses in an assessment process that applies the systematic approach to health improvement presented in Healthy People 2010 (U.S. Department of Health and Human Services, 2000, p. 6) with specific emphasis placed on the determinants of health and health status. In addition, the PHNAT directs the reader to use the intervention wheel interventions because they identify community healthcare needs, goals, plans, and evaluations. This chapter sees assessment as fluid process, and the PHNAT offers the user a kaleidoscopic view of this process.

In Chapter 4, "Fundamentals of Epidemiology and Social Epidemiology," Susan Moscou presents the science of epidemiology. Moscou begins the chapter with a discussion of the history of epidemiology that highlights two epidemiological revolutions. The chapter covers the terms descriptive epidemiology, analytic epidemiology, the epidemiologic triad, and the chain of infection. The author then introduces social epidemiology and the social determinants of health in the second part of the chapter. Comparison between epidemiology and social epidemiology provide the reader with an understanding between the two and allows for greater application of the concepts.

Joanne K. Singleton, Teresa Haines, Rona F. Levin, and Jon Barone contribute their expertise to Chapter 5, "Evidenced-Based Practice From a Public Health Nursing Perspective." This chapter defines the meaning of evidence-based practice, specifically focusing on public health nurses. Through the examples and case study, the authors describe a systematic approach to finding best available evidence. Specifically, they explore the application of evidence-based practice to public health issues of health literacy and tobacco use. The case study allows the reader to gain insight into how a public health nurse can use an evidence-based approach to improve the health of a local community.

Chapter 6, "Applying Technology in Public Health Nursing," approaches technology in public health nursing from the perspective of how public health nurses use technology in their practice. Martha Kelly with Lewenson and Truglio-Londrigan begin the chapter with the rational for including technology in practice. They define the various concepts needed to understand nursing informatics and explore the use and acceptance of technology in public health nursing practice. The authors use case studies from nurses who work in public health and have firsthand experience adapting to technology in the workplace. The case studies highlight issues related to introducing laptops, pagers, nursing informatics systems, and other forms of technology into practice. Their case studies give insight into how technology can be incorporated into practice.

Astrid Hellier Wilson and Mary de Chesnay contributed Chapter 7, "Considerations of Culture in the Health of the Public." In this chapter Wilson and de Chesnay define the subconcepts associated with culture. They compare and contrast public health issues in terms of cultural influences and provide analysis of public health nursing interventions for selected cases in terms of cultural competence. Wilson and de Chesnay explore the meaning of culture, ethnocentrism, xenophobia, and ritual and what it means to be a participant observer and relate to the meaning of culturally competent care in public health. Throughout this chapter they ask the reader to participate in "field observations" that allow for active learning and self-reflection.

The next five chapters address the strategies found on the intervention wheel. These intervention strategies have been separated out into five themes: Hitting the Pavement, Running the Show, Working It Out, Working Together, and Getting the Word Out. One of the assumptions of the intervention wheel includes the idea that public health nurses apply the nursing process to the multiple levels of practice including the individual/family, community, and systems (Keller, Strohschein, & Briske, 2008). Each intervention chapter explains a particular portion of the wheel and includes a vignette or case study that highlights the interventions and levels of practice.

Chapter 8, "Hitting the Pavement," refers to the outreach, case finding, screening, surveillance, and disease and health event investigation strategies that are found on the red wedge of the intervention wheel. The authors of this chapter, Margaret Macali, Karen Galanowsky, Monte Wagner, and Truglio-Londrigan, divide the chapter into several sections. The first section describes the key intervention strategies. The second section demonstrates the application of these intervention strategies within the context of several public health issues. The third provides a case study to help the reader understand the process of these interventions as they are applied to the various levels of practice including individual/family, community, and system.

In Chapter 9, "Running the Show," Janna Dieckmann addresses three important public health interventions found in the green wedge of the intervention wheel: referral and follow-up, case management, and delegated functions. Dieckmann writes that these interventions have similarities, may overlap, and may be addressed toward similar working objectives. All three interventions draw the public health nurse to stretch beyond the nurse–client dyad, as the nurse seeks to add the contributions of other community services and health providers to improve the system for client support and change. At the community practice level, this means the public health nurse participates in initiating services or expanding availability/access to meet an identified need. At the systems practice level, the public health nurse modifies organizations and policies that shape systems of care. At the individual/family practice level, the public health nurse uses interventions designed to change knowledge, attitudes, beliefs, practices, and behaviors (Rippke, Briske, Keller, Strohschein, & Simonetti, 2001).

In Lin Drury's Chapter 10, "Working It Out," the reader returns to the modern-day Henry Street Settlement where Lillian Wald first introduced the idea of public health nursing in 1893. Drury focuses on the blue wedge of the intervention wheel, specifically focusing on intervention strategies that include counseling, consultation, and health teaching. The chapter defines and describes these strategies, then identifies an issue in public health practice, and finally demonstrates via a case study the "applying" and the "doing" of these interventions. The case study refers to the Henry Street Settlement, now a not-for-profit social service institution located on the Lower East Side of Manhattan in New York City. This settlement supports the needs of the vulnerable populations who live in the community, expanding over the years to include 19 sites such as day care centers, youth groups, work force training, homeless shelters, mental health centers, summer camps, senior centers, and in the performing arts. Drury uses the Henry Street Settlement and the multicultural community it serves as a case study for public health nursing interventions that she and her students at Pace University in New York City have brought back to Henry Street.

In Chapter 11, "Working Together," author Adrienne Wald presents the strategies found in the orange wedge of the intervention wheel. The chapter explores the interventions of collaboration, coalition building, and community organizing. This chapter devotes a separate section to each of the three interventions and then as a collective action. As in all the chapters, this chapter describes the best evidence-based practices that address the issue of physical inactivity. The application of these interventions to this important 21st century public health crisis illustrates how each intervention strategy works and reinforces key concepts.

In Chapter 12, "Getting the Word Out," Susan Moscou addresses the interventions found on the yellow wedge of the intervention wheel. These strategies include advocacy, social marketing, and policy development and enforcement of public health nursing interventions. Moscou identifies obesity as one of the major public health issues in the United States. Moscou focuses specifically on obesity in children, primarily in junior high school, using a case study that highlights this public health issue. The case study depicts how the public health nurse engages in the application and the doing of the three interventions—advocacy, social marketing, and policy development—and enforcement through the three levels of public health practice.

The final chapters move the reader from the intervention wheel to issues reflecting global perspectives, disaster nursing, economic issues, and finally public health nursing education. Here the text draws from history, economics, and education to provide a unique way of presenting the content to the reader.

Christine Hallett, in Chapter 13, "Protecting, Sustaining, and Empowering: An Historical Perspective on the Control of Epidemics," traces the means by which humans have attempted to eradicate certain of those "bugs" they consider harmful: the bacteria and viruses that cause epidemic and endemic infections. Hallett uses three case studies showcasing specific diseases appearing at specific historical moments: bubonic plague, as it appeared in the Early Modern Italian city states during the 16th and 17th centuries; Spanish influenza as it appeared in the cities of the United States in 1918 and 1919; and AIDS as it appeared in the United Kingdom during the 1980s. From this historical perspective the reader explores the ways in which human societies have attempted to combat global epidemics. They learn the role the nurse has played working alongside governments, doctors, and scientists in the prevention of epidemic diseases. In addition, Hallett explores the nurse's role in the treatment and care of patients with life-threatening infectious diseases at different historical moments and in different places.

In Chapter 14, "Historical Highlights in Disaster Nursing," Barbara Mann Wall and Arlene Keeling continue to use an historical perspective as they examine the role of public health nurses in disasters. Wall and Keeling state that "evidence for practice for disaster management logically comes from history." They turn to history to gain an understanding of what has worked in the past and recognize that nurses' contributions in the past are "often overlooked" and seen as "routine." Wall and Keeling presents nurses' response to several late 19th and 20th century disasters, including the yellow fever epidemic of 1888, the Johnstown flood of 1889, the 1900 Galveston hurricane, the 1918 influenza pandemic, the 1947 Texas City ship explosion, and the 1964 Alaska earthquake. The experiences learned during these disasters become a rich source of evidence for nurses today addressing modern-day disasters.

Public health nursing does not exist in a vacuum and is responsive to economic factors that all citizens experience. In Chapter 15, "Public Health: Costs, Challenges, and Considerations," Mary Alice Donius discusses the present state of the U.S. healthcare system with regard to cost and care. Donius describes the five principle participants ("the 5 P's") in the healthcare delivery system as the (1) purchasers, (2) payers, (3) providers, (4) patients or populations, and (5) policymakers. Donius also explains how the often-competing interests of these 5 P's create negative healthcare outcomes. The chapter looks at how federal dollars support the public health infrastructure, and they use case studies in both the public and private section to examine the ways and means public health nurse may reconsider the delivery of health care from a public health perspective.

In the final chapter, Cathleen Shultz and Karen Kelley address the need to include public health in nursing curricular. Chapter 16, "Nursing Education and Public Health Nursing," challenges nurse educators to respond to the public health needs of society both locally and globally. Shultz and Kelley use their own institution, Hardy University in Searcy, Arkansas, as an example where faculty must create the clinical experiences that integrate public health nursing concepts into the curriculum. Some of the student clinical experiences that Shultz and Kelley present include wellness screening, simulation experiences, disaster drills, mass immunization drill, service learning, faith-based clinic, and school health screening. The chapter explores the shift from a local to a global world view and looks at concepts of social justice and the culture of poverty. This final chapter shows how the various issues and intervention strategies found throughout *Public Health Nursing: Practicing Population-Based Care* can be brought into the classroom to create the nurses we need in the future.

Public Health Nursing: Practicing Population-Based Care offers the reader a broad view of public health nursing, encouraging all nurses to consider themselves public health nurses. It is only through the applying and doing of public health nursing that society may attain the goal expressed in the historic 1978 Declaration of Alma-Ata of "Health for All" (International Conference on Primary Health Care, 1978). This call to action reverberates throughout nursing's rich history then and now. As early public health nursing leader, Edna Foley wrote the following in 1921:

> Public Health means health for all. . . . Good health is the inalienable right of every citizen, man, woman, or child, and since this vague, almost unknown quality is the right of every citizen, should not good public health nursing be the concern of the laity, as well as of the handful of nurses who are struggling with this big problem? (1991/1922, p. 135)

References

Abrams, S. E. (2007). Nursing the community, a look back at the 1984 dialogue between Virginia Henderson and Sherry L. Shamansky. *Public Health Nursing, 24*(4), 382–386.

Foley, E. L. (1991/1922). Main issues in public health nursing. In N. Birnbach & S. B. Lewenson (Eds.), *First words: Selected addresses from the National League for Nursing 1894–1933* (pp. 133–137). New York: National League for Nursing.

International Conference on Primary Health Care. (1978). *Declaration of Alma-Ata.* Retrieved January 28, 2009 from www.who.int/hpr/NPH/docs/declaration_almaata.pdf

Keller, L., Strohschein, S., & Briske, L. (2008). Population-based public health nursing practice: The intervention wheel. In M. Stanhope & J. Lancaster (Eds.), *Public health nursing: Population-centered health care in the community* (pp. 186–214). St. Louis, MO: Mosby Elsevier.

Minnesota Department of Health, Division of Community Health Services, Public Health Nursing Section. (2001). *Public health interventions: Applications for public health nursing practice.* St. Paul: Minnesota Department of Health..

Rippke, M., Briske, L., Keller, L. O., Strohschein, S., & Simonetti, J. (2001). *Public health interventions: Applications for public health nursing practice.* Public Health Nursing Section, Division of Community Health Services, Minnesota Department of Health. Retrieved December 15, 2008 from http://www.health.state.mn.us/divs/cfh/ophp/resources/docs/phinterventions_manual2001.pdf

U.S. Department of Health and Human Services. (2000). *Healthy people 2010* (Vol. 1). Washington, DC: U.S. Government Printing Office.

Wald, L. D. (1915). *The house on Henry Street.* New York: Henry Holt and Company.

ACKNOWLEDGMENTS

One lesson in life that I have learned is that support and guidance from others is essential. Others let you see what you can do and also how to do it. As I reflect on my life I see that throughout my professional practice there were transitional periods, and in those periods there were people, nurses, who showed me what I could do and how to do it. During my undergraduate studies it was Mathy Mezey. As I moved on and transitioned into an academic setting it was Geraldine Valencia-Go. These individuals were icons to me and showed me what I could do as a woman and as a nurse.

The most recent transition presented another professional nurse, Sandy Lewenson. Sandy has shown me the importance of collegiality, professionalism, and friendship. It was Sandy who suggested the partnership in which we began and completed our first book, *Decision-Making in Nursing: Thoughtful Approaches for Practice*. It was she who opened this door. She assured me that I could do this, that I had the ability, and that she would not let me fail. It was Sandy who permitted me to see that my dream of writing a public health text was not only a dream but could be a reality. I wish to thank her for this. I never would have attempted such a challenge if it was not for her unwavering support. It is amazing what two "girls" from "the Bronx" can do.

I also want to thank my family, in particular my husband, Michael Londrigan, for always being there for me, especially those nights when I was absolutely sure that I could not do one more ounce of work and when I would begin to doubt myself. It was his support, comfort, strength, and love that gave me the energy I needed as well as the peace. Finally, I want to also thank my children, Paul and Leah. I have one message for you both. As you are presently engaging in your own transitions, moving out into the world and embarking on your own professional endeavors, always remember to look and observe what is transpiring around you and reflect on these observations. These reflections are sometimes the best educational life experiences.

Marie Truglio-Londrigan

My participation in the writing of this book on public health nursing began as Marie Truglio-Londrigan convinced me that this was an important and much-needed text. While the market showcased many public health/community health texts already in use, Marie convinced me that there was nothing out there that covered what we planned to cover. She appealed to my love of public health nursing, nursing education, and nursing history, suggesting that all three could be combined in this work.

My love of public health nursing began when I went to Hunter College-Bellevue School of Nursing between 1967 and 1971. I was never quite sure why I was becoming a nurse. The hospital was filled with sick people that sometimes died, nurses were overworked and understaffed, and there was little time left for teaching patients, never mind families, about healthy lifestyles. It was not until my public health course in my senior year with Marjorie Martin that it all came together. My first exposure to public health nursing was as a visiting nurse in the central Harlem office of the Visiting Nurse Service of New York. I was in love. There were never too many people to visit, never too many stairs to climb, and never too many blocks to walk. After graduation I worked a short while on a medical–surgical unit per the advice some professors gave me until I felt that I needed to be out in the community. My years as a public health nurse included giving parenting classes, offering nutritional counseling, doing wound care, assessing the health status of families in their homes, monitoring lead level screening, and an assortment of other public health nursing activities.

These skills translated in later years to my work in nursing education. It was at the various schools where I worked that I honed the skills of educating future public health nurses. I integrated nursing history into all aspects of my teaching because the history of nursing speaks of nurses' rich contributions to the public health movement in the United States.

Living a healthy lifestyle has always been an important part of my life and my family's. Why wait to eat heart-healthy foods and exercise after you have a stroke when you could be have been doing so all along? My husband Richard Lewenson agreed with my philosophy and led our family through running marathons, gym memberships, low-fat diets, and a healthy lifestyle that we have managed to maintain for many years. Our daughters and their families, Jennie, Chris, Sarah, Nicky, Jeff, and Georgia, have made healthy lifestyle a way of life as well. My brother's family, Billy, Cindy, Heather, Ross, and Barbara also participate in finding a healthy balance in their busy lives. My sister, Michelle, an educator and my real "editor," who also ascribes to a healthy lifestyle, faces her husband Michael's descent into dementia and has become one of the many Americans facing this growing public health concern. Our mother Pearl's own battle with dementia continues to challenge us all to live life to the fullest. The lessons I learn from all of my family, such as the importance of helmet laws, the essence of prenatal and postnatal care, planning healthy diets, skiing in Vermont, fishing on the Delaware River, and witnessing the developmental milestones of one-year-old and four-month-old granddaughters affirm the need for public health nurses. The lessons I learn at home through my family have supported my work on this text.

 I am indebted to all those who touched my life during my early years as a public health nurse as it led me in the direction to learn more, teach, and write. I acknowledge all of my colleagues that have supported my love of public health, nursing education, and nursing history. I am especially appreciative of my family and friends who listen, suggest, critique, edit, and encourage me to grow. I want to thank my coeditor for convincing me to reflect and to participate in this project.

Amy Sibley and Rachel Shuster, both at Jones and Bartlett, also need to be acknowledged, for they understood the need for another public health nursing text that addressed the goal for all of us to live a healthier lifestyle. We also must thank Lisa Cerrone for helping us through the daunting editing process. We both would like to thank the following individuals: Georgina Atuahene, Doris Asante, Michael Tawiah, and Emma Kariuki. These individuals were students at The College of New Rochelle in the RN/BSN program and they graciously agreed to use the Public Health Nursing Assessment Tool in their final community course. Their input was greatly appreciated.

And, finally, we want to acknowledge the many wonderful contributors that added their knowledge and wisdom to the text. Thank you all for making *Public Health Nursing: Practicing Population-Based Care* a reality!

Sandra B. Lewenson

Contributors

Carole A. Baraldi, MS, RN
Consultant, Public Health Nurse
   Educator
New York, New York

Jon Barone, MS, RN, FNP-BC
Family Nurse Practitioner
Spine Surgery Service
Department of Orthopaedics
Hospital for Joint Diseases
NYU Langone Medical Center
New York, New York

Madeline R. Cafiero, MS, RN, FNP,
   CWOCN
Assistant Professor
The Sage Colleges—Nursing
Troy, New York

Lois O. Carnochan, MS, RN
Coordinator Clinical Undergraduate
   Programs
School of Nursing
The College of New Rochelle
New Rochelle, New York

Marisa A. Cortese-Peske, RN, MS, PNP
Lienhard School of Nursing
Pace University
New York, New York

Mary de Chesnay, DSN, PMHCNS-BC,
   FAAN
Director
WellStar School of Nursing
Kennesaw State University
Kennesaw, Georgia

Janna L. Dieckmann, PhD, RN
Clinical Associate Professor
School of Nursing
University of North Carolina at
   Chapel Hill
Chapel Hill, North Carolina

Mary Alice Higgins Donius, EdD, RN
Dean and Associate Professor
School of Nursing
The College of New Rochelle
New Rochelle, New York

Lin Drury, PhD, RN
Associate Professor
Lienhard School of Nursing
Pace University
New York, New York

Anny M. Eusebio, RN, MSN, FNP-BC
New York-Presbyterian Hospital
Columbia Medical Center Associates
   in Internal Medicine
New York, New York

Stephen A. Ferrara, MSN, RN, FNP-BC
Private Practice
White Plains, New York

Shirley Franco, MSN, FNP
President
NP in Family Health, PC
Mahopac, New York

Karen Galanowsky, MPH, BSN, RN
Nurse Consultant
New Jersey Department of Health and
   Senior Services Tuberculosis Program
Trenton, New Jersey

Teresa M. Haines, DNP, RN, FNP-BC
Assistant Professor of Nursing
Lienhard School of Nursing
Pace University
Pleasantville, New York

Christine E. Hallett, PhD, RGN
Senior Lecturer
School of Nursing, Midwifery
   and Social Work
Director
UK Centre for the History of Nursing
   and Midwifery
University of Manchester
Manchester, England

Arlene Keeling, PhD, RN, FAAN
Centennial Professor of Nursing
Director for the Center of Historical
   Nursing Inquiry
University of Virginia
Charlottesville, Virginia

Karen Kelley, MSN, RN
Assistant Professor
College of Nursing
Harding University
Searcy, Arkansas

Martha Kelly, EdD, RN
Assistant Professor of Nursing
Lienhard School of Nursing
Pace University
Pleasantville, New York

Rona F. Levin, PhD, RN
Professor, Chair
Department of Graduate Studies
Lienhard School of Nursing
Pace University
New York, NY

Margaret Macali, MS, RN, CS
Director of Public Health Nursing Service
Clinical Specialist, Public/Community
   Health Nursing
Bergen County Department of Health
   Services
Paramus, New Jersey

Susan Moscou, FNP, PhD, MPH
Associate Professor
Mercy College
Dobbs Ferry, New York

Eileen T. O'Grady, PhD, RN, NP
Visiting Professor
Lienhard School of Nursing
Pace University
New York, New York

Irene S. Rempel, BS, RN, LMSW
Instructor
School of Nursing
Long Island College Hospital
Brooklyn, New York

Lisa Seiff, RN, BSN
Prime Care
New York, New York

Cathleen M. Shultz, PhD, RN, CNE, FAAN
Dean, Professor of Nursing
College of Nursing
Harding University
Searcy, Arkansas

Joanne K. Singleton, PhD, RN, FNP-BC
Professor, Program Director
Family Nurse Practitioner
Doctor of Nursing Practice Program
Lienhard School of Nursing
Pace University
New York, New York

Monte Wagner, MPH, MS, FNP-BC
Clinical Assistant Professor
The College of New Rochelle
New Rochelle, New York

Adrienne Wald, EdD(c), MBA, RN
Director of Wellness Education and Programs
The College of New Rochelle
New Rochelle, New York

Barbara Mann Wall, PhD, RN
Associate Professor, Associate Director
Barbara Bates Center for the Study of the
  History of Nursing
School of Nursing
University of Pennsylvania
Philadelphia, Pennsylvania

Doreen Gallagher Wall, MS, RN, BC
Psychiatric Nurse
Assertive Community Treatment Team
Visiting Nurse Service of New York
New York, New York

Astrid Hellier Wilson, DNS, RN
Professor
WellStar School of Nursing
Kennesaw State University
Kennesaw, Georgia

Reviewers

Kimberly Balko, MS, RN
Empire State College
Saratoga Springs, New York

Emily Barey, MSN, RN
Epic Systems Corporation
Verona, Wisconsin

Angeline Bushy
University of Central Florida College
   of Nursing—Daytona Campus
Daytona Beach, Florida

Jennell P. Charles, PhD, RN
Clayton State University
Morrow, Georgia

Kim Clevenger, MSN, RN, BC
Assistant Professor of Nursing
Morehead State University
Morehead, Kentucky

Arlene Rosen, EdD, RN
Assistant Professor
College of New Rochelle
New Rochelle, New York

CHAPTER 1

WHAT IS PUBLIC HEALTH AND PUBLIC HEALTH NURSING?

Marie Truglio-Londrigan
Sandra B. Lewenson

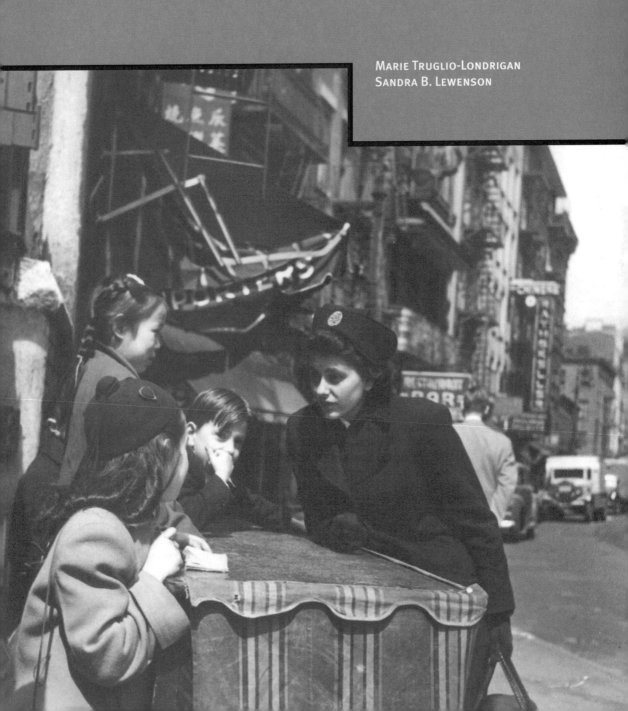

Recognizing limits to what the health service professions can now do, in relation to common health problems faced everyday, by no means negate the fact that as conditions essential for health are more fully known and are provided and used by individuals and communities, more and more individuals will be enabled to experience greater health (Peplau, 1952, p. 15).

LEARNING OBJECTIVES

At the completion of this chapter, the reader will be able to

- Define the meaning of public health and public health nursing.
- Describe what is meant by the terms "care of the public" and "population-based care."
- Describe the goals and objectives of Healthy People 2010.

- Examine the 10 essential public health services in relation to the core functions of public health practice.
- Examine the role of the public health nurse within the larger context of public health.

KEY TERMS

- Assurance
- Core functions of public health
- Essentials of public health
- Health promotion
- Healthy People 2010

- Maintaining health
- Preventing disease
- Public health
- Public health nursing
- Risk reduction

It never fails. Sit around a table and discuss the health of the public or population-based care and one frequently receives blank stares. What is **public health**? What do we mean when we speak about the health of the "public" or "population-based care?" What is the role of the public health nurse within this larger framework? And, who pays for public health? These questions need to be answered for those in practice. This chapter presents information that provides answers to these questions, thus enhancing practitioners' working knowledge of the scientific discipline known as public health. Creating a professional nursing workforce that demonstrates a vigorous practice integrating cultural congruent nursing actions based on evidence and recognizing the funding streams lay the groundwork for a strong public health infrastructure that will ultimately enhance and sustain the public's health.

PUBLIC HEALTH DEFINED

To fully understand the concept of public health, it is important to review the definitions put forth over time by those in practice. This exercise will assist the reader in knowing and understanding the important characteristics and features of this discipline.

"Public health work is as old as history," wrote J. Howard Beard in 1922. Beard's article, published in *The Scientific Monthly*, charts the early progress of public health starting with the early Egyptians, who filtered mud from the Nile River to create a safer water source for citizens. Throughout history the health of the public has been a concern for local and national governments and all members of society. The public health movement in the United States had its origins in Boston, Massachusetts, in the mid-1800s where Lemuel Shattuck's noted reports on the healthcare needs of the community became the "blueprint for American health organization" (Beard, 1922; Scheele, 1949, p. 293). A noted public health leader in the early 20th century, C. E. Winslow (1920) defined public health as follows:

> [T]he science and the art of preventing disease, prolonging life, and promoting physical health and efficiency through organized community efforts for the sanitation of the environment, the control of community infections, the education of the individual in principles of personal hygiene, the organization of medical and nursing service

for the early diagnosis and preventive treatment of disease, and the development of the social machinery which will ensure to every individual in the community a standard of living adequate for the maintenance of health. (p. 30)

The definition of public health changed over time to accommodate the needs of American society.

In 1988 a more recent definition of public health was presented by the Institute of Medicine (IOM). The IOM defined public health as "what we, as a society, do collectively to assure the conditions in which people can be healthy" (IOM, 1988, p. 1). Society collectively works together to provide services. These services are generally provided to a population to prevent disease and to maintain health (Buttery, 1992). The American Public Health Association Web site includes the following definition for public health: "the science and art of protecting and improving the health of communities through education, promotion of healthy life styles, and research for disease and injury prevention" (n.d., para. 1). The Association of Community Health Nursing Educators builds on the IOM definition and states that the conditions under which people can be healthy "are assured by government and community activities to prevent disease and promote health" (Levin et al., 2007, p. 6).

Populations

When one considers the above definitions on public health, one comes to understand that the discussion of health moves beyond the health of the individual, family, or community to the health of the population. For example, Hurricane Katrina hit the Gulf Coast in Louisiana in the

United States on August 29, 2005. In the weeks that followed, healthcare professionals cared for individuals and their family members who were evacuees without shelter and suffered from physical and emotional distress. Brodie, Weltzien, Altman, Blendon, and Benson (2006) surveyed the experience of the Hurricane Katrina evacuees. Their results provided valuable information for public health professionals "highlighting challenges of effectively evacuating cities' most at-risk residents during a disaster and providing for long-term health needs of vulnerable populations in the aftermath" (p. 1407). The outcomes of this research also provided valuable information for public health officials as they engaged in discussions for future planning with regard to evacuation when disasters hit and how to ensure the protection of the public during this evacuation. **Table 1-1** gives additional examples of how a specific public health intervention, such as education, may vary depending on whether the focus is on individuals, families, populations, or communities.

The concept of caring for populations can be difficult to understand and perhaps serves as a barrier to the way nurses or other healthcare workers are educated and approach care. The noted 20th century nursing leader, Virginia Henderson, when questioned how one could nurse an aggregate said, "I think it impossible to nurse an aggregate effectively until you have effectively nursed individuals and acquired considerable judgment as to what helps clients or patients prevent disease, cope with it, or die with dignity when death is inevitable" (Abrams, 2007, p. 384). This question has been raised many times in hopes of understanding what a population means and what it means to care for a population. Definitions of "populations" illustrate characteristics and features specific to public health. Williams and Stanhope (2008) define a population or aggregate as "a collection of individuals who have one or more personal or environmental characteristics in common" (p. 11). The Association of Community Health Nursing Educators uses the same definition as Williams and Stanhope in the work completed by Levin et al. (2007). The American Nurses Association (2007) builds on the definition of population as "those living in a specific geographic area (e.g., a neighborhood, community, city, or county) or those in a particular group (e.g., racial ethnic, age, disease) who experience a disproportionate burden of poor health care outcomes" (p. 5).

Henderson's concern about nursing populations versus nursing individuals may stem from her concern of the division in health care when we separate the care of populations and care of individuals. Henderson asked, "Should we have one category of health workers treating disease and another preventing it? Or should we all be trying primarily to prevent disease, and, even while treating it, to be helping the victim to prevent a recurrence?" (Abrams, 2007, p. 384). The separation of public health care between the individual and aggregate is discussed in Chapter 2, where the changing definitions of **public health nursing** explore this dichotomy.

Preventing Disease and Maintaining Health

Other important characteristics of public health are **preventing disease** and **maintaining health**. These concepts illustrate where the emphasis is placed on care.

Table 1-1 Examples of the "Educational" Interventions for Individuals, Families, Populations, and Communities

	Individual	Family	Population	Community
	Refers to individual clients, who may be part of a family, a population, and live in a community.	Refers to a family system, which may be defined as any or all individuals who live in what they consider a family system.	Refers to a defined number of people.	Refers to individuals, families, populations, and organizations (profit and not-for-profit) that may or may not share the same ideas, values, beliefs, and/or physical location, but do intervene and network with each other.
Lyme disease prevention and early detection programs	Target the client (e.g., young adult gardeners) and provide education about Lyme disease, its cause, and methods of prevention, such as pulling socks over pants and wearing repellent. This education can be provided in a pamphlet and placed in areas where individuals may pick it up and read it, such as pharmacies and gardening supply stores.	Target families and provide education for caretakers of children about the cause of Lyme disease and methods of prevention. This information may be developed and delivered in magazines available in primary care practitioner offices or at organizations such as Boys and Girls Clubs of America.	Target the population and provide education for the public about Lyme disease. This information may be developed and delivered on signs in high-risk areas (such as hiking trails) or in special service announcements on the radio.	A healthy community ensures that a hiking trail in their geographical community is clear of brush and that appropriate signs are posted warning of high-risk areas. A healthy community will also ensure that funding is available to sustain these endeavors.
Child car seat prevention programs	Target the child, using developmentally appropriate play strategies that illustrate use of child car seats and booster seats.	Target caretakers (e.g., parents, grandparents, day care workers), educating them about the importance of using child car seats with pamphlets and videos in preschools.	Target populations through the use of billboards highlighting the importance of appropriate use of child car seats.	A healthy community will have strong organizations that provide programs to support use of child car seats. For example: a local hospital may stage a "drive-through" child car seat safety check; a fire department may install safety car seats for newborns.

The emphasis of care in public health is placed on maintaining health or **health promotion** and on preventing disease and **risk reduction**. To explain these concepts in greater detail and to fully understand these concepts, we turn to the historic work of Leavell and Clark (1965), who noted, "The ultimate objectives of all medical, dental, and public health practice, whether carried out in the office, the clinic, the laboratory, or the community at large, are the promotion of health, the prevention of disease, and the prolongation of life" (p. 14). According to Leavell and Clark (1965), there are three levels of prevention. The first level, primary prevention, includes interventions designed to promote health via health promotion strategies and to specifically protect the individual from disease "by providing immunizations and reducing exposure to occupational hazards, carcinogens, and other environmental health risks" (Greiner & Edelman, 2006, p. 17). Thus these interventions take place before the presence of disease and disability known as the prepathogenesis period. The second level of prevention, known as the period of pathogenesis, takes place once disease is present. Interventions include screening activities and providing treatment early, thereby preventing the consequences of advanced disease such as disabilities. Finally, the third level of prevention includes rehabilitation intervention strategies. "This is more than stopping a disease process; it is also the prevention of complete disability. . . . Its positive objective is to return the affected individual to a useful place in society and make maximum use of his remaining capacities" (Leavell & Clark, 1965, p. 26). **Figure 1-1** offers a pictorial view of the natural history of any disease.

Today, public health nursing activities in primary, secondary, and tertiary prevention have evolved and take into consideration that health is not linear. In fact, if a person requires tertiary rehabilitative services, health promotion strategies are still important. Henderson's question raised above speaks to this nonlinear approach and encourages us to think about providing care for disease while simultaneously promoting health.

Multiple Disciplines

Additional review of the above definitions on public health demonstrates the collective nature of public health and the need for multiple disciplines to work together in ensuring the health of the public. **Figure 1-2** is a visual depiction of this.

What does this mean? The IOM (2003) speaks to this collective endeavor as a process that must involve multiple individuals and multiple organizations. "The concept of a public health system describes a complex network of individuals and organizations that have the potential to play critical roles in creating the conditions for health. They can act for health individually, but when they work together toward a health goal, they act as a system—a public health system" (IOM, 2003, p. 28). The IOM further describes these participants as "actors" in the public health system. These actors include the governmental public health infrastructure such as local and state departments of health, the healthcare delivery system, academia, and communities. These communities may include schools, religious organizations, and other not-for-profit organizations, just to name a few. In addition, businesses and corporations are considered important actors

FIGURE **1-1**   **Levels of prevention.**

Source: Leavell & Clark, 1965.

because they too play an important role in how they influence population health with regard to working conditions and the healthcare benefits they provide. Finally, the IOM identifies the media as an important actor in this healthcare system. Consider the impact that media plays just in its ability to reach populations through the various media streams available. Ultimately, these actors and their integrative and participatory roles serve as a reminder of the Declaration of Alma-Ata International Conference (1978) that recognized primary health care as a major strategy for achieving health for all. At this historic interna-

tional conference, participants expressed a need for all governments and other international organizations to engage in actions that would ensure the implementation of primary health care around the world. The Declaration of Alma-Ata International Conference (1978) described and explained primary health care as follows:

[R]equires and promotes maximum community and individual self-reliance and participation in the planning, organization, operation and control of primary health care, making fullest use of local, national and other

FIGURE **1-2**   The intersectorial public health system.

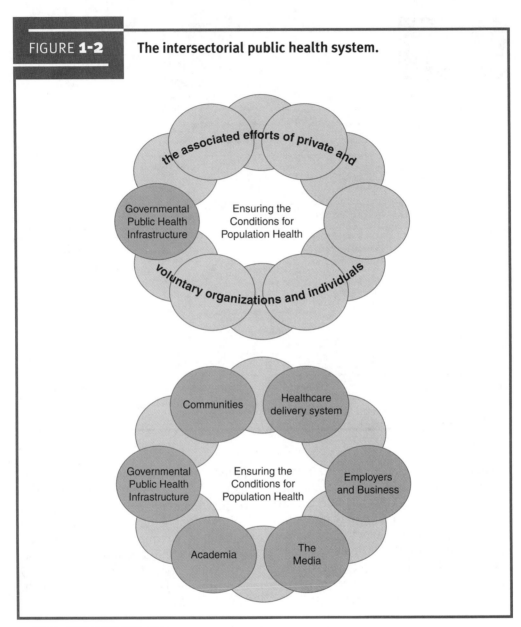

Source: Institute of Medicine, 2003.

available resources; and to this end develops through appropriate education the ability of communities to participate. (para. 12)

Ensure the Public Health

Working together as actors is important, but it is the ability to *ensure* the health of the public that is critical. How does one ensure the health of the public? The involvement and the role of the government are important in this regard. The

IOM ... o this very issue:

es, the government's
the health of its citi-
t, from the nature of
Health officials are
:ted or appointed by
cted officials. To the
:hat citizens place a
ealth, these elected
countable to ensure
it is able to monitor
ealth and intervene
hrough laws, poli-
and expenditure of
;sary for the health
blic. (p. 101)

e healthy without
support of the ser-
blic healthy. Late
.... early 20th century public health nursing leaders, like Lillian Wald and Mary Brewster, who began the Henry Street Settlement in the Lower East Side of New York City, recognized the need to garner the help of the government to support their efforts to improve the health of the immigrant population that flooded the streets of New York during this period. Wald and Brewster's public health nurses wore the official badges they received showing endorsement by the New York

Board of Health as they visited the homes of the families in the community (Buhler-Wilkerson, 2001). Wald, along with the other public health nurses, continued to advocate for playgrounds for children in the community, school nurses in the public schools, and votes for women as a means of ensuring the public's health (Lewenson, 2007). Suffragist and public health nurse Lavinia Dock equated the ability to vote with the ability to improve health. In an early *American Journal of Nursing,* Dock (1908) asked nurses to consider the value of the women's vote, saying, ". . . take the present question of the underfed school children in New York. How many of them will have tuberculosis? If mothers and nurses had votes there might be school lunches for all those children" (p. 926).

Service

Finally, the above definitions mention the types of services provided. For example, mention is made about the importance of education as a service. How does one provide this service to a population? There are many ways this may be approached, and it is for the readers and practitioners of public health to creatively define the types of services. There are also other services that may be directed to a population. This text, for example, features the application of the Minnesota Department of Health Population-Based Public Health Nursing Practice Intervention Wheel Strategies. This wheel contains 17 intervention strategies or services that are population-focused and may be applied to the levels of practice including individuals, families, communities, and systems.

The definitions of public health presented in this chapter highlight certain

---

BOX **1-1**   **Overview of Key Characteristics and Features of Public Health**

Key Characteristics and Features of Public Health

Population-based

Preventing disease

Maintaining health

Multiple disciplines

Assurance

Services

---

key characteristics and features. **Box 1-1** presents an overview of these key characteristics and features that are further exemplified in later chapters.

PUBLIC HEALTH NURSING

Public health nurses play a central role in supporting the health of the public. Chapter 2 is entirely dedicated to the history of public health nursing, showing the development of this role over time. Public health nursing, a term first coined in the late 19th century by nursing leader Lillian Wald (Buhler-Wilkerson, 1993), included the roles of "health visitor, health teacher, social worker and even health *inspector*" (Crandall, 1922, p. 645). Crandall wrote that these roles evolved based on the rich foundation of nursing (Crandall, 1922). This strong nursing background continues today as public health nursing serves the health of the public.

The Missouri Department of Health and Senior Services (2006) uses the following contemporary definition of public health nursing:

[P]ractice of promoting and protecting the health of populations using knowl-

edge from nursing, social, and public health sciences. More specifically public health nursing is a systematic process by which the health and the health care needs of a population are: 1) assessed in order to identify individuals, families, and populations health care needs, 2) a plan for intervention is developed with the community to meet the identified needs, 3) evaluations are conducted to determine the extent to which the intervention has an impact on the health status of the individual, family, and the population, and 4) the results of the process are used to influence and direct the current delivery of care. (p. 8)

What we may glean from this definition is that public health nursing by definition mirrors the general definitions of public health, with emphasis on the systematic process that nurses use to "do" their work. This process is the nursing process. Therefore throughout this text the reader will note that the nursing process is the guiding framework for assessing the needs of the population, diagnosing the needs of the population, planning interventions based in evidence using the intervention wheel, implementing those strategies, and ultimately evaluating outcomes of the population. The definition of public health nursing above also notes how results of the process are used to influence and direct the current healthcare delivery system, therefore making assurances to the public when results and outcomes are positive that these outcomes will be sustained over time.

PUBLIC HEALTH NOW

For centuries, diseases such as the Black Plague, leprosy, smallpox, tuberculosis, and influenza terrorized the population with extraordinary death tolls. Similarly, for centuries it was assumed that nothing could be done about these little-understood outbreaks because they were a message from the supernatural who in some way was dissatisfied with us. Since these earlier times, the scientific discipline of public health has made remarkable strides, noted by the decrease in communicable diseases along with the marked improvements in our sanitation efforts (Beard, 1922).

Recent years have seen a resurgence in communicable and infectious diseases such as H1N1, along with a renewed cry to strengthen the public health infrastructure in the United States. Problems such as chronic illnesses, obesity, a healthcare system whose cost of care is out of control coupled with populations holding no health insurance or limited insurance, health disparities, the stripping of the environment, rising mental health issues, and violence and terrorism clearly inform public health professionals of the need for a call to action. The Institute of Medicine (2003) spoke about the IOM 1988 report and stated that the earlier report "presented strong evidence to indicate that

the governmental public health infrastructure was in disarray" (IOM, 2003, p. xi).

Ten Essential Public Health Services

Historically, public health professionals have responded to the call to action as noted by changes and progress in meeting the needs of the public. One more recent outcome to this call was the development of the 10 essential public health services by the Public Health Functions Steering Committee (U.S. Department of Health and Human Services [DHHS] Public Health Service, 1994). This steering committee included representatives from U.S. Public Health Service agencies and other major public health organizations. The 10 **essentials of public health** provide a guiding framework for the responsibilities of local public health systems and the foundation for strategy building toward a healthy, integrated public health system capable of ensuring the health of the public. **Box 1-2** presents these 10 essential public health services. A review of these essential services again illustrates for us the key characteristics and features noted in the previous definitions of public health.

Three Core Functions

Each of these 10 essential services falls under one of the three **core functions of public health**: assessment, policy development, and **assurance** (IOM, 1988). The skills included in assessments by a public health agency require the systematic collection and analysis of data on the health of the population for early identification of health problems and/or the identification of potential problems. Policy development recommends that public health agencies serve the public by developing

---

BOX **1-2**   **The Ten Essential Public Health Services**

Monitor health status to identify community health problems.

Diagnose and investigate health problems and health hazards in the community.

Inform, educate, and empower people about health issues.

Mobilize community partnerships to identify and solve health problems.

Develop policies and plans that support individual and community health efforts.

Enforce laws and regulations that protect health and ensure safety.

Link people to needed personal health services and ensure the provision of health care when otherwise unavailable.

Ensure a competent public health and personal healthcare workforce.

Evaluate effectiveness, accessibility, and quality of personal and population-based health services.

Conduct research to attain new insights and innovative solutions to health problems.

Source: U.S. Department of Health and Human Services Public Health Service, 1994.

---

public health policies based on evidence for the correction of an issue or problem. Finally, assurance requires that public health agencies provide services directly or by other private or public agencies. In addition, assurance guarantees services for those unable to afford them. These three core functions guide the public health professional in the development, implementation, and evaluation of various public processes that assist the professional in meeting the healthcare needs of the public (**Figure 1-3**).

Healthy People 2010

The three core functions of public health and the ten essential public health services provide the foundation for the health agenda for the nation known as **Healthy People 2010**. Healthy People 2010 is a continuation of a previous initiative that began in 1979 when the *Healthy People: The Surgeon General's Report on Health Promotion and Disease Prevention* was released, providing national goals for reducing premature deaths and preserving independence for older adults. "Healthy People 2010 presents a comprehensive, nationwide health promotion and disease prevention agenda. It is designed to serve as a roadmap for improving the health of all people in the United States during the first decade of the 21st century" (U.S. DHHS, 2000, p. 1). This map serves as a guide for healthcare professionals and their partners as they make collective decisions about what types of health initiatives to engage in and how to implement and evaluate these initiatives. These partners are central to the success of the Healthy

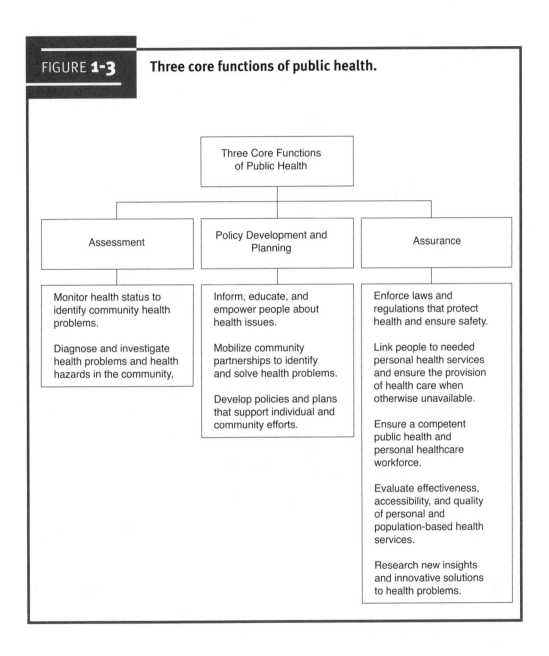

FIGURE 1-3   **Three core functions of public health.**

Three Core Functions of Public Health

Assessment

Policy Development and Planning

Assurance

Monitor health status to identify community health problems.

Diagnose and investigate health problems and health hazards in the community,

Inform, educate, and empower people about health issues.

Mobilize community partnerships to identify and solve health problems.

Develop policies and plans that support individual and community efforts.

Enforce laws and regulations that protect health and ensure safety.

Link people to needed personal health services and ensure the provision of health care when otherwise unavailable.

Ensure a competent public health and personal healthcare workforce.

Evaluate effectiveness, accessibility, and quality of personal and population-based health services.

Research new insights and innovative solutions to health problems.

People 2010 agenda. "Addressing the challenge of health improvement is a shared responsibility that requires the active participation and leadership of the Federal Government, States, local governments, policy makers, health care providers, professionals, business executives, educators, community leaders, and the American public itself (U.S. DHHS, 2000, p. 4). This resonates with the earlier work mentioned above that addresses intersectorial and collective work of

FIGURE **1-4**   **Systematic approach to health improvements.**

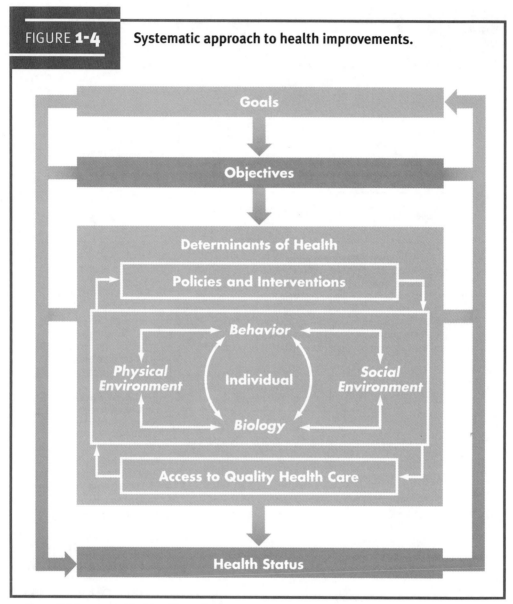

Source: U.S. Department of Health and Human Services, 2000.

public health practitioners. Public health nurses are important actors in this collective work and have historically been present in public health initiatives. The launching of Healthy People 2020 is expected. Information on this may be found at http://www.healthypeople.gov/HP2020.

Within Healthy People 2010 a systematic approach to health improvement is presented as a model in **Figure 1-4**. It is from this model that the authors developed in

Chapter 3 an assessment tool for public health nurses to use in their practice.

There are four key elements in this systematic approach, the ultimate outcome being the improvement of the health for the general public:

1. Goals
2. Objectives
3. Determinants of health
4. Health status

GOALS

Two goals are documented in Healthy People 2010: increase quality of years of healthy life and eliminate health disparities. The first goal addresses life expectancy as well and considers this as "the average number of years of people born in a given year are expected to live based on a set of age-specific death rates" (U.S. DHHS, 2000, p. 8). This goal, however, not only speaks to the need for achieving a longer life but a healthy life with quality. The second goal reviews the evidence and tells us about the health disparities evident among various demographic groups in the United States. These demographic groups include "gender, race or ethnicity, education or income, disability, geographic, location, or sexual orientation" (U.S. DHHS, 2000, p. 11). To discuss specific examples in each of these demographic groups goes beyond the scope and purpose of this chapter. It is, however, an awareness of the very existence of these disparities and an understanding of their etiology that is critical for public health professionals and their partners in the development of initiatives to create a balanced healthcare system where health parity is the rule rather than health disparity.

FOCUS AREAS AND OBJECTIVES

The nation's progress in achieving the two goals of Healthy People 2010 is measured through 467 objectives in 28 focus areas (**Box 1-3**). The objectives are written in specific measurable terms so that improvement in health status for

---

BOX **1-3**   **Healthy People 2010 Focus Areas**

1. Access to Quality Health Services
2. Arthritis, Osteoporosis, and Chronic Back Conditions
3. Cancer
4. Chronic Kidney Disease
5. Diabetes
6. Disability and Secondary Conditions
7. Educational and Community-Based Programs
8. Environmental Health
9. Family Planning
10. Food Safety
11. Health Communication
12. Heart Disease and Stroke
13. HIV
14. Immunization and Infectious Diseases
15. Injury and Violence Prevention
16. Maternal, Infant, and Child Health
17. Medical Product Safety
18. Mental Health and Mental Disorders
19. Nutrition and Overweight
20. Occupational Safety and Health
21. Oral Health
22. Physical Activity and Fitness
23. Public Health Infrastructure
24. Respiratory Diseases
25. Sexually Transmitted Diseases
26. Substance Abuse
27. Tobacco Use
28. Vision and Hearing

Source: U.S. Department of Health and Human Services, 2000.

a particular objective in a specific focus area is capable of being tracked. For example, if you as a public health nurse have conducted an assessment and have identified that tobacco smoking among a population of adolescents in a particular community is a major problem, you would identify the area of focus to be number 27 (tobacco use). If you examine Healthy People 2010 further, you will note a specific goal for tobacco use. The goal states, "Reduce illness, disability, and death related to tobacco use and the exposure to second hand smoke" (U.S. DHHS, 2000, p. 27). What then follows is a series of objectives with targets set for 2010, many of which are specific to adolescents.

DETERMINANTS OF HEALTH

The third key element in this systematic approach is determinants of health. These determinants include biology, behaviors, social environment, physical environment, policies and interventions, and access to quality health care. An individual's biology, inclusive of genetic make-up, along with the individual's responses or behaviors to particular experiences and/or situations influence his or her health along with the individual's social and physical environment. Additional important determinants include policies and other interventions that may affect the health of the population. Finally, access to health care influences health and quality of life. Chapter 3 further defines these determinants and uses this systematic approach for the development of a population-based nursing assessment tool.

HEALTH STATUS

What is the health of the population? This is the question that public health nurses and other professionals ask as they engage in this systematic approach. To answer this question these public health-care professionals must, using available technology, monitor and evaluate what happens to the population as a result of experiencing or living the determinants of health. Many public healthcare professionals monitor and evaluate the health of the population by monitoring, analyzing, and evaluating birth and death rates, morbidity, and mortality rates as an example. The leading health indicators, such as tobacco use, injury and violence, or immunizations, are also an appropriate means to monitor and evaluate the health of the population. **Box 1-4** illustrates these leading health indicators. As with the 28 focus areas, these leading health indicators each have specific objectives that are written in measurable and objective terms so that progress may be tracked and thus the health of the nation monitored and evaluated.

BOX **1-4** **Ten Leading Health Indicators**

Physical activity

Overweight and obesity

Tobacco use

Substance abuse

Responsible sexual behavior

Mental health

Injury and violence

Environmental quality

Immunization

Access to health care

Source: U.S. Department of Health and Human Services, 2000.

Application to Communities

How does one apply this systematic approach presented in Healthy People 2010 to one's individual community? To answer this question public health nurses and their partners may apply *Healthy People in Healthy Communities.* This document was developed by the U.S. DHHS (2001) in an attempt to enlist communities to use Healthy People 2010 as a tool that can be applied to ensure a healthy population locally. A healthy community is defined as "one that embraces the belief that health is more than merely an absence of disease; a healthy community includes those elements that enable people to maintain a high quality of life and productivity" (U.S. DHHS, 2001, p. 1). *Healthy Communities* uses the set of 10 priorities known as the leading health indicators previously noted. These 10 leading health indicators are a smaller set of priorities for communities to use in the development of their specific local initiatives. "Motivating individuals to act on just one of the indicators can have a profound effect on increasing the quality and years of healthy life and on eliminating health disparities—for the individual as well as the community overall" (U.S. DHHS, 2001, p. 4).

To become a healthy community the public health nurse and the members of the community must work together in a partnership using multiple strategies. One such strategy is to use the MAP-IT technique, a mnemonic for **M**obilize, **A**ssess, **P**lan, **I**mplement, and **T**rack (U.S. DHHS, 2001).

Mobilizing key individuals and organizations within the community is the first crucial step as one applies the MAP-IT technique. One way to mobilize such a group is through partnering with others and developing a coalition. Truglio-Londrigan (2008) noted, "this coming

together to work *together* brings the notion of making decisions *together*. Group decision-making, therefore, allows individual to come *together* in a partnership to work toward a goal and ultimately achieve their vision" (p. 131). In this case the vision is a healthier community.

The next step in the MAP-IT technique is to *assess* the community of interest. This assessment is discussed in detail in Chapter 3. What is important to point out here is that this assessment is the collection of data to identify the priority needs of the community. This then becomes the vision that the mobilized coalition works on. See **Box 1-5** for examples of Web sites that may assist the public nurse obtain these data.

BOX **1-5**   **Relevant Web Sites for Public Health Nurses**

http://www.cdc.gov/od/ocphp/nphpsp/EssentialPHService.htm

This Web site delves into the 10 essential public health services in great detail.

http://www.health.gov/healthypeople

This Web site offers Healthy People 2010 documents.

http://www.cdc.gov/nchs/about/otheract/hpdata2010/abouthp.htm

This Web site offers detailed information on objectives and data systems.

http://www.healthypeople.gov

This Web site offers detailed information on the Healthy People 2010 document. It also offers links for the reader to learn about the Healthy People 2020 initiative.

The third step in the MAP-IT technique is the development of the *plan*. What is the plan of action to address the issue that was identified as a result of the assessment in step 2? This plan needs to take into consideration resources such as funding, people, technology, and time. Specific steps need to be developed along with time frames and the clear identification of who is responsible for what portion of the plan. It is very important to remember that in the development of this plan, the population must be included that accounts for various social, political, economic, and cultural factors that impact this plan. For plans to be successful, they must be culturally congruent with the values, beliefs, and needs of the population in addition to being based in evidence. The development of this plan uses the intervention strategies found on the Minnesota Department of Health Population-Based Public Health Nursing Practice Intervention Wheel Strategies.

Once the plan has been identified, the next step in the MAP-IT technique is to *implement* the plan. Again, clear communication between and among all members of the coalition is important so that every member knows who is responsible for what activities. For this communica-tion to be effective, one must remember that "There is no 'power over' in a coali-tion, only 'power with'. . . . This requires equal empowerment of all members of the coalition in order for the members to communicate and work together" (Truglio-Londrigan, 2008, p. 135).

The final step in the MAP-IT technique is to *track* the progress of any and all ini-tiatives and inform all members of the community of the outcomes.

CONCLUSION

This chapter serves as a guiding frame-work for the reader. It considers a discus-sion of public health along with a presentation of the nation's agenda of "Health for All" (U.S. DHHS, 2000). Within this framework materials demonstrate how to incorporate our public health nursing agenda into the nation's agenda. Chapter 3 uses this guiding framework to design the public health nursing assess-ment tool. Chapters 8 through 12 are based on the Minnesota Department of Health Population-Based Public Health Nursing Practice Intervention Wheel Strategies, which serve as templates for action for our profession and models by which we may guide our own practice.

References

Abrams, S. E. (2007). Nursing the community, a look back at the 1984 dialogue between Virginia Henderson and Sherry L. Shamansky. *Public Health Nursing, 24*(4), 382–386.

American Nurses Association. (2007). *Public health nursing: Scope and standards of practice.* Silver Springs, MD: American Nurses Association.

American Public Health Association. (n.d.). What is public health? Retrieved May 24, 2008, from http://www.whatispublichealth.org

Beard, J. H. (1922). Progress of public health work. *Scientific Monthly, 14*(2), 140–152.

Brodie, M., Weltzien, E., Altman, D., Blendon, R., & Benson, J. (2006). Experiences of hurricane Katrina evacuees in Houston shelters: Impli-cations for future planning. *American Journal of Public Health, 96*(8), 1402–1408.

Buhler-Wilkerson, K. (1993). Bringing care to the peo-ple: Lillian Wald's legacy to public health nurs-ing. *American Journal of Public Health, 83*(12), 1778–1786.

Buhler-Wilkerson, K. (2001). *No place like home: A his-tory of nursing and home care in the United States.* Baltimore: Johns Hopkins University Press.

Buttery, C. M. G. (1992). Provision of public health services. In J. M. Last & R. B. Wallace (Eds.), *Public health & preventive medicine* (13th ed., pp. 1113–1128). Norwalk, CT: Appleton & Lange.

Crandall, E. P. (1922). An historical sketch of public health nursing. *American Journal of Nursing, 22*(8), 641–645.

Declaration of Alma-Ata International Conference on Primary Care. (1978). Primary health care. Retrieved June 8, 2008, from http://www.who.int/publications/almaata_declaration_en

Dock, L. (1908). The suffrage question. *American Journal of Nursing, 8*(11), 925–927.

Greiner, P., & Edelman, C. (2006). Health defined: Objectives for promotion and prevention. In C. Edelman & C. Mandle (Eds.), *Health promotion throughout the life span* (pp. 3–22). St. Louis, MO: Elsevier Mosby.

Institute of Medicine [IOM]. (1988). *The future of public health*. Washington, DC: National Academy Press.

Institute of Medicine [IOM]. (2003). *The future of the public's health in the 21st century*. Washington, DC: National Academy Press.

Leavell, H., & Clark, A. E. (1965). *Preventive medicine for doctors in the community* (3rd ed.). New York: McGraw-Hill.

Levin, P., Cary, A., Kulbok, P., Leffers, J. Molle, M., & Polivka, B. (2007) Graduate education for advanced practice public health nursing: At the crossroads. Association of Community Health Nursing Educators (ACHNE), 1–24, Retrieved November 23, 2009, from http://www.achne.org/files/public/GraduateEducationDocument.pdf

Lewenson, S. B. (2007). A historical perspective on policy, politics and nursing. In D. J. Mason, J. K. Leavitt, & M. W. Chaffee (Eds.), *Policy and politics in nursing and health care* (5th ed., pp. 21–33). St. Louis, MO: Saunders Elsevier.

Missouri Department of Health and Senior Services. (2006). Public health nursing manual. Retrieved April 4, 2009, from http://www.dhss.mo.gov/LPHA/PHNursing/PHN_Manual.pdf

Peplau, H. (1952). *Interpersonal relations in nursing*. New York: G. P. Putnam's Sons.

Scheele, L. A. (1949). Anniversary program—150th year U.S. Public Health Service. *American Journal of Public Health and the Nation's Health, 39*(3), 293–302.

Truglio-Londrigan, M. (2008). Flattening the field: Group decision-making. In S. B. Lewenson & M. T. Truglio-Londrigan (Eds.), *Decision-making in nursing: Thoughtful approaches for practice* (pp. 131–144). Sudbury, MA: Jones and Bartlett.

U.S. Department of Health and Human Services [DHHS] Public Health Service. (1994). *The public health workforce: An agenda for the 21st century*. A report of the Public Health Functions Project. Retrieved August 27, 2009, from http://www.health.gov/phfunctions/pubhlth.pdf

U.S. Department of Health and Human Services [DHHS]. (2000). *Healthy people 2010* (Vol. 1). Washington, DC: U.S. Government Printing Office.

U.S. Department of Health and Human Services [DHHS]. (2001). *Healthy people in healthy communities*. Washington, DC: U.S. Government Printing Office.

Williams, C., & Stanhope, M. (2008). Population-focused practice: The foundation of specialization in public health nursing. In M. Stanhope & J. Lancaster (Eds.), *Public health nursing: Population-centered health care in the community* (pp. 2–21). St. Louis, MO: Mosby Elsevier.

Winslow, C.-E. A. (1920). The untilled fields of public health. *Science, New Series, 51*(1306), 22–33.

PUBLIC HEALTH NURSING IN THE UNITED STATES: A HISTORY

SANDRA B. LEWENSON

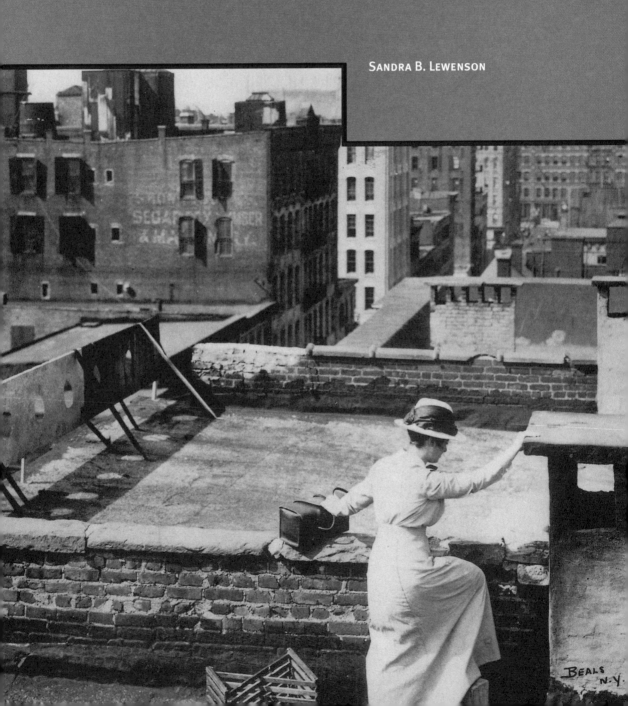

The history of public health nursing is continuous. What we are, we have become through those that have gone before, and the great leaders are of no country, but of the world (Gardner, 1933, p. 15).

LEARNING OBJECTIVES

At the completion of this chapter, the reader will be able to

- Define the various terms used to describe the work of nurses who have practiced in public health nursing over time.

- Describe the history of public health nursing.
- Explain the relevance of the history of nursing to current issues in public health nursing.

KEY TERMS

- Community health nurse
- District nurse
- Home care nurse

- Population
- Public health nurse
- Visiting nurse

H iestand (1982) called for the historian to reflect on "practice as it changed over time" because of its relevance to "understanding the nurses' experience" (p. 11). The purpose of this chapter is to reflect on the practice of public health nursing by examining the nurse's evolving experience in this role. This experience has been influenced by the type of agency where nurses worked, the community in which they served, the economic climate, the advances made in the sciences and technology, and other social-political factors that shaped the kind of work being done (Bryant, 1968; Stewart & Vincent, 1968). The evolution of public health nursing reflects the response to these factors and the transformation that these nurses made in meeting the needs of individuals, families, **populations**, and communities (American Nurses Association [ANA], 2007). As the public health nursing role evolved, so did the nomenclature, leading some to question what a **public health nurse** is. This chapter examines public health nursing and the shift in roles as the names changed throughout the late 19th century until today. It also highlights the educational requirements for the public health nurse because as the titles and responsibilities changed to meet the needs of society, so did the educational requirements and expectations. Although this chapter seeks to explain the history of public health nursing and to address the question of what is a public health nurse, it raises more questions for the reader to consider than provides answers.

WHAT IS A PUBLIC HEALTH NURSE?

Early public health nursing leader Mary Gardner raised the question of what to call the nurse who provided care in the home in the preface of her 1933 book, *Public Health Nursing*. She decided on using the term "public health nurse" throughout her book instead of the other possible terms attributed to this role. Gardner (1933) explained as follows:

> Certain questions of nomenclature have arisen, chief among them the name to be given to the nurse and to her work as described in these pages. In view of the present tendency toward more generalized methods of administration, and also because the functions of the various nurses are now so closely interwoven, the names "visiting nurse" and "visiting nursing association" have not been used in this book. "Public health nurse" and "public health nursing" have been substituted throughout to describe all types of nurses and organizations. (p. x)

Others questioned who was considered to be a public health nurse and the activities of this nurse. For example, Welsh (1936) wrote an article entitled, "What Is Public Health Nursing?," where she exclaimed that the very need for public health nursing to define itself after 50 years of organized activity was in itself an "indication of the lack of unity within the field itself" (p. 452). Confusion about who and what a public health nurse was stemmed from the increasing specializations that public health nurses were branching into other areas, such as tuberculosis nurses, maternity nurses, infant welfare nurses, and other specialty areas aside from **visiting nurses**.

The change in names used to describe the person who provided the care in the home has perpetually confused those in health care as well as consumers of care (Geis, 1991; Humphrey & Milone-Nuzzo, 1996; Jones, Davis, & Davis, 1987; Levin et al., 2007; Roberts & Heinrich, 1985; Welsh, 1936). In schools of nursing, for example, students take courses in public health that are often labeled community health. Faculty members debate what they consider a "good" community clinical experience. This debate usually includes whether a visiting nurse experience ("carry the bag") or working in a health department or incorporating public health initiatives in a shopping mall or any number of combination of experiences allow the student to understand the full dimension of public health nursing. This confusion stems from the faculty's orientation to this specialty and from the terminology used to describe the course: Is it public health or community health or both? Clark (2008) poignantly asks what's in a name and tries to explicate the meaning of the various terms used to describe this specialty.

As the public health nursing role evolved, so did the names of this role. The changing names reflected the tensions between and among the stakeholders that shaped the work of public health nurses. The lack of cohesiveness of the various volunteer and public

Visiting nurse with a young boy. *Source:* Courtesy of the Visiting Nurse Service of New York.

organizations and the separation of the preventative care from the curative aspects of the public health nurse's role led Buhler-Wilkerson (1993) to write, "it is little wonder, then that the question, 'What is a public health nurse' has been debated for more than 80 years" (p. 1783). The history of public health nursing provides the reader with the origins of the various names, the educational requirements for these roles, and insight into the debate that continues today as to what a public health nurse is.

EVOLUTION OF THE PUBLIC HEALTH NURSE

District Nurses

District nursing began in 1859 as part of an experiment where a hospital-based, trained nurse was sent to provide nursing care to the poor in "a small district" in Liverpool, England (Hughes, 1893/1949). From that early success the promoter of this experiment, William Rathbone,

expanded this work, dividing Liverpool into 18 districts and supplying each district with its own **district nurse** (Hughes, 1893/1949). The adoption of this successful form of nursing spread, and various agencies began to use district nurses throughout England.

English nursing leader Dacre Craven (1889/1984) wrote about the work of the district nurse in England and attributed Rathbone's experiment as the defining incident in identifying the distinct work of the district nurse. In Craven's description of the district nurse, she includes the care of the sick poor in their homes as the main focus of a district nurse. The responsibilities of the district nurse were carefully explained in Craven's work entitled, *A Guide to District Nursing,* first published in 1889. Craven was considered one of the first superintendents of the central home where district nurses lived together. These nurses were drawn together from "the class of gentlewomen, with a view to bringing women of higher education and refinement to grapple with the special difficulties of the work" (Hughes, 1893/1949, p. 113).

District nurses addressed the health of the poor in the community and needed to have a "real love for the poor and a desire to lessen the misery" (Craven, 1889/1984, p. 1) that was found in the homes. Concern for the family and bringing cleanliness to the patient, the family, and the environment in which the family lived was part of the district nurse's role. The district nurse needed to know about the sanitary and charitable organizations in the district where the patients lived. In this way when sanitary problems arose, such as a defective water supply, or "untrapped" cesspools or "unemptied dustbins," the nurse would notify the appropriate "sanitary committee of the district . . . who [would] take legal steps, if necessary, to compel the landlord to put the premises into a proper sanitary condition" (Craven, 1889/1984, p. 11). The daily work consisted of care of the sick poor and enabled the nurse to observe the sanitary conditions in the home that affected the health of the patient, the family, and the community (or district) in which the patient lived. Craven (1889/1984) gave the following examples of the sanitary work of the district nurse:

> Sometimes there is a plague of flies in the room, which can be traced to some foul or decaying animal or vegetable refuse. When the nurse carries down the dust and ashes to the dustbin she sees whether it ought to be emptied, and ascertains when this was last done. As she fetches water for the kettle she can find out whether it is from an impure and uncovered cistern, and as she empties the slops of her patient she ascertains whether the w.c. is in a good sanitary condition, and with a separate cistern from that used for drinking purposes (and she can herself occasionally flush the pan of the w.-c). (pp. 11–12)

Another important role of the district nurse was to educate patients, friends, and family about the need for a sanitary environment. The nurse taught about the need for personal cleanliness and hygiene, and she herself was expected to be a role model of both. The nurse's uniform, as Craven (1889/1984) described, reflected a clean and neat appearance. The district nurse was to be a paragon of excellence in the way she cared for the sick poor, managed the sanitation of the environment, and educated those about cleanliness and sanitary principles. She also assumed the responsibility for the care of the dying patient and the dead. Craven (1893/1949) wrote that district nurses were instructed on the "best positions in which to place the dying, according to their ailment . . . so that they might breathe to the last without unnecessary effort of pain" (p. 133).

As the district nurses that Craven (1889/1984) wrote about carried on their work, they also were responsible for keeping records of what they did. Each district nurse spent time on paperwork documenting her caseload, the time she spent, and the care she provided in each home. This the nurses shared with the superintendent of the district nurses who collated their reports into a monthly report. The superintendent kept a log of all the cases the nurses managed. Based on the district nurses' work, reports included the number of new cases per month, the length of visits, and the number of visits required by the patients (Craven, 1889/1984, p. 131). Superintendents rated the work done and the data collected. For example, they would use ratings such as "excellent," "good," "moderate," "imperfect," or "nil" to rank such things as the patient's status; the cleanliness of the patient, the room, utensils, and beds; and the various kinds of treatments, like sponge baths, mouth care, precautions against bed sores, wound care, and other treatments. Records of various types of cases such as typhoid fever, diphtheria, puerperal disease, scarlet fever, obstetrical cases, and care of the newborn were also kept. The superintendent's report also included an evaluation of the probationers, who acted as the district nurses, on their ability to observe the sick and manage the care of the sick (Craven, 1889/1984).

Knowledge about the work of these early district nurses in England spread to the United States. In 1893 Amy Hughes, Superintendent of Nurses at the Metropolitan and National Nursing Association, one of the agencies to form in London, came to the United States to speak before the International Congress of Charities, Correction and Philanthropy in Chicago. She explained to the American audience that "district nursing is the technical name for the work of nursing the sick poor in their own homes" (p. 111). Interest in district nursing spread as trained nurses from the early Nightingale-influenced training schools sought ways to improve the health of those who lived in the community. Miss C. E. Somerville, from Lawrence General Hospital in Massachusetts, said, "the last quarter of the century was well advanced when America caught the reflection of England's light, and the era of trained nursing for the poor began in this country" (Somerville, 1893/1949, p. 119).

Early district nursing associations, also called visiting nurse associations, organized in the United States. Some were established along religious missionary lines that expected the care of the sick to include a religious concern for the well-being of the patient. An early example of this was the Woman's Branch of the New York City Mission and Tract Society that in 1877 used trained nurses to provide care to the sick in the home in New York City (Lewenson, 1993; Somerville, 1893/1949). Two years later the Ethical Culture Society offered a nondenominational visiting nurse service that rendered care to the sick poor. Both associations began almost 20 years before the secular visiting nurse service was founded by Lillian Wald and Mary Brewster in 1893 at the Henry Street Settlement. Other early district and visiting nurse associations opened in Boston, Chicago, Philadelphia,

and other cities across the United States, offering care to the sick poor and those of moderate means. They shared a common goal and assumed many of the same roles as their counterpart district nurses did in England (Somerville, 1893/1949).

Nightingale's paper "Sick Nursing and Health Nursing," presented at the Chicago World Fair in 1893, described the district nurse as providing care to the sick at home as well as someone who assumed the work as a health missioner. A health missioner required additional training in how to teach healthy behaviors to mothers in the community and in the home. Nightingale outlined some of the content that was included in their additional training in areas such as sanitary conditions in the home, management of health of adults, women in childbearing years "before and after confinement," and infants and children (Nightingale, 1893/1949, p. 41).

Nightingale (1893/1949) believed that to improve the health of infants and babies, mothers needed to learn about healthier lifestyle behaviors. Nightingale used a population focus to explain why these health missioners needed to be concerned about the health of infants and babies. She wrote that, "The life duration of babies is the most 'delicate test' of health conditions. What is the proportion of the whole population of cities or country which dies before it is five years old? We have tons of printed knowledge on the subject of hygiene and sanitation. The causes of enormous child mortality are perfectly well known: they are chiefly, want of cleanliness, want of fresh air, careless dieting and clothing, want of whitewashing . . . in one word, want of household care of health" (p. 29). Nightingale's idea about health nursing extended to the community, and she summarized this in her paper by saying, "The health of the unity is the health of community. Unless you have the health of the unity there is no community health" (Nightingale, 1893/1949, p. 35).

The concept of health missioners or health nursing was embedded in the work of the expanding role of the visiting nurse in the United States as these nurses added to their work the ideas generated by the public health movement that was calling for ways to keep communities healthy. The public health movement was ongoing in the United States since the mid-1800s when the Shattuck commission identified the need for the creation of local health boards that would collect statistical data on the population, including records of marriages, births, and deaths. States were called on to investigate "the cause of disease, abatement of the smoke nuisance, adoption of means for public health education, and other far-reaching measures" (Beard, 1922, p. 142). Scientific discoveries about the causes of the spread of certain diseases like yellow fever, malaria,

tuberculosis, or poliomyelitis further advanced public health initiatives. Visiting nurses cared for the sick at home and provided the families they visited with information about how to keep their families and communities healthier.

Public health nursing leader Lillian Wald attended the Chicago exposition and was greatly influenced by Nightingale's paper describing health nursing (Haupt, 1953). Haupt (1953) wrote that Wald had "accepted Florence Nightingale's concept of 'health nursing' and put the word 'public' in front of it so that all the people would know that they could use it" (p. 81). The nurses at the Henry Street Nurses Settlement, for example, cared for the sick at home and offered classes to mothers on how to keep their families healthier. Although the term "health missioner" is rarely seen in the literature describing public health nursing in the United States, the dimension of health promotion and disease prevention continued to be imbued in the work of public health nursing.

Lillian Wald (left) and friends, 1915. *Source:* Courtesy of the Visiting Nurse Service of New York.

Visiting Nurse

Public health nursing leader Lavinia Dock addressed the issue of nomenclature in her text, *A Short History of Nursing* (Dock & Stewart, 1938). Dock wrote that the first evidence of the term "visiting nursing" was found in the early records of St. John's House, England, which began in 1848. During that period cholera and smallpox were rampant in England and the United States, and "Anglican and Catholic sisters spent their lives in visiting the poor and caring for the sick under the most terrible conditions" (Dock & Stewart, 1938, p. 305). By the 20th century, however, the role of the visiting nurse expanded into what was to become part of the larger "public health movement." Dock wrote, "In the twentieth century visiting nursing became one part of the broadening field of 'public health nursing,' as an ideal of the visiting nurse who was teacher, sanitarian and public-spirited citizen as well as nurse, gradually took form" (Dock & Stewart, 1938, pp. 305–306). This new expanding field of public health nursing, Dock believed, was to become the "nursing of the future" (p. 306).

As mentioned earlier, public health nurses were closely aligned with the

Philadelphia visiting nurse with a family. *Source:* Courtesy of the Barbara Bates Center for the Study of Nursing History, University of Pennsylvania.

public health movement that flourished during the early 20th century. Fitzpatrick (1975a) described the noted public health expert Charles Winslow's identification of three phases of the public health movement: "the phase of empirical environmental sanitation, the bacteriological phase, and the educational phase" (p. 6). The fact that nurses were already engaged in providing both health care and health education within communities led Winslow and others to acknowledge the value public health nurses brought to the larger public health movement (Fitzpatrick, 1975a).

Modern Nursing Movement

The history of the modern nursing movement in the United States began in 1873 as Nightingale influenced the opening of schools for nurses in New York, Connecticut, and Massachusetts (Lewenson, 1993). It was a time of great change for women who sought a way to financially support themselves in some kind of labor outside of the home. Women read a description about one of the new training schools that had started at Bellevue Hospital in New York City in *The Century Magazine* (North, 1882), describing nursing as a "new profession for women" (p. 38). Once a nursing student completed the apprenticeship training at one of these hospital schools, however, she was sent out as a "trained nurse" into the community without the security of hospital employment. Instead of hiring their graduates, hospitals typically used their next class of nursing students to staff the hospital. A trained nurse consequently had to find employment elsewhere and usually worked as a private duty nurse, caring for one patient in the home setting, or as a public health nurse, working in public or privately

funded organizations with responsibilities for visiting patients in their homes and promoting health in the community.

By 1893, 20 years after the first few Nightingale-influenced training schools began, nursing superintendents of the schools that had already opened joined together with other women from around the world at the now famous Chicago World's Fair. It was at this international conference that professional nursing organizations in the United States began. The first organization to form was the American Society of Superintendents for Nurses. This group was started by pioneering nursing superintendents who wanted to establish standards and control over the education and practice of nursing. These leaders banded together in 1893 and by 1912 became known as the National League of Nursing Education, which changed its name again in 1952 to the current title, the National League for Nursing (NLN). As this group formed, the leaders, Isabel Hampton Robb, Lavinia Dock, and others, saw the need to organize nurses working at the bedside. The need to control practice; lobby for state nursing registration laws, which were nonexistent at the time; and support those nurses in financial trouble led to the formation of the Nurses Associated Alumnae of the United States and Canada in 1896, which in 1911 became known as the American Nurses Association.

This need to control and standardize nursing education and practice extended to another group of nurses marginalized because of racial bias. Many African American nurses were excluded from joining the ANA as a result of a shift to statewide membership in the organization. Once that occurred in 1916, individual nurses no longer could join and relied on membership through their state nurses associations (Carnegie, 1991; Lewenson, 1993). Racist policies of many states, particularly in the south, prohibited African American nurses from membership and left them without the support of a professional organization. This meant issues such as control of education in their nursing schools and control of practice through state registration laws that often discriminated against them would be left unattended until 1908, when the National Association of Colored Graduate Nurses (NACGN) formed. Nursing leader Martha Franklin sought support from other African American nurses to establish this organization to support the needs of black nurses in the United States. This organization lasted from 1908 until 1952 when integration into the ANA was achieved (Carnegie, 1991).

Sophia Palmer, first editor of the *American Journal of Nursing*, wrote that, "Organization is the power of the age. Without it nothing great is accomplished" (Palmer, 1897/1991, p. 297). Organizations formed throughout the country, addressing many of the Progressive Era issues touching on the social, economic, and political welfare of the population. Nurses, by virtue of their education and practice, were aware of the connection between a healthy society and the right to vote (Lewenson, 1993). Concern for women's rights extended into the discussions of the NLN and the ANA, leading to organizational support of a woman's right to vote by 1912. The NACGN also supported women's rights initiatives as evidenced by its support of the work of the International Council of Nurses in that area. The NACGN had sent a delegation years ahead of both the NLN and the ANA to participate in discussions related to women's rights around the globe (Lewenson, 1993).

Public Health Nursing Emerges

Throughout the late 1800s and early 1900s, Lavinia Dock advocated suffrage for women and wrote extensively about this issue in the *American Journal of Nursing* and other journals of that period. Dock aligned the vote with health care and said that without it, nurses would not be able to effectively improve the health of society (Lewenson, 1993). Concern for the public's health was shared by others like Lillian Wald and Mary Brewster, who founded the Henry Street Settlement in New York City's Lower East Side in 1893 to address the health of the people who lived there. Graduates and friends from the New York Hospital training school, Wald and Brewster opened the nurses' settlement house in 1893 (2 years after they had graduated from the training school) to care for the population of immigrants who flooded into the United States during the late 19th and early 20th centuries. Concern for the spread of illness became a real threat to many Americans who lived in the overcrowded cities and experienced firsthand the diversity of those who immigrated here (Fitzpatrick, 1975a; Lewenson, 1993).

Buhler-Wilkerson (1985) said the impetus of the wealthier parts of society to improve the health of the poor stemmed, in part, from an understanding of the germ theory along with the idea that infectious diseases could be spread easily to their own families and communities by those immigrants who "sewed clothes in their filthy tenement homes or who processed food" (p. 1155). Early visiting nurses were hired by philanthropic women who sought to provide the urban poor with assistance during times of illness. According to Buhler-Wilkerson (1985), the nurses hired by these lady philanthropists were to bring their shared vision of the "good society" by bringing "care, cleanliness, and character to the homes of the sick poor" (p. 1155). Nurses were to teach the families they visited about the ways of American life that would lead to the prevention of disease and promotion of health. Fear of the spread of illness prompted some of the concerns of those nurses and their benefactors in bringing health care to the homes of the sick poor (Buhler-Wilkerson, 1985).

Dock worked at the Henry Street Settlement alongside Wald and other colleagues, engaging in what we now call primary healthcare activities, including visiting homes of those who needed care related to an illness, participation in well-

baby clinics, case finding, health-promoting activities, surveillance, and school nurse activities. They lived within the Henry Street settlement in the same community in which they provided nursing care. It was the comprehensive visiting nurse services like the ones delivered at Henry Street that proliferated throughout the country and offered another way for nurses to support themselves while caring for individuals, families, populations, and communities. Nursing care included the care of the sick at home and offered well-baby classes and other health-promoting courses to the community.

Most nurses who graduated from the nursing schools in the late 1800s worked in private duty, providing nursing services to one patient in the home. This focus

Henry Street nurses, 1903. *Source:* Courtesy of the Visiting Nurse Service of New York.

differed somewhat from that of the visiting nurse. Visiting nurses saw several patients in a day, and depending on the agency in which they worked, variable fees were attached to their visit based on the patients' ability to pay. While caring for the sick at home, they also provided much needed health education. Often, the ability to care for the sick at home fostered a level of trust among the families and community they served, which in turn provided them easier access to these same groups as they sought to provide health education. The work of the visiting nurse evolved into what became known as public health nursing and became a viable specialization for the graduate trained nurse. Having coined the term "public health nurses," Wald and other nursing leaders recognized a need to control the practice of this emerging specialization in nursing and founded the National Organization for Public Health Nursing (NOPHN) in 1912 (Buhler-Wilkerson, 2001).

National Organization for Public Health Nursing

The NOPHN grew out of a desire by public health nurses to control the practice and standards of the emerging field of public health nursing. By 1912 the number of public health nurses had grown to over 3,000 and their work was supported through private and public funding (Gardner, 1933). The work was accepted by the community and extended far beyond the care provided to the sick at home. The public health nurses' role had expanded to meet the needs of a growing American urban and rural population. Public health nurses visited patients in the home and provided additional primary healthcare services. In 1933, Gardner described the

increasingly expanded and valued role of the public health nurse as follows:

We find other agencies counting not only on her help in individual cases, but upon the knowledge which she has gained from her unique position. We see that she has had her effect on state and city legislation, and has influenced public opinion to effect non-legislative reform. We find her valued as a preventive agent and health instructor by municipalities and state bodies, and the usefulness of her statistics acknowledged by research workers. We find her acting as probation officer, tenement house and sanitary inspector, county bailiff, domestic educator, and hospital social workers. She is found in the juvenile courts and the public playgrounds, in the department stores and the big hotels, in the schools and factories, in the houses of small wage-earners and in the swarming tenements of the poor. We find her in the big cities, the small towns, the rural districts and the lonely mountain regions. We find her dealing with tuberculosis, babies, mental cases, industrial workers, expectant mothers, midwifery and housing conditions. (p. 25)

The expansion of the public health nurse's role in all facets of life grew in response to the needs of society. Visiting nurse associations proliferated throughout the early 20th century. Public health nurses worked for these newly forming visiting nurse associations throughout the country in both rural and urban settings. They provided care to the sick in their homes, educated the public on healthcare measures that would prevent illnesses like tuberculosis and other communicable diseases, and promoted healthy behaviors. Each of these associa-

Nurse teaching a nutrition class to a family, 1928. *Source:* Courtesy of the Visiting Nurse Service of New York.

tions developed its own guidelines and was mostly organized by lay boards that did not have the same background as public health nurses who founded some of the earlier visiting nurse associations, such as the Chicago Visiting Nurses Association or the Cleveland Visiting Nurse Association (Fitzpatrick, 1975a). Fitzpatrick (1975a) explained that, "Until the rapid extension of public health nursing associations took place, there had been some success in upholding higher ethical and professional practices as well as a certain degree of conformity among the largest associations. This was due, in part, to the exceptional leadership ability

and ideals of the early pioneers in the movement" (pp. 18–19). Yet as public health nursing associations expanded in the early 1900s, the lack of appropriate supervision and the misplaced understanding by the lay boards that ran the newly organized visiting nurse associations caused many in nursing to be worried about a real "threat to sound nursing practice itself" (Fitzpatrick, 1975a, p. 19).

Without clarity about the nursing role in public health, without understanding what the educational requirement of this nurse should be, and without standards regarding the practice, public health nursing leaders believed it imperative to organize. Public health nursing educator Ella Crandall contacted several of her peers between 1910 and 1911 asking them for their thoughts on the need for another nursing organization that specifically focused on public health nurses. Crandall found support among her colleagues; however, support for the format of such an organization varied. Although all agreed that an organization was needed and all agreed to lay members being included, some favored becoming a committee of the already-existing ANA. Crandall's idea, however, was for a separate organization that focused on setting standards and guidelines for public health nursing practice and education (Fitzpatrick, 1975a).

In 1912 Crandall's idea for a separate organization prevailed and the NOPHN formed. Leaders in nursing, like Lillian Wald, Mary Beard, Mary Gardner, Edna Foley, Jane Delano, and Anna Kerr, participated in the organization of this newly formed group. They addressed the issues of standardizing public health nurse requirements, such as requiring them to be graduates of nurse training schools and registered nurses in states that required registration, and supported the idea of agency membership, which meant that non-nurses could be members of the organization, an idea that had not yet been practiced by the ANA or the National League of Nursing Education (forerunner of the NLN). The purpose of the NOPHN was to promote "sound public health nursing for the people of this country, who would be the recipients of the service" (Fitzpatrick, 1975a, p. 24).

The architects of this new organization struggled with what to name the group. Some wanted to reflect the name of the visiting nurse, whereas others, like Cran-

dall, sought to use the term "public health nursing" in the title. Public health nursing was considered to be broader than the earlier term of visiting nurse. The leaders debated the name, and when they finally came up with the title, "National Association of Public Health Nurses," again Crandall argued that the name needed to reflect more than nurses. Edna Foley, another public health nursing leader, suggested the name, "National Organization for Public Health Nursing," which was unanimously agreed upon (Fitzpatrick, 1975a). Wald was elected as the organization's first president.

One of the early NOPHN pamphlets (1914) described the public health nurse as follows:

A Public Health Nurse is a product of evolution. She has developed from the old-fashioned district or visiting nurse, who visits and nurses the sick, poor patient in his home. She is still that same visiting nurse and also, according to the demands of the community in which she serves, a public school nurse, an infant welfare nurse, a tuberculosis nurse, a hospital social service nurse, a sanitary inspector, a truant officer, a social worker, a visiting dietician, and even a midwife. Adequate preparation means special training and experience for each worker.

The idea that public health nursing evolved from the various terms to date— district nurse, visiting nurse—represented the full scope of practice that public health nurses were expected to provide. Public health nurses initially engaged in the wide range of practice, knowing that providing care in the home as visiting nurses afforded them access where health-promoting behaviors could take place. Who paid for the care, whether the public or a privately run voluntary or business association, often determined the types of services the nurse could provide. The earlier public health nurse found employment as school nurses, industrial nurses, visiting nurses, and in other settings where they could impact the health of a particular population. For example, they worked with mothers and babies and people with communicable diseases like tuberculosis. Providing preventative and health promotional education in the community was all part of the work of public health nurses regardless of particular setting or agency for whom they worked.

As public health nurses became more valuable to society, their numbers and the number of settings where they worked increased. Yet the tension between the privately funded visiting nurse services, which offered more of the care of the sick at home, compared with publically run health departments, which assumed more of the activities like surveillance of communicable diseases and health education, created a separation, perhaps a false separation, of the work of the public health nurse. The frequently seen overlap of the public health nurse's role created confusion in both the public and the profession's understanding of that role (Buhler-Wilkerson, 1985).

The term "public health nurse" was continually being defined and refined. For example, in 1919, 5 years after the formation of the NOPHN, Executive Director, Ella Crandall, wrote to George Vincent at the Rockefeller Foundation where she sent him a "corrected report" of a previously shared description of the term "public health nurse." Crandall (1919) wrote the following:

Term public health nurse considered for past five or six years by public health nurses and people administering visiting nurse associations as applicable to work of modern visiting nurse because (1) any nurse giving bedside care should realize opportunities for teaching health protection and hygiene; (2) individual illness not solely individual matter but lowers health standard for family, hence for community; consequently visiting nurse is a public health nurse; although usually supported by private funds, ultimate goal to have all public health nursing supported by public funds as are public school teachers,

A public health nurse weighing children, 1930. *Source:* Courtesy of the Visiting Nurse Service of New York.

nurses employed by municipality not allowed time for bedside cared; hence dependent on visiting nurse to round out her service; impossible to employ both kinds of workers in small and rural communities, therefore rural nurse must be trained in both.

There was a distinction in the work of the public health nurse based on the setting, the specialization, and the environment in which the public health nurse practiced. If the public health nurse worked in an urban setting, there were more resources in the community that addressed the various healthcare needs of the population. As a result, visiting nurses, in many instances, focused more on the care of the sick at home, whereas nurses who worked in public health departments focused more on the preventive and health-promoting kinds of education the public required. In rural settings where healthcare resources were more limited, the public health nurse would offer the full range of public health services, including the preventive and the curative.

In 1919 the NOPHN published a book presenting a description of the public health nurse that recognized that "public health nursing is a profession still in process of evolution" (Brainard, 1919, p. v). Anna Brainard (1919) wrote that although public health nurses worked in both publically and privately funded organizations, "It does not necessarily mean nursing done under the direction of a public department of health: it means nursing done for the health of the public. It does not mean merely bedside care; it means nursing care with an eye to the social as well as the medical aspects of the case" (p. 4). Her definition of a public health nurse included "any graduate nurse who is doing any form of social work in which the health of the public is concerned, and in which her training as a nurse comes into play or is recognized as a valuable part of her equipment" (p. 4).

The idea that public health nurses were found providing bedside care in the home as well as dispensing health information to the public continued to create tension as to the role of the public health nurse throughout the 20th and 21st centuries. The public health nurse found herself dependent on the resources in the community. The division of the type of care the organization provided continued to be a source of concern for those in public health because it was viewed as necessary for the public health nurse to offer a full range of services to improve the health of the public.

Early Experiments in Public Health Nursing

METROPOLITAN LIFE INSURANCE COMPANY

In 1909, just before the founding of the NOPHN, the Metropolitan Life Insurance Company linked visiting nurses with home care services that were offered to millions of their policyholders. Wald was instrumental in setting the stage for the expanded role of public health nurses. Evidence of the efficacy of that care was collected by nurses through the statistics they kept of their work (Gardner, 1933). The public, as well as the company, valued the work of the visiting nurses who participated in this program that lasted from 1909 until 1952. Almost 20 years before this successful experiment was to end, Gardner (1933) wrote, "the tendency of the Company towards an increase in the use of the nurse's time for instructive work in the home is an interesting comment on

the value of such work in the actual con-
servation of life" (p. 24).

The visiting nurse brought health care
and healthcare education into the homes
of the families she visited. The number of
visits to the home of policyholders
throughout the United States rose to one
billion home visits, making Wald's experiment one of the "first national system of
insurance coverage for home-based care"
(Buhler-Wilkerson, 1993, p. 1782) The
demise of the Metropolitan Visiting Nurse
experiment, however, came about
because of many factors, one of which
Hamilton (1988) related to tension created by two different approaches to care:
an economic concern for cost containment, as espoused by the Metropolitan
Life Insurance Company, and the other
embodying the concern to provide nursing services to those in need regardless of
the need to contain costs (Hamilton,
1988). In addition, by 1952, the decline in
policyholders coupled with the increasing
cost of nursing service led the company
to close this program (Buhler-Wilkerson,
1993). Although historians like Hamilton,
Buhler-Wilkerson, and others critique the
experiences of the past from a vantage
point of time, Alma Haupt, who was the
director of Nursing Bureau of Metropolitan Life Insurance Company from 1935
until it closed in 1952, expressed her
more immediate and perhaps personal
view of the program, highlighting the
success of the program. Haupt (1953)
wrote the following:

> "Metropolitan Nursing Service" has
> provided an example of how a profes-
> sion and a business organization can
> work together for a common goal—
> better health, less sickness and death,
> and better business. It has shown that
> maintaining a high standard of nursing

service depends on the availability and
use of the cooperation, leadership, and
standards of a profession. It has
shown the advantages of having the
prestige, leadership, and financial and
organizational backing of the Metropolitan, a company whose contributions have had marked influence on
the health of a nation. (p. 84)

AMERICAN RED CROSS PUBLIC HEALTH NURSING SERVICE

Wald's insight into the needs of populations in both the urban and rural communities led to another important
experiment in public health nursing. Buhler-Wilkerson (1993) describes this experiment as the founding of the American
Red Cross Public Health Nursing Service
(also known as Red Cross Town and
Country Nursing Service) in 1912. Public
health nurses were used to bring public
health care to rural communities around
the country. The Red Cross organized and
standardized the work of these public
health nurses to function in the community, providing an expanded role of public
health nursing services that included
home care and preventative care.

In keeping with the need to engage
communities in the care of their health,
the Red Cross published in 1913 a small
text that accompanied a course that was
given to mothers in the community. The
purpose of this book was to promote
healthy behaviors and prevent serious
illness by involving the family, in most
cases mothers, to support the work of
public health nurses. In the preface of the
book, Mabel Boardman, Chairman of the
National Relief Board of the American
Red Cross, wrote, "work as hard as they
might, neither the medical nor nursing
professions could alone accomplish
much along sanitary lines until the

people in general became aroused to the importance of such matters. Knowledge that personal health depends largely upon the health conditions of the community brings home to each individual a serious personal interest and sense of responsibility" (Delano & McIsaac, 1913, p. v). Nursing leaders Jane Delano and Isabel McIsaac, authors of this text, sought to educate the public about health as part of a broader public health initiative by the American Red Cross. This text was republished several times during the 20th century with different titles. In 1941 the title of the course offered to mothers was called "Red Cross Home Nursing," and a subsequent text was published in 1942 with that same title. In the preface of this version, Mary Beard, Director of Nursing Service at the American Red Cross, again made the strong connection between science and health and illness, stressing the need for healthcare professionals to be supported in their work by educating the homemaker about health. "The individual in the home—particularly the mother or homemaker—continues to hold a responsible place in relation to health. Her part is one of keeping herself and her family in good health, of assisting in giving proper care to members of her household when they are ill, and of supporting community action for the promotion of health" (Trott, 1942, p. v).

The American Red Cross National Nursing Service lasted until 1947 when fewer than 100 Red Cross services remained. The nurses who served in these rural areas provided both the nursing care at home and the health promotion and disease prevention activities that designated the ideal role of the public health nurse. This dichotomy of the two roles, although combined in most rural settings because of lack of services, was mostly reflected in urban settings where the split between the visiting nurse hired by voluntary agencies and the public health nurse hired in public agencies segmented the care that nursing could have more seamlessly provided (Roberts & Heinrich, 1985). Buhler-Wilkerson (1993) speaks in depth about the repercussions of this public health nursing experiment and the reasons for its demise. Although this discussion is beyond the scope of this chapter, the reader is encouraged to explore the reasons for this change as it relates to the lack of a cohesive plan of care that would translate Wald's vision of public health nursing to the American public. The division between the curative care provided to the sick at home and the activities of health promotion and disease prevention by competing healthcare agencies contributed to the end of this experiment and perhaps contributes to the continued confusion about the role of the public health nurse.

The Evolution Continues: Public Health Nursing in the 1930s

The 1930s saw the economic depression where unemployment in all communities permeated the well-being of those who lived during this period of time. Between 8,000 and 10,000 nurses were unemployed as well during this period (Abrams, 2007a). Nurses lost private duty positions and public health employment and found relatively few hospital jobs available (Ashmun, 1933; Fitzpatrick, 1975b). Public health nurses saw their salaries cut and their jobs lost (Abrams, 2007a). The New Deal, however, brought government-funded healthcare programs to American communities to improve economic conditions, hiring unemployed graduate nurses with or without public health experience in programs like the Children's Bureau. Both the public health movement and the need for communities to determine their health-care needs faced the challenging economic downturn of the 1930s. Public health nurses, however, with help from various governmental programs, endured this economic crisis, continuing to find meaning in their work in both the public and private settings.

Toward the end of the depression, in 1938, a revised copy of the *Board Members' Manual for Board and Committee Members of Public Health Nursing Services* was published by the NOPHN. The purpose of such a manual was to offer guidance to the many local community advisory boards comprised of lay and professional people that formed in communities around the country to provide support "for public health activities of municipal and state governments" (NOPHN, 1938, p. vi). The preface of the manual reminded the reader that "at a time when some despairing folk would turn over all social activities to tax-supported agencies, it is well to remind ourselves that voluntary associations still have essential things to contribute: flexibility and willingness to experiment, standards of efficiency . . . creation of public opinion, discovery of community leaders" (NOPHN, 1938, p. vi). Community boards undertook a variety of public health services in the community, including managing finances, determining public health policies, and deciding on the right type of public health nursing programs that were needed in a community, such as "public health nursing associations, American Red Cross chapters, and tuberculosis associations" (NOPHN, 1938, p. ix). The *Board Members' Manual* supported these community advisory boards as both a guide and a reference because they served both public and private organizations engaged in public health activities.

The NOPHN (1938) *Board Members' Manual* also provided a definition of the term "public health nursing," stating that public health nursing includes "all nursing services organized by a community or an agency to assist in carrying out any or all phases of the public health program. Services may be rendered on an individual, family, or community basis in home, school, clinic, business establishment, or office of the agency" (NOPHN, 1938, p. 4). The role of the public health nurse by the late 1930s still included both the care of the sick at home and the broader work of community education and health promotion activities. The idea of separating the services of the public health nurse, according to the *Board Members' Manual,* would fly in the face of "efficiency and economy" (NOPHN, 1938, p. 6). The range of functions that the public health nurse was responsible for were maternity health, infant and preschool health, school health, industrial nursing, adult health, communicable diseases, tuberculosis, syphilis and gonorrhea, noncommunicable diseases, orthopedic services, vital statistics, sanitation, mental hygiene, nutrition, reports and records, and medical standing orders (NOPHN, 1938). The care moved from the concern for individuals to concern for the health of the larger community. It was recommended that each community have public health agencies to engage in some, if not all, of the above activities as part of a planned approach to provide a comprehensive public health nursing program in the community.

C.E.A. Winslow (1938a), a professor of public health at the Yale School of Medicine, recognized the need for communities to organize all nursing care in the community to meet the health needs of the public. He spoke about the need for voluntary organizations to continue to be part of communities' planned public health resources. Winslow (1938a) wrote that "good public health nursing by its very nature is a generalized family service and the ideal toward which we are working is that of a single public health nurse in a given area providing both bedside care and health education to the families under her charge. Any administrative plan which tends to separate bedside care from health instruction, or nursing for the poor from nursing for the rich is undesirable" (p. 2). Winslow saw public health nurses as providing a wide range of nursing services, all for the purpose of fostering health.

The need for more public health nurses in the community required financial support from both the public and private sector. Winslow (1938a) saw a need to coordinate all nursing services in the community, including those in the hospital, private duty, and public health:

> Under an organized community plan it should be possible to develop effective coordination of all the nursing forces of the community. It is obvious that duplications of work by different agencies should be avoided, unfilled needs discovered and met, and the public informed as to the role of each agency . . . planning should make possible better service for the home and far more economical use of community resources. The respective fields of the hospital and public health nursing agency could be adequately defined and provision made for continuity of treatment upon discharge from the institution. (p. 4)

Simplistically, the coordination of community nursing services could ultimately enhance the health care of the public and could lead to such innovations as insuring the middle class with home healthcare service benefits, increasing the income of public health nurses, and ultimately supporting a "modern public health program" (Winslow, 1938a, p. 7). The need for public support of nursing education was also considered a part of the plan that Winslow saw as essential to improving and increasing the number of public health nurses.

Through the evolutionary development of community advisory boards and councils as well as the three nursing organizations (NLN, ANA, and NOPHN) and organizing the Joint Committee on Community Nursing Service (in 1934), coordination of public health nursing needs throughout the country was a goal that some believed could be established (Winslow, 1938a, 1938b). Winslow, along with others, looked toward these local

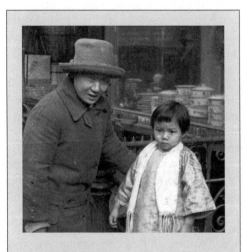

A public health nurse with a child in Chinatown. *Source:* Courtesy of the Visiting Nurse Service of New York.

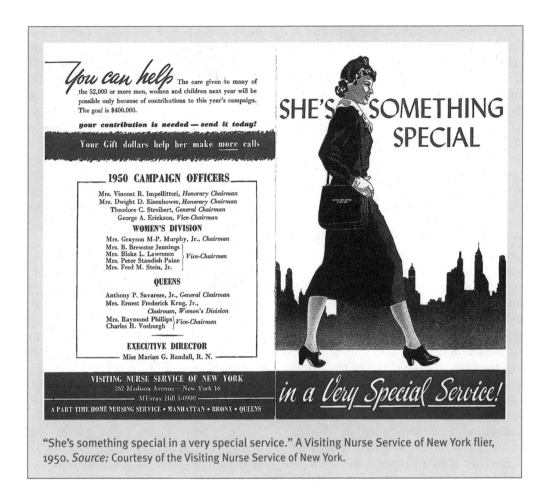

"She's something special in a very special service." A Visiting Nurse Service of New York flier, 1950. *Source:* Courtesy of the Visiting Nurse Service of New York.

and organizational councils to solve the concerns about providing for the health of the public. Winslow (1938a) wrote, "I am convinced that the development of a fully coordinated and truly effective system of community nursing, in home and in hospital, for rich and for poor, including health instruction and bedside care, is one of the most vital social problems of the present day . . . but the community councils of nursing can solve it if they have the courage and vision" (p. 8). Nurses needed to organize and bring together the various stakeholders, hospitals, community agencies, and private

duty nurses to coordinate and advance the public health nursing services in the community.

Public Health Nursing in the Second Half of the 20th Century

By the middle of the 20th century, the kinds of nursing services that communities would need as public health and public health nursing evolved in response to advances in science, new technologies, and social legislation. The advent of new drugs, like penicillin in the 1940s, created different challenges for public health nurses. Nurses working in the community had to address the healthcare issues presented by an increasing aging population as people lived longer, caring for the chronically ill, and responding to cardiac diseases and cancer (Winslow, 1945, p. 989). The dramatic communicable illnesses at the beginning of the 20th century gave way to the increase of disabilities of chronic illnesses later on in the century. Even though the cost of care in the home was less than institutional-based care, the institution offered families some support from the daily responsibilities of providing care in the home (Buhler-Wilkerson, 2001).

In the 1950s the nursing profession underwent a transformation as many of the earlier nursing organizations reorganized. The NOPHN, for example, was subsumed under the NLN. Public health nursing issues became part of the larger organization that may or may not have sufficiently addressed the needs of this important evolving nursing role. Nursing sought to break down racial and gender bias in nursing, and the NACGN became extinct as it merged with the ANA in 1952. The profession also sought to move nursing education into institutions of higher learning and to encourage more men and women of diverse backgrounds into the profession (Brown, 1948). Esther Lucille Brown, author of the noted study about nursing, also acknowledged that health care was changing and the existing barriers between healthcare institutions within the community and hospital were breaking down. Brown (1948) wrote that, "The hospital is moving *out* into the larger community; the community is moving *into* the hospital" (p. 30). The public health agencies that up to the 1940s had successfully focused on reduc-

ing morbidity and mortality rates were now poised to focus on diseases of middle age. Increasing amounts of federal funding in various statewide public health initiatives addressing the control of "venereal disease, tuberculosis, cancer, mental health, and maternal child health" (Brown, 1948, p. 31) added to a changing public health environment in which public health nurses worked. Nurses needed to meet different challenges that public health nursing afforded.

HOME HEALTH NURSING

The social upheaval of the 1960s challenging women's rights, civil rights, as well as the U.S. military responsibility in Vietnam also brought with it sweeping social reforms. Medicare legislation in 1965 included a home healthcare benefit to constituents that "increased the reach and visibility of home care and led to its significant growth" (ANA, 2008, p. 2). The 2008 ANA publication regarding the evolution of home health nursing refers the reader back to the founder of the modern nursing movement, Florence Nightingale, and to William Rathborn's district nursing. The evolution of the term "home health nursing" included similarly expressed ties to the history of public health nursing in the ANA (2007) description of public health nursing. These two terms, home health nursing and public health nursing (and this may be too simplistic), diverged as more people were discharged earlier from hospitals by the 1970s as a result of a Medicare benefit offering home care support. Acute care in the home, offered 24 hours a day, 7 days a week, was an outcome of the increased home care benefits reaped by this new social legislation.

A public health nurse teaching a baby class, 1942. *Source:* Courtesy of the Visiting Nurse Service of New York.

By the 1980s home care services became essential for those people being discharged earlier and earlier from hospitals as a result of the institution of diagnosis-related groups in hospitals across the United States. Home health nursing focused on acute care of individual patients in the home similar to the focus of early district nurses on care of the sick in the home. Two national nursing organizations formed in the 1980s to address the needs of **home care nurses**, the Visiting Nurse Associations of America and the National Association for Home Care (ANA, 2008).

The ANA published the first standards in home care in 1986 that were subsequently revised in 1992, 1999, and more recently in 2008. Although the definition of home health nursing differs greatly from that of the more recent definition of public health nurse (ANA, 2007), they both share a similar history. However, this history diverged in the 1960s because of the social and political changes in healthcare benefits. The ANA (2008) definition of home health nursing describes it as providing nursing care to the "acutely ill, chronically ill, and well patients of all ages in their residences" (p. 3). The definition goes on to include that the home health nurse focuses on "health promotion and care of the sick while integrating environmental, psychosocial, economic, cultural, and personal health factors affecting an individual's and family's health status" (p. 3). This varies from the ANA (2007) definition of public health nursing, which states that "public health nursing is the practice of promoting and protecting the health of populations using knowledge from nursing, social and public health science" (p. 5). The ANA (2007) further delineates the practice of public health nursing as "population-focused with the goals of promoting health and preventing disease and disability for all people through the creation of conditions in which people can be healthy" (p. 5). According to the ANA (2008), home health nurses assume a greater responsibility in "managing the financial cost of care," and it is this aspect of their role that differentiates this specialty from other nursing specialties (p. 4). Because home health nurses work directly with both public and private payers of care, they must have knowledge of the financial systems that pay for this care to support the individuals and families within their care. The striking difference between the two nursing specialties seems to be the breadth in which they approach the care as well as the target of their care and yet there seems to be overlap.

COMMUNITY HEALTH NURSE
A term of more recent origin and coined by the ANA refers to all nurses who work outside of an institutional setting

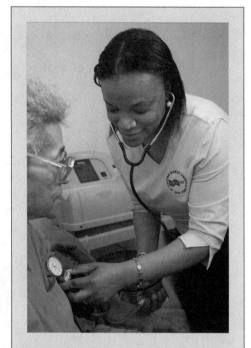

A public health nurse of today. *Source:* Courtesy of the Visiting Nurse Service of New York.

such as the hospital (Clark, 2008). The term "**community health nurse**" refers to nursing services in the community and encompasses the work of the public health nurse (Jones et al., 1987). In the 1980s some viewed the terms "community health nurse" and "public health nurse" as interchangeable, whereas some interpreted public health nursing to be a specialty encompassed by the term "community health nurse" (Levin et al., 2007). In 1985 the term "community health nurse" meant that any nurse who worked in a community setting, whether or not he or she was educationally prepared for public health nursing, was considered a community health nurse (Levin et al., 2007). Public health nurses, however, needed advanced education at the master's or doctoral level that was based on public health science (Levin et al., 2007). A distinction between public health nursing and other community health nurses was made in 1992 calling for public health nurses to be "community-based and population focused" (Williams as cited by Levin et al., 2007, p. 6). The noted nursing leader of the second half of the 20th century, Virginia Henderson, questioned how one could separate "home care from public health nursing . . . and is puzzled at the change that has come about in the public image of the community nurse" (Abrams, 2007b, p. 385).

Public Health Nurse in the 21st Century

The title of public health nurse was used since Lillian Wald claimed the name for the work of the visiting nurse who provided both sick care in the home and the full range of health promotion and disease-preventing activities in the community in the early part of the 20th century. Wald collected statistical data on the work of the public health nurse of Henry Street. She served as an advocate for healthcare policy reforms and refined the work of the public health nurse to include school nursing and led the many early experiments in public health nursing as mentioned earlier in this chapter. As the 20th century progressed and public and private agencies divided the kinds of nursing services provided, the role of the public health nurse was often segmented into either the care of the sick or the population-based health-promoting and dis-ease-prevention activities. By the 1970s (and perhaps beginning earlier in the 1960s), community health nursing was the term that was frequently used instead of public health nursing, and in 1973 the ANA published for the first time a standards of community health nursing practice (ANA, 2007). In 1986 the ANA defined the community health nursing practice as promoting and preserving the "health of populations by integrating the skills and knowledge relevant to both nursing and public health" (ANA, 2007, p. 56). The glossary of the 1986 document (that was reprinted in the 2007 edition of the *ANA Public Health Nursing: Scope and Standards of Practice*) stated that the terms "*public health nursing* and *community health nursing* are synonymous" (ANA, 2007, p. 57).

The ANA (2007) described the distinguishing characteristic of public health nursing as population focused with "goals of promoting health and preventing disease and disability as well as improving the quality of life" (p. 11). Public health nurses still cared for the sick at home as well as maintained an expanded role in the care of the public's health. Public health nurses were involved in eight content domains, including "informatics, genomics, communication, cultural competence, community-based participatory research, policy and law, global health and ethics" (ANA, 2007, p. 2). The increasing complexity of the role was noted by the ANA (2007) as a result of societal and political events that signify challenges to the stability of a community, whether it be local, national, or global. The ANA (2007) identified the threats to the "health of populations as including a re-emergence of communicable diseases, increasing incidence of drug-resistant organisms, overall concern about the structure of the health care system, environmental hazards, and the challenges imposed by the presence of modern public health epidemics such as obesity- and tobacco-related deaths" (p. 3). Public health nurses are now involved with "syndromic surveillance, mass casualty planning and the handling of biological and chemical agents" (ANA, 2007, p. 4). Partners in the community now include law enforcement officers, communication experts, postal workers, and others involved in the safety of the community-at-large. According to the ANA (2007), the public health nurse has a greater emphasis on population-based services than ever before. The level of understanding is greater and the demands for higher education more profound. Evidence-based practice guides public health nurses in their work with populations under duress. The current definition of the public health nurse described by the ANA (2007) has evolved into the following:

> Public health nursing is the practice of promoting and protecting the health of populations using knowledge from nursing, social, and public health sciences (American Public Health Association, Public Health Nursing Section, 1996). The practice is population-focused with the goals of promoting health and preventing disease and disability for all people through the creation of conditions which people can be healthy. (p. 5)

This text applies the Minnesota Department of Health Population-Based Public Health Nursing Practice Intervention Wheel as a model to guide public

A public health nurse of today. *Source:* Courtesy of the Visiting Nurse Service of New York.

health nursing practice. Public health nursing, according to the Minnesota Department of Health (2007), is defined as "the synthesis of the art and science of public health and nursing" (p. 2). This science and art focuses on the development of interventions to the population as opposed to the individual. This population may be defined as a population at risk or those with a common risk factor leading to the threat of a particular health issue. It also may be defined as a population of interest known as a healthy population who may in fact improve their

Mothers and a public health nurse with babies. *Source:* Courtesy of the Visiting Nurse Service of New York.

health by making certain choices that will further promote health and/or protect against disease or injury. For example, an adolescent population that engages in alternative sports and chooses to wear protective gear avoids serious injury. Although public health nurses' primary focus is working with populations, their work often extends beyond this. Minnesota Department of Health (2001) noted the following:

Public health nurses work in schools, homes, clinics, jails, shelters, out of mobile vans and dog sleds. They work with communities, the individuals and families that compose communities and the systems that impact the health of those communities. Regardless of where public health nurses work or whom they work with, all public health nurses use a core set of interventions to accomplish their goals. (p. 1)

Public health nursing still maintains the need to provide care to those in the community, and the evolution of the term continues and seems to be the term that now describes the role of those nurses who work within the community.

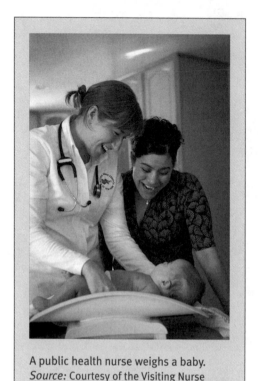

A public health nurse weighs a baby.
Source: Courtesy of the Visiting Nurse Service of New York.

EDUCATION OF PUBLIC HEALTH NURSES

Although the nomenclature of public health nurses changed over time, the one constant that can be found in the literature was the need for advanced education for those who worked in this specialization. From the inception of public health nursing in the United States, early nursing leaders recognized the need for public health nurses to have more education than the three-year diploma training provided to support the work they did in this specialization. Programs such as the postgraduate course at the Instructive District Nursing Association of Boston in 1906 and the one started at Teachers College in 1910 were designed to better prepare nurses to take up the work of nursing in the community (Gardner, 1933; Haupt, 1939). By 1915 there were approximately four postgraduate programs in public health that grew to over 15 by 1922. By 1952 there were over 28 programs set within colleges and universities approved by the NOPHN (NLN, 1952). The various studies that examined nursing in the early 20th century, like the Goldmark report, examined the kinds of advanced education required of public health nurses, above and beyond the training they received in the three-year programs (Crandall, 1922). Later studies, such as Brown's 1948, *Nursing for the Future,* recognized that "as collegiate schools of nursing have developed . . . it has come to be believed that preparation designed for beginning positions in public health nursing can and should be built into the basic curriculum" (p. 96). Nurses entering the public health nursing field would be prepared at the baccalaureate level.

In 1952 a joint committee consisting of the NOPHN and the U.S. Public Health Service studied the curricular needs of the public health nurse. The number of public health nurses had increased to over 24,000 in 1952 from 3,000 in 1912 (Gardner, 1933; NLN, 1952). This increase in numbers constituted a "potent force in translating public health science into service" (NLN, 1952, p. iii). As before, public health nurses were responding to the changing concepts of public health that extended into all facets of life. The joint committee developed a public health nursing curriculum guide that reflected the current thinking of that period, which was that public health was "to provide, through community effort, those services for the saving of life, the prevention of disease, and the restoration to health which the individual or family is unable to provide, or to provide as well, by individual effort" (NLN, 1952, p. iii).

The joint committee noted that the profound changes in the science of medicine, public health, psychology, education, social organization, social sciences, and public health administration called for a new and more comprehensive curriculum guide than had previously existed. Recognizing the need for public health nurses to be responsive to future changes, the curriculum guide was designed to develop the professional skills of the individual to meet the needs for the "immediate future" as well as "be able to adjust to changing situations" (NLN, 1952, p. 2). The joint committee recognized the need for advanced content to be included in their guide; however, they seemed ambivalent about specifying the level in which the public health curriculum would be instituted (NLN, 1952):

> While the Central Committee decided that an adequate basic nursing education in accordance with generally accepted standards would be assumed in the preparation of the Guide, the Committee recognized that this raised certain practical questions. The actual curriculum content that is needed to produce the knowledge and skill required of the public health nurse today or tomorrow is of course conditioned by the students' previous educational and professional background. It has not been found possible nor deemed necessary to specify at each point in the Guide where the learning should take place—in the school of nursing, in the postgraduate program of study, or through a variety of other processes of education and professional experience. (p. 6)

Associate degree programs in nursing that originated in the early 1950s, with the intent of preparing the "technical" nurse, began to include community and home care in the curriculum in the 1990s (NLN, 1993). In 1993 the NLN published a booklet claiming a vision for nursing education that called for a population-based focus for all nursing programs. All nursing programs accredited by the organization, including baccalaureate, associate, diploma, and practical nursing programs, would ensure that all nurses, "are prepared to function in a community-based, community-focused health care system" (NLN, 1993, p. 3). The idea that all types of entry into practice programs would include community content in their curriculum challenged the idea that this content had usually been reserved for baccalaureate and higher degree programs. Although the level of content may have varied, according to the ANA (2007) the "baccalaureate degree in nursing is the educational credential for entry into public health practice" and the master's level prepares a "nurse specialist level with specific expertise in population-focused care" (p. 10). The ANA (2007), however, acknowledges the role that the associate degree and diploma graduate registered nurse as well as the licensed practical nurse have in a community setting. The graduates of these programs also practice in a community setting "where care is directed toward the health or illness of individuals or families, rather than populations" (ANA, 2007, p. 10).

The ANA (2007) describes the term "advanced practice public health nurse" as a master's prepared public health nurse who functions as a clinical nurse specialist or a nurse practitioner using a population-focused care model. Doctoral education also affords additional opportunities for public health nurses to function in roles such as informatics, clinical practice, epidemiology, and education. Here too the coursework at the doctoral level would have a population focus that translates into the work of the public health nurse.

In 2006 Erie County, New York State, advertised for a public health nursing position on the Internet. Anyone responding to this ad had to have a bachelor's or master's degree in nursing. Other states and counties may have different criteria for hiring, but for many agencies the bachelor's degree is the minimum requirement for public health nurses. In most literature about public health nurses, the bachelor's is the minimum requirement. In a recent press release, the American Association of Colleges of Nursing again reiterated that one of the essentials of baccalaureate education is "health promotion and disease prevention at the individual and population levels are necessary to improve population health" (2008, p. 2). Yet in keeping with the vast social and economic changes that fostered a shift from hospital-based care to more home-based care, nursing care at all educational levels adjusted to accommodate to the care needed in the home.

CONCLUSION

The history of public health nursing tells the story of an extraordinary group of professionals who over time adapted to the healthcare needs of the public. Whether they cared for the sick poor or those who could pay, whether they worked in voluntary visiting nurses' organizations or in municipal health departments; whether they were educated in postgraduate programs or in baccalaureate degree programs, these nurses provided both curative and preventive services to the population living in the community. Changing names from district nurse to public health nurse to community nurse and back again to public health nurse only typified the efforts of nurses to adjust to changes that social, political, and economic factors required. The ability to continue to work in public health, regardless of the term applied to their work, shows the resiliency of public health nursing. The tradition whereby a need to redefine itself and reflect on the kinds of care they can provide in both the public and private sector continues with us today. As we read further in the text, it is important to remember the origins of the public health nurses' role as the intervention wheel is applied. Consider the many iterations of this role and how nursing continues to evolve, serve its present day populations, and learn from its past.

References

Abrams, S. E. (2007a). For the good of a common discipline. *Public Health Nursing, 24*(3), 293–297.

Abrams, S. E. (2007b). Nursing the community, a look back at the 1984 dialogue between Virginia Henderson and Sherry L. Shamansky. *Public Health Nursing, 24*(4), 382–386.

American Association of Colleges of Nurses. (2008, October 30). Press release: Nursing schools move to transform baccalaureate education in response to patient care needs and the changing nature of the registered nurse. Retrieved in a blast e-mail to Sandra Lewenson from the AACN on October 30, 2008; reader was directed to the following Web site for additional information: http://www.aacn.nche .edu/Education/pdf/BaccEssentials08.pdf

American Nurses Association [ANA]. (2007). *Public health nursing: Scope and standards of practice.* Silver Springs, MD: American Nurses Association.

American Nurses Association [ANA]. (2008). *Home health nursing: Scope and standards of practice.* Silver Spring, MD: American Nurses Association.

Ashmun, M. (1933). The cause and cure of unemployment in the nursing profession. *The American Journal of Nursing, 33*(7), 652–658.

Beard, J. H. (1922). Progress of public health work. *Scientific Monthly, 14*(2), 140–152.

Brainard, A. M. (1919). *Organization of public health nurses.* New York: Macmillan.

Brown, E. L. (1948). *Nursing for the future: A report prepared for the National Nursing Council.* New York: Russell Sage Foundation.

Bryant, Z. (1968). The public health nurses' expanding responsibilities. In D. M. Stewart & P. A. Vincent (Eds.), *Public health nursing* (pp. 3–9). Dubuque, IA: Wm. C. Brown Company.

Buhler-Wilkerson, K. (1985). Public health nursing: In sickness or in health? *American Journal of Public Health, 75*(10), 1155–1161.

Buhler-Wilkerson, K. (1993). Bringing care to the people: Lillian Wald's legacy to public health nursing. *American Journal of Public Health, 83*(12), 1778–1786.

Buhler-Wilkerson, K. (2001). *No place like home: A history of nursing and home care in the United States.* Baltimore: Johns Hopkins University Press.

Carnegie, M. E. (1991). *The path we tread: Blacks in nursing 1854–1990.* New York: National League for Nursing Press.

Clark, M. J. (2008). *Community health nursing* (5th ed.). Upper Saddle River, NY: Pearson-Prentice Hall.

Crandall, E. P. (1919). Letter dated January 9, 1919, from Ella Crandall, Executive Secretary, National Organization for Public Health Nursing, to Dr. George E. Vincent at the Rockefeller Foundation. Collect RC, Record Group 1.1, Series 200, Box 121, Folder 1494, Rockefeller Archives, Pocantico, NY.

Crandall, E. P. (1922). An historical sketch of public health nursing. *American Journal of Nursing, 22*(8), 641–645.

Craven, D. (1889/1984). *A guide to district nursing.* London: Macmillan and Company. (Originally published in 1889.) In S. Reverby (Series Ed.),

The history of American nursing, A Garland Series. New York: Garland Publishing.

Craven, D. (1893/1949). On district nursing. In I. A. Hampton and others, *Nursing of the sick 1893: Papers and discussions from the International Congress of Charities, Correction and Philanthropy, Chicago* (published in 1949 under the sponsorship of the National League of Nursing Education, pp. 127–133). New York: McGraw-Hill.

Delano, J. A., & McIsaac, I. (1913). *American Red Cross textbook on elementary hygiene and home care of the sick.* Philadelphia: P. Blakiston's Son & Co.

Dock, L. L., & Stewart, I. M. (1938). *A short history of nursing: From the earliest times to the present day* (4th ed. illustrated). New York: G. P. Putnam's Sons.

Fitzpatrick, M. L. (1975a). *The National Organization for Public Health Nursing, 1912–1952: Development of a practice field.* New York: National League for Nursing Press.

Fitzpatrick, M. L. (1975b). Nurses in American history: Nursing and the Great Depression. *American Journal of Nursing, 75*(12), 2188–2190.

Gardner, M. S. (1933). *Public health nursing* (2nd ed., completely rev.). New York: Macmillan.

Geis, M. J. (1991). Differences in technology among subspecialties in community health nursing. *Journal of Community Health Nursing, 8*(3), 161–170.

Hamilton, D. (1988). Clinical excellence, but too high a cost: The Metropolitan Life Insurance Company Visiting Nurse Service (1909–1953). *Public Health Nursing, 5*(4), 235–240.

Haupt, A. C. (1939). Thirty years of pioneering: In public health nursing. *American Journal of Nursing, 9*(36), 619–626.

Haupt, A. C. (1953). Forty years of teamwork in public health nursing. *American Journal of Nursing, 53*(1), 81–84.

Hiestand, W. C. (1982). Nursing, the family, and the "new" social history. *Advances in Nursing Science*, April:1–12.

Hughes, A. (1893/1949). The origin and present work of Queen Victoria's Jubilee Institute for Nurses. In I. A. Hampton and others, *Nursing of the sick 1893: Papers and discussions from the International Congress of Charities, Correction and Philanthropy, Chicago* (published in 1949 under the sponsorship of the National League of Nursing Education, pp. 111–119). New York: McGraw-Hill.

Humphrey, C. J., & Milone-Nuzzo, P. (1996). *Orientation to home care nursing.* Gaithersburg, MD: Aspen.

Jones, D. C., Davis, J. A., & Davis, M. C. (1987). *Public health nursing: Education and practice.* Springfield, VA: U.S. Department of Health and Human Services, Public Health Service, Health Resources and Services Administration, Bureau of Health Professions, Division of Nursing.

Levin, P., Cary, A., Kulbok, P., Leffers, J. Molle, M., & Polivka, B. (2007). Graduate education for advanced practice public health nursing: At the crossroads. Association of Community Health Nursing Educators, 1–24.

Lewenson, S. B. (1993). *Taking charge: Nursing, suffrage, and feminism in America, 1873–1920.* New York: Garland Publishing.

Minnesota Department of Health. (2001). Public health interventions: Applications for public health nursing practice. Retrieved August 28, 2009, from http://www.health.state.mn .us/divs/cfh/ophp/resources/docs/ phinterventions_manual2001.pdf

Minnesota Department of Health. (2007). Cornerstone of public health nursing. Retrieved January, 1, 2009, from http://www.health.state .mn.us/divs/cfh/ophp/resources/docs/ cornerstones_definition_revised2007.pdf

National League for Nursing [NLN]. (1952). *Public health nursing curriculum guide.* New York: National League for Nursing Press.

National League for Nursing [NLN]. (1993). *Vision for nursing education.* New York: National League for Nursing Press.

National Organization for Public Health Nursing [NOPHN]. (1914). Pamphlet attached to a letter sent by Ella Crandall to John D. Rockefeller on October 13, 1914, requesting funding for the organization. Collect RC, Record Group 1.1, Series 200, Box 121, Folder 1498, Rockefeller Archives, Pocantico, NY.

National Organization for Public Health Nursing [NOPHN]. (1938). *Board members' manual for board and committee members of public health nursing services* (2nd ed., revised and reset). New York: Macmillan.

Nightingale, F. (1893/1949). Sick nursing and health nursing: Addendum. District nursing. In I. A. Hampton and others, *Nursing of the sick 1893: Papers and discussions from the International Congress of Charities, Correction and Philanthropy, Chicago* (published in 1949 under the sponsorship of the National League of Nursing Education, pp. 24–43). New York: McGraw-Hill.

North, F. N. (1882). A new profession for women. *The Century Magazine, 25*(1), 38–47.

Palmer, S. (1897/1991). Training school alumnae associations. In N. Birnbach & S. B. Lewenson (Eds.), *First words: Selected addresses from the National League for Nursing 1994–1933* (pp. 293–297). New York: National League for Nursing Press.

Roberts, D. E., & Heinrich, J. (1985). Public health nursing comes of age. *American Journal of Public Health, 75*(10), 1162–1172.

Somerville, C. E. M. (1893/1949). District nursing. In I. A. Hampton and others, *Nursing of the sick 1893: Papers and discussions from the International Congress of Charities, Correction and Philanthropy, Chicago* (published in 1949 under the sponsorship of the National League of Nursing Education, pp. 119–127). New York: McGraw-Hill.

Stewart, D. M., & Vincent, P. A. (1968). *Public health nursing.* Dubuque, IA: Wm. C. Brown Company.

Trott, L. L. (1942). *American Red Cross textbook on Red Cross home nursing.* Prepared under the direction of nursing service, American Red Cross. Philadelphia: The Blakiston Company.

Welsh, M. S. (1936). What is public health nursing? *American Journal of Nursing, 36*(5), 452–456.

Winslow, C.-E. A. (1938a). Nursing and the community. *Public Health Nursing,* April. Reprint.

Winslow, C.-E. A. (1938b). Organizing for better community services. *American Journal of Nursing, 38*(7), 761–767.

Winslow, C.-E. A. (1945). Postwar trends in public health and nursing. *American Journal of Nursing, 45*(12), 989–992.

ASSESSMENT: USING THE PUBLIC HEALTH NURSING ASSESSMENT TOOL

MARIE TRUGLIO-LONDRIGAN
SANDRA B. LEWENSON

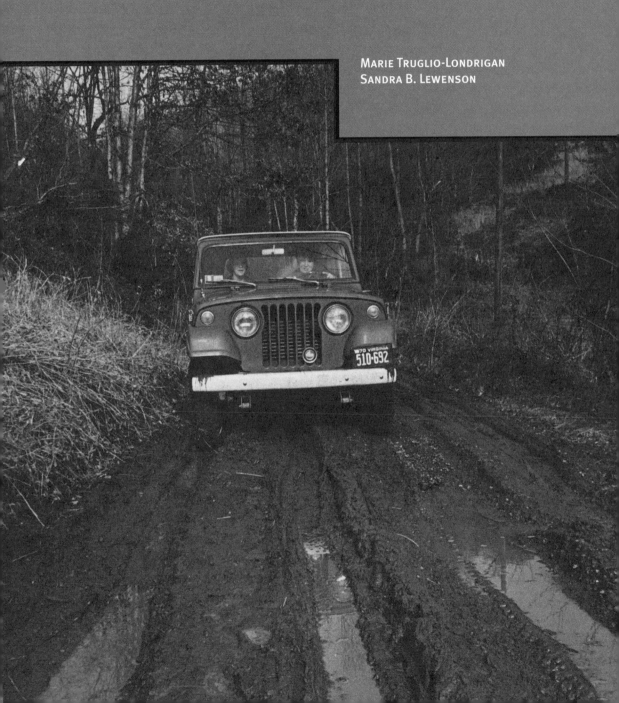

The public health movement did not create the public health nurse, it found her at work in her district nursing the sick, watching over their families, and the neighborhood, and teaching in the homes those sanitary practices, those measures of personal and home hygiene, which do much to prevent disease and to promote health (Nutting, 1923/1991, p. 361).

LEARNING OBJECTIVES

At the completion of this chapter, the reader will be able to

- Identify the importance of a public health nursing assessment.

- Describe the components of the public health nursing assessment tool.
- Apply the public health nursing assessment tool.

KEY TERMS

- A Systematic Approach to Health Improvement
- Assessment
- Determinants of health
- Health status

- Minnesota Department of Health Population-Based Public Health Nursing Practice Intervention Wheel Strategies

---

Assessment supports decision making in health care by providing information about the health of the individual, family, community, system, and population. Shuster and Goeppinger (2008) state that "community assessment is one of the three core functions of public health nursing and is the process of critically thinking about the community" (p. 351). Public health nurses recognize that communities in which the individual, family, system, or population reside influence the health and well-being of all stakeholders. Likewise, the individual, family, system, and population affect the health of the community and each other. An assessment tool guides the public health practitioner through the process of discovery.

This chapter presents the public health nursing assessment tool (PHNAT), newly designed by Lewenson and Truglio-Londrigan, that uses the concepts found in Healthy People 2010 (**Figure 3-1**) and the **Minnesota Department of Health Population-Based Public Health Nursing Practice Intervention Wheel Strategies** as its organizing framework.

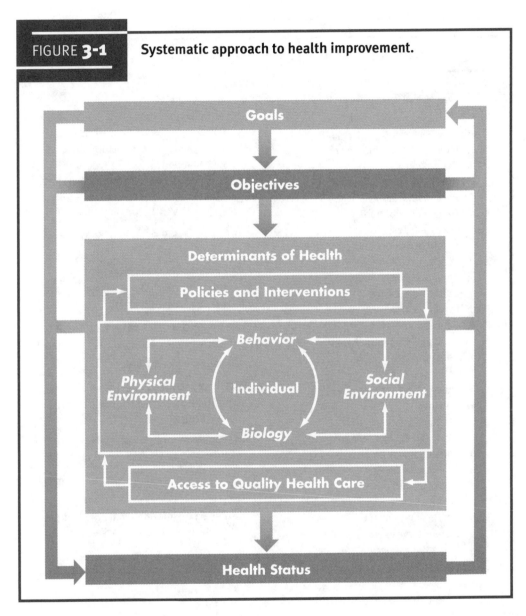

FIGURE **3-1**   **Systematic approach to health improvement.**

Source: U.S. Department of Health and Human Services, 2000.

Specifically, the PHNAT uses the **determinants of health** (biology, behavior, social environment, policy and interventions, and access to care) and **health status** identified in the schematic, "A System-atic Approach to Health Improvement" (U.S. Department of Health and Human Services [DHHS], 2000, p. 6), to organize the assessment process. Using the determinants of health and health status helps

---

BOX 3-1   Public Health Nursing Assessment Tool Schematic

PART I: ASSESSMENT OF DETERMINANTS
OF HEALTH

1. Biology—Assess:
   a. Individual client or family
   b. Population
   c. Age distribution
   d. Race distribution
   e. Gender distribution
2. Behavior—Assess:
   a. Health behaviors in the individual or family
   b. Employment distribution
   c. Leading industries
   d. Family income
   e. Educational level
3. Physical Environment—Assess:
   a. Community (windshield survey)
   b. Other observations
4. Social Environment—Assess:
   a. Housing
   b. Transportation
   c. Workplace
   d. Recreational facilities
   e. Educational facilities
   f. Places of worship
   g. Social services
   h. Health services
   i. Library services
   j. Law enforcement

   k. Fire safety
   l. Communication
5. Policy and Interventions—Assess:
   a. Organizational structure of community
   b. Political issues in community
6. Access to Care—Assess:
   a. The Seven A's

PART II: ANALYSIS OF HEALTH STATUS

A. Vital statistics
B. Communicable diseases
C. Noncommunicable diseases
D. Leading causes of death

PART III: PRIORITIZE PUBLIC HEALTH
ISSUES

A. Issues in priority order

PART IV: PLAN, IMPLEMENT, AND EVALUATE
USING MINNESOTA INTERVENTION
STRATEGIES

A. Population-Based Public Health
   Intervention Strategies and Levels of
   Practice

PART V: REFLECTION

A. Reflect on information learned during
   Public Health Nursing Assessment

---

the public health nurse determine the priority needs of the community and then develop, implement, and evaluate a plan using the intervention wheel strategies as its guide. The PHNAT also asks the public health nurse to reflect on the experience of doing a public health nursing assessment. **Box 3-1** provides an outline of the organization of the PHNAT. It does not include all the detail

that is found in the PHNAT but rather provides a quick schematic.

OVERVIEW OF THE PHNAT

Unique Qualities of PHNAT

The PHNAT offers a *kaleidoscopic* way to view the individual, family, community, system, and population. The authors see this kaleidoscopic capability as essential to public health nurses' practice as they work with a wide spectrum of clients. In the public health nurse's practice, clients include individuals, families, communities, systems, and populations. Therefore a tool that permits the public health nurse to focus on each of these clients must be flexible. The PHNAT permits the public health nurse to assess the individual as well as simultaneously assess the community, population, and system. This flexibility permits the public health nurse to shift his or her view back and forth depending on the area of focus and the priority needs at that moment in time. The application of "A Systematic Approach to Health Improvement" facilitates this shifting back and forth (U.S. DHHS, 2000).

The design of the PHNAT guides the user throughout the process, including the data gathering, analysis, plan, implementation, evaluation, and reflection with tables and questions. Each part of the tool includes space for responses to questions, tables where data can be organized, and definitions for each determinant of health. The PHNAT prompts the user to analyze and reference the data collected. As the user becomes more familiar with the PHNAT, additional information and data may be sought, new tables formed, and original ones revised depending on the needs of the user. For example, if the user wants to compare the findings with national or global data, he or she can do so. An online version of the PHNAT found in this text further facilitates the use of this tool because it can be more easily manipulated and implemented in that format. The comprehensiveness of the PHNAT also suggests that the completion of a public health nursing assessment would lend itself to group work in a course or in the practice setting.

The Internet provides a wealth of data that can be incorporated into the study. Information such as geography and history of a community as well as census track boundaries and data are also found on the Internet and facilitates the assessment of the community. Online databases, such as those found in **Box 3-2**, are examples of important resources the public health nurse may use when completing the PHNAT. The data needed for many of the suggested tables on the PHNAT can be found through the Internet and the various electronic databases. The public health nurse should be sure to select reliable and valid sources on the Internet.

Part I and II of the PHNAT can be completed in any sequence. This flexibility permits the group to work on this tool, collect the data, and, when they are ready, take the next step. Assessment is not a linear process and allows for the public health nurse to complete the process based on expediency, interest, time, and efficiency.

The PHNAT is designed to assist those who study the needs of a community. It can be used by faculty to teach graduate and undergraduate nursing students the method of assessing a community by

---

BOX **3-2** **Examples of Online Database and Web Sites**

http://www.census.gov

http://www.fedstats.gov

http://cdc.gov/nchs

http://health.gov/nhic

http://www.cdc.gov/BRFSS/

using a population-based focus. It is meant to be used by public health nurses who work in all types of community settings such as home care, visiting nurse service, health departments, neighborhood health centers, schools, or industry. Because the PHNAT encourages the collaboration of partnerships within a community, this tool will be shared and used by others in the community. The ethics of public health practice warrant the public health nurse collecting the data to be mindful and respectful of those being assessed. For example, students assessing a community must schedule appointments with the various stakeholders rather than showing up unannounced. They also should carry identification and a letter of introduction from their school in some instances. An assessment is never a static process, nor is the PHNAT a final product. The designers of the PHNAT consider the need for it to be responsive to the needs of public health nurses engaged in the assessment process.

Part I: Determinants of Health

In part I of the PHNAT the public health nurse collects information pertaining to those factors that determine the health of individuals, families, and the population living in a community. The health determinants that organize this section include biology, behavior, physical environment, social environment, policy and interventions, and access to care (U.S. DHHS, 2000).

BIOLOGY

In "A Systematic Approach to Health Improvement," the depiction of the determinants of health places the individual in the center of the model (U.S. DHHS, 2000). This individual's health is determined by biology and behaviors both affecting and

being affected by the other. Biology includes the nonmodifiable factors such as family history, age, race, gender, and genetics (U.S. DHHS, 2000). Modifiable factors that influence health include choices made by individuals with regard to rest; exercise; diet; use of harmful substances such as tobacco, drugs, and alcohol; and/or the use of protective equipment or not, such as helmets (U.S. DHHS, 2000). In this first section the public health nurse who is working with an individual and family conducts an assessment of the individual and family. The public health nurse gathers the information on the individual and family as a client using whatever health assessment tool he or she uses in the particular academic or clinical setting. It is from this focused view that the public health nurse then turns the kaleidoscope and looks outward to the community and asks those questions that inform his or her practice pertaining to the health of the community. Questions to be considered and answered throughout the assessment process include the following:

- What is the health of the client?
- What are the client's health behavior and choices?
- Do these choices support health and a healthy lifestyle?
- What are the resources in the community that facilitate the health of the client?
- Does the client have access to these resources?
- What part of the population does that client represent?
- What is the status of their health?

Aside from the individual and family assessment, this section also asks the user to look at the population that makes up the community being studied, such as the age, race, and gender statistics of that community. The databases in Box 3-2 help the public health nurse complete this section.

BEHAVIOR

The data to be collected in this section of the PHNAT look at the behaviors of individuals and families. The U.S. DHHS (2000) defines behaviors as "individual responses or reactions to internal stimuli and external conditions . . . and have a reciprocal relationship to biology" (p. 19). Every time a person smokes, for example, the lung tissue is altered, leaving the person with a greater risk for shortness of breath, cancer, or emphysema. These alterations may lead the person to change his or her behavior and stop smoking. Families may alter the way they approach diet and exercise when they have a family history of heart disease. The public health nurse collects data on the individual and family that reflect their behavior and again turns the kaleidoscope to look outward to the community. Some of the questions that provide insight into behavior are as follows:

- What does your assessment of the client tell you about his or her behavior?
- What types of choices does he or she make?
- How does family support health choices?
- How does the community support health choices or not?

In addition to these questions, behaviors about the population living in the community are assessed. The following data to be collected in this section include information about the work done by the population, identifying the leading industries in the community, seeking the income levels in the community, and ascertaining the educational level of those

25 years and older. These data provide the user with a broad spectrum of behaviors that affect the health of the individual, family, and population living in the community. In this section as well, electronic databases yield important data.

PHYSICAL ENVIRONMENT

The U.S. DHHS (2000) determinants of health look beyond the individual and family and challenge the public health nurse to assess the physical and social environment of the community at large. These same physical and social environmental factors inform the public health nurse as to the health of the community and the population that reside within that community. The physical environment is defined as follows (U.S. DHHS, 2000):

> [A]s that which can be seen, touched, heard, smelled, and tasted. However, the physical environment also contains less tangible elements, such as radiation and ozone. The physical environment can harm individual and community health, especially when individuals and communities are exposed to toxic substances; irritants; infectious agents; and physical hazards in homes, schools, and worksites. The physical environment also can promote good health, for example, by providing clean and safe places for people to work, exercise, and play. (p. 19)

Collecting assessment data on the physical environment includes what is often referred to as a "windshield survey" (Anderson & McFarlane, 1988; Stanhope & Lancaster, 2008). The windshield survey reflects what one can view from a car window as one drives through a community and contains observations of various components in the community such as housing, open spaces, transportation, race, ethnicity, restaurants, and stores. In urban areas where the use of cars is limited and limiting, walking through the community yields similar results. As the public health nurse walks or drives through a community, she assesses the physical environment using the five senses (Matteson, 1995). Does she see trees, flowers, blue sky, trash, cracked asphalt, smokestacks, or garbage? Does she hear birds, dogs, rain, car horns, screams, or traffic? Does she smell flowers, grass, gas, or sewerage? And, finally, what does she taste? In other words is the environment clean and safe for the people or are there hidden dangers such as radiation, ozone, carbon monoxide, and lead in their homes? The PHNAT asks the public health nurse to identify the boundaries of the community, the physical characteristics in relation to typography and terrain, the history of the community, sanitation services such as garbage pickup and recycling, and environmental programs that protect air, food, water, and animal and vector control. Here the public health nurse can obtain the data by using the Internet and electronic databases, by walking or driving through a community, or by interviewing members of the community.

SOCIAL ENVIRONMENT

The public health nurse assesses the client's interactions and connections with family, friends, and others in ones' community. These interactions are important for positive health outcomes in individuals/families and a population. Social support may be viewed as the type of supportive behavior that is offered to an individual/family or population by another person, family, or agency/organization. That support may be emotional support, instrumental support as in services provided, information support such as knowledge, and appraisal support

such as feedback to a person (House, 1981). These social supports may be offered informally, as in the type of support offered to an individual by a family member or a friend, or they may be more formal, as in the support offered by an agency such as Meals on Wheels. The social environment assessment section of the PHNAT asks for information about formal and informal support systems in the community. Some of the areas that the public health nurse assesses include housing, transportation, work, recreation, education, places of worship, health care, social services, library, law enforcement, fire, and communication (U.S. DHHS, 2000).

POLICY AND INTERVENTIONS

The public health nurse must also assess the policies and interventions that influence the health of the community under study. Examples include policies on seat belt use, helmet use, and child car seats. Each of these policies has had a positive influence on the health and well-being for individuals and the population at large, resulting in a decrease in disabilities and injuries. The public health nurse must be knowledgeable about how his or her community functions with regard to the political infrastructure and as such must assess this infrastructure to be familiar with how it works: who are the political formal leaders; how can they be reached; what initiatives have they supported in the past; what are the laws that affect the individual/family, population, and community with regard to the public's health; are these laws upheld; are there issues that have not been addressed; and, if so, what can be done to address these issues? The data collected in this section include the organizational structure of the community, a description of the political issues in the community, and an identification of some of the public health laws that impact the community and its members' health. As the public health nurse conducts this portion of the assessment, it is important to explore what the local newspapers report, to meet with the local government, and check out the school boards or any of the governing bodies in that area. Meet the candidates if it is an election year and listen to what the community is saying. Using the Internet, here and throughout the PHNAT, assists the user to obtain the necessary data and learn about the community.

ACCESS TO CARE

Finally, access to quality care is another important part of the PHNAT. Whereas other community assessment tools have included many of the above health determinants, the inclusion of access to care using the seven A's is unique to the PHNAT:

- **A**ccess: What good is a particular resource in a community if the members of that community cannot access the service?
- **A**wareness: For access to take place one must have knowledge or awareness that there is a need and that there is a service to meet that need.

In addition to access and awareness, there are five additional components to consider. Each of these five components also influences the health and well-being for the individual/family and the population that reside in a particular community. These five additional components are (Krout, 1986; Truglio-Londrigan & Gallagher, 2003; Williams, Ebrite, & Redford, 1991):

- **A**vailability
- **A**ffordability
- **A**cceptability

- **A**ppropriateness
- **A**dequacy

Specifically, each of these key seven components is essential to assess and analyze.

As the public health nurse conducts the assessment, he or she must also analyze the particular section as he or she proceeds. For example, is the community service or agency that supports health education in the community adequate or inadequate? Does the client have access to the transportation that may be available in the community? This ongoing analysis during the assessment provides necessary information about the health of the community in question. The seven A questions can assist the public health nurse in analyzing his or her findings:

- Is the population *aware* of their needs and the services in the community?
- Can the population gain *access* to the services that they need?
- Is the service *available* and convenient to the population in terms of time, location, and place for use?
- How *affordable* is the service for the population in question?
- Is the service *acceptable* to the population in terms of choice, satisfaction, and cultural congruence?
- How *appropriate* is the service for the specific population or is there a fit?
- Is there *adequacy* of service in terms of quantity or degree?

Part II: Analysis of Health Status

Part II of the PHNAT involves gathering census data that provide the public health nurse with evidence about the overall health status of the population living in a particular community. The public health nurse may already have some idea as to the health of the population by asking the critical questions related to the determinants of health; however, gathering the health status data provides additional quantitative evidence. The public health nurse examines the most recent health status data and compares the data with earlier census data. The purpose of this comparison is to look for trends in health status. Many times the public health nurse will go back even further in the census data to see patterns that have emerged over time. This information may be gathered by looking at the demographics such as population by number and percentage for age and sex, race, and ethnicity. In addition, numbers and percentages for family types and marital status are included. Vital statistics such as birth and death as well as the number and percentages for deaths by selected causes are gathered. Additional information gathered includes life expectancy and risk factors. Here, too, as throughout the assessment, the Internet and electronic databases provide important avenues for the demographic and epidemiological data that are sought.

Part III: Prioritize Public Health Issues

Once the public health nurse conducts the assessment and analysis in parts I and II, the data elucidate what priority public health issues exist within the community. In determining the priority health issues, the public health nurse, using a population-based focus, collaborates with other public health practitioners, key informants in the community, and any organization or agency who may have a voice with regard to the population and public health issue. In population-based care it is partnerships that form the nec-

essary bonds to make sustainable change necessary for health in the particular targeted population. The public health nurse must first communicate and share the assessment data with these individuals/organizations, and this begins the process. Those involved in the partnership work together to form a common understanding of the issue. All involved, including the population of interest residing in the community, agree on the priority issue identified. This is essential for a positive outcome.

Part IV: Plan, Implement, and Evaluate Intervention Using Minnesota Intervention Strategies

In this section of the PHNAT, the public health nurse, along with any members of the partnership established during the assessment process, develops a plan of action using the intervention wheel strategies, implements that plan, and evaluates the outcome of these strategies. The PHNAT involves the application of the intervention wheel, which identifies 17 nursing interventions applied to three levels of practice: individual/family, community, and system. The intervention wheel began in the mid-1990s as part of a "grounded theory process carried out by the public health nurse consultants at the Minnesota Department of Health" (Keller, Strohschein, & Briske, 2008, p. 189). Questioning the contribution public health nurses made in population-based care, the consultants held a series of workshops that informed them of the work of public health nurses. They analyzed the input of public health nurses who worked in a variety of community settings using a systematic evidenced-based review of the literature. This enabled the consultants to construct the wheel graph depicting the 17 intervention strategies applied to the three levels of practice (Stanhope & Lancaster, 2008). The 17 intervention strategies visually depicted and color coded on the wheel are case finding, surveillance, disease and health event investigation, outreach, screening, referral and follow-up, case management, delegated functions, health teaching, counseling, consultation, collaboration, coalition building, community organizing, advocacy, social marketing, and policy development and enforcement. The intervention wheel was "conceived as a common language or catalog of general actions used by public health nurses across all practice settings" (Keller et al., 2008, p. 193).

For the purposes of this text, these intervention strategies have been separated out into five themes addressed in specific intervention chapters:

1. *Hitting the pavement* includes the strategies case finding, surveillance, disease and health event investigation, outreach, and screening (Chapter 8).
2. *Running the show* includes the strategies referral and follow-up, case management, and delegated functions (Chapter 9).
3. *Working it out* includes the strategies health teaching, counseling, and consultation (Chapter 10).
4. *Working together* includes the interventions collaboration, coalition building, and community organizing (Chapter 11).
5. *Getting the word out* includes the interventions advocacy, social marketing, and policy development and enforcement (Chapter 12).

Using case studies, Chapters 8 through 12 focus on each of these themes using examples from public health nurses who use the intervention wheel strategies to address public health problems experienced by individuals, families, and populations within their communities. The reader is asked to refer to these chapters when using the PHNAT.

When selecting the intervention strategy and developing a plan of action, the public health nurse works in concert with others in the community and considers:

- The audience to be targeted for the plan
- Short-term goal(s), long-term goal(s), and outcome
- Community resources
- Financing of the implementation and evaluation of the plan
- Evidence that supports the intervention for this population
- Best place to implement the strategy
- Best person to implement the strategy
- How to evaluate whether or not the outcomes are met

Part V: Reflection

This final section of the PHNAT reminds the public health nurse to be reflective in his or her practice. Self-reflection aids in the decision-making process (Truglio-Londrigan & Lewenson, 2008). The table in this section asks that a record be kept of the experience. The person who conducts the assessment may use this chart to record when he or she worked on the assessment, how he or she responded to the various parts of the assessment, reflect on the group experience if the assessment was conducted in a group, or any personal or professional reflection observed during the assessment process.

CONCLUSION

This chapter explains how to conduct a public health nursing assessment process using the author-designed PHNAT. The unique qualities of the PHNAT include the use of the U.S. DHHS (2000) determinants of health and health status, application of the intervention wheel strategies, and self-reflection. The application of the PHNAT provides the public health nurse with the information that needs to be analyzed and ultimately determine the priority health care issues for a specific population within a community. To carry out the assessment, the public health nurse uses a variety of methods to obtain the data, including observation, interviews, Internet, census tracks, govern-

ment reports, newspaper accounts, and evidence of best practice. The public health nurse both collaborates and shares his or her findings with other public health practitioners, key informants in the community, and other agencies in the specific community of interest to determine the priority. Once this priority is identified, the public health nurse works toward the development and implementation of a culturally congruent initiative based in evidence. The evaluation of the initiative is part of the plan, as is the reflective piece by the public health nurse. Both the outcomes of the evaluation and the reflections provide rich feedback to the community and the public health nurse as he or she continues the ongoing assessment process.

References

Anderson, E. T., & McFarlane, J. (Eds.). (1988). *Community as client: Application of the nursing process.* Philadelphia: Lippincott.

House, J. S. (1981). *Work stress and social support.* Reading, MA: Addison-Wesley.

Keller, L. O., Strohschein, S., & Briske, L. (2008). Population-based public health nursing practice: The intervention wheel. In M. Stanhope & J. Lancaster (Eds.), *Public health nursing: Population-centered health care in the community* (7th ed., pp. 186–214). St. Louis, MO: Mosby Elsevier.

Krout, J. A. (1986). *The aged in rural America.* Westport, CT: Greenwood.

Matteson, P. S. (1995). *Teaching nursing in the neighborhoods: The Northeastern University Model.* New York: Springer.

Nutting, A. (1923/1991). Thirty years of progress in nursing. In N. Birnbach & S. B. Lewenson (Eds.), *First words: Selected addresses from the National League for Nursing 1894–1933* (pp. 358–369). New York: National League for Nursing Press.

Shuster, G. F., & Goeppinger, J. (2008). Community as client: Assessment and analysis. In M. Stan-

hope & J. Lancaster (Eds.), *Public health nursing: Population-centered health care in the community* (7th ed., pp. 339–372). St. Louis, MO: Mosby Elsevier.

Stanhope, M. & Lancaster, J. (Eds.). (2008). *Public health nursing: Population-centered health care in the community* (7th ed.). St. Louis, MO: Mosby Elsevier.

Truglio-Londrigan, M., & Gallagher, L. (2003). Using the seven A's to determine older adults' community resource needs. *Home Healthcare Nurse, 21*(12), 827–831.

Truglio-Londrigan, M., & Lewenson, S. B. (2008). Know yourself: Reflective decision-making. In S. B. Lewenson & M. Truglio-Londrigan (Eds.), *Decision-making for nurses: Thoughtful approaches to practice* (pp. 1–11). Sudbury, MA: Jones and Bartlett.

Williams, M., Ebrite, F., & Redford, L. (1991). *In-home services for elders in rural America.* Kansas City, MO: National Resource Center for Rural Elderly.

U.S. Department of Health and Human Services. (2000). *Healthy people 2010* (Vol. 1). Washington, DC: U.S. Government Printing Office.

PUBLIC HEALTH NURSING ASSESSMENT TOOL

DESIGNED BY
SANDRA B. LEWENSON
AND MARIE TRUGLIO-LONDRIGAN

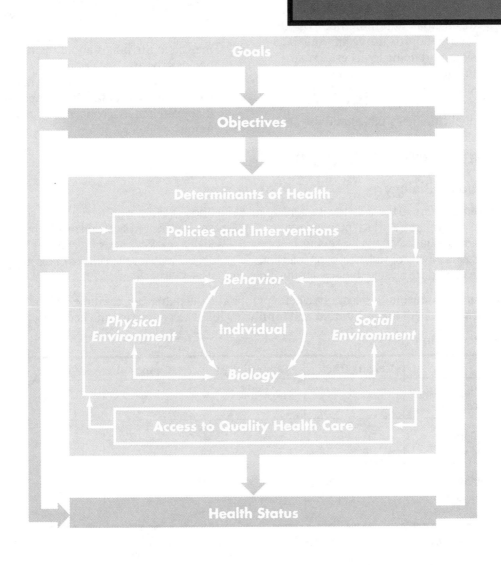

Suggestions for table use:

1. Read all horizontal and vertical columns. These will give cues about the key questions to ask.
2. Fill in the vertical column for each table that requests information on the Seven A's. When filling in these boxes, include the most pertinent information that you feel informs the assessment.
3. When completing Part I, Section 6: Access to Care, you will note that it is a summary of the work that you did throughout Part I. Reflect on this information to arrive at your decisions pertaining to access to care.
4. In some instances you need to consider collecting data on multiple years to identify trends. You can duplicate these tables and use them to collect the data on different years, such as the 1990 and 2000 censuses, or the upcoming 2010 census.
5. Remember, this is a working document that you, the public health nurse, can adjust and revise to meet the needs of the community being assessed. The collection of data is more important than filling in the boxes or cutting and pasting informaiton from the Web site. You may need to compile additional data in a particular area, depending what you learn as you go. For example, you may fill in the boxes about the number of schools in a community, but you may also want to know the number of students per faculty member, if that was cited as a concern by a community collaborator.

PART I: DETERMINANTS OF HEALTH

Section 1. Biology

"**Biology** refers to the individual's genetic makeup (those factors with which he or she is born), family history (which may suggest risk for disease), and the physical and mental health problems acquired during life. Aging, diet, physical activity, smoking, stress, alcohol or illicit drug abuse, injury or violence, or an infectious or toxic agent may result in illness or disability and can produce a "new" biology for the individual" (U.S. DHHS, 2000, p. 19).

A. Assessment: In this section, when appropriate, the public health nurse will include an assessment of the **individual** and **family**. Include the genogram and ecogram.

B. Population

	Census track	Community	County	State
Population at last census				
Population density				
Population changes in the last 10 years				

Sources of evidence: _____

C. Age

Years (include years as per data)	Census track		Community		County		State	
	#	%	#	%	#	%	#	%

Sources of evidence: _____

D. Race

	Census track		Community		County		State	
	#	%	#	%	#	%	#	%
White								
Black/ African American								
Hispanic								
Asian								
Native American								
Other								

Sources of evidence: _____

E. Gender

	Census track		Community		County		State	
	#	%	#	%	#	%	#	%
Female								
Male								

Sources of evidence: _____

Section 2. Behaviors

"**Behaviors** are individual responses or reactions to internal stimuli and external conditions. Behaviors can have a reciprocal relationship to biology; in other words, each can react to the other. For example, smoking (behavior) can alter the cells in the lung and result in shortness of breath, emphysema, or cancer (biology) that then may lead an individual to stop smoking (behavior). Similarly, a family history that includes heart disease (biology) may motivate an individual to develop good eating habits, avoid tobacco, and maintain an active lifestyle (behaviors), which may prevent his or her own development of heart disease (biology)" (U.S. DHHS, 2000, p.19).

In this section the public health nurse will consider:

- What does your assessment of the individual client tell you about your individual client's behavior?
- What types of choices does he or she make?
- How do family members help your client make healthy choices or not help him or her make healthy choices?
  - Exercise
  - Diet
  - Sleep/rest
  - Stress reduction
- How does the community support healthy choices or not?
  - Smoking bans in restaurants
  - Vending machines in schools with healthy choices
  - Recreational spaces for populations

A. Employment

	Number in census track	Number in community	Number in county	Number in state
Employed persons				
Unemployed persons				

Sources of evidence: _____

B. Leading Industries in the Community (*Name at least 2*)

Name	Address	Type	Number employed

Sources of evidence: _____

C. Family Income (*Percent of population*)

	Census track	Community	County	State
$0–5,000				
$5,000–9,999				
$10,000–14,000				
$15,000–24,999				
$25,000–34,999				
$50,000–64,000				
$65,000–79,000				
$80,000 or more				
	100%	100%	100%	100%

Sources of evidence: _____

D. Educational Level of People Over 25 Years of Age (*Percent of population*)

	Census track	Community	County	State
9th grade and below				
High school graduate				
Some college				
College graduate (Associate and Baccalaureate)				
Median number of years completed				

Sources of evidence: _____

Section 3. Physical Environment

"**Physical environment** can be thought of as that which can be seen, touched, heard, smelled, and tasted. However, the physical environment also contains less tangible elements, such as radiation and ozone. The physical environment can harm individual and community health, especially when individuals and communities are exposed to toxic substances; irritants; infectious agents; and physical hazards in homes, schools, and worksites. The physical environment also can promote good health, for example, by providing clean and safe places for people to work, exercise, and play" (U.S. DHHS, 2000, p. 19).

In this section the public health nurse writes a brief narrative description of the community including the topography, climate, history, and boundaries. This is where you should do a windshield survey. Include the reason for selecting this community and your impressions of the physical environment of this community.

   a. Topography and climate
       Terrains
       Climate—seasonal variations in temperature, humidity, and rainfall
       Unusual topographical features
   b. History of community
       Write a brief historical account of the selected community
   c. Boundaries
       Geographical boundaries
       State
       County

Community district board
Village
Census track

d. Reports of toxic substances or exposure to other environmental hazards, such as lead and carbon monoxide.

e. Home assessment of individual, client, and family (if applicable)

f. Identify what you observed with regard to the following:
- Waste disposal, sanitation, litter
- Air quality, incinerators
- Stagnant water
- Insects, rodents
- Stray dogs and cats
- Signs of decay
- Limited open spaces for recreation
- Quality of food (e.g., open food stands with insects, expiration dates on canned foods outdated)
- Condition of roads, sidewalks, playgrounds, public spaces, parks
- Other observations of the physical status of the community indentified in your windshield survey

A. Sanitation

Service	Description of services (*Include whether it is community based, state, or national*)	Analysis of the Seven A's
Water supply		
Sewage supply		
Solid waste disposal		
Provisions or laws for recycling		
Air contaminants		
Vector control programs for deer, ticks, rabid animals, rodents		
Other		

Sources of evidence: _____

Section 4. Social Environment

"**Social environment** includes interactions with family, friends, coworkers, and others in the community. It also encompasses social institutions, such as law enforcement, the workplace, places of worship, and schools. Housing, public transportation, and the presence or absence of violence in the community are among other components of the social environment. The social environment has a profound effect on individual health, as well as on the health of the larger community, and is unique because of cultural customs; language; and personal, religious, or spiritual beliefs. At the same time, individuals and their behaviors contribute to the quality of the social environment" (U.S. DHHS, 2000, p. 19).

A. Housing Conditions

Housing characteristics	Total number of units	Owner occupied	Renter occupied	Vacant	Housing subsidies/ homeless provisions

Sources of evidence: _____

B. Transportation

Service	Description of services (*Cost, destination of service, quality of service, condition of services and/or roads, handicap accessible*)	Analysis of the Seven A's
Train		
Bus		
Taxi including private services		
Major roads		
Minor roads		
Volunteers providing transportation		
School buses		

Sources of evidence: _____

C. Workplace

Places of employment	Description of workplace (*Professional, industry, factories, schools, town, city, county, businesses*)	What is the workplace environment for safety? What is the estimated yearly salary range of employees?

Additional questions to ask:

- Do most people who reside in the community work in the community, or do they commute?

- If they commute, what is their mode of transportation?

- What is the cost of that commute?

- What is the time of the commute?

- Does this commute impact quality of life?

Sources of evidence: _____

D. Recreational Facilities: Parks, Playgrounds, and Athletic Fields

Recreational facilities	Area served/services provided (*Cost, population served, hours, maintenance of facilities*)	Analysis of the Seven A's

Sources of evidence: _____

E. Educational Facilities

Facility	Number of public	Number of private (Religious)	Number of private (Secular)
Preschool			
Elementary			
Junior high			
Senior high			
Colleges/universities			
Early morning programs			
Recreational programs within school system			
After school programs			

Sources of evidence: _____

F. Places of Worship

Name, address, phone	Denomination	Services

Sources of evidence: _____

G. Social Services (*e.g., food and clothing banks, homeless shelters, adult day care, child care*)

Agency name, address, phone	Area served, services provided, cost of services	Analysis of the Seven A's

Sources of evidence: _____

H. Health Services (*e.g., public, acute, home care, community, long term, occupational*)

Agency name, address, phone	Area served, services provided (*Cost, hours, population served*)	Analysis of the Seven A's

Sources of evidence: _____

I. Library Services

Library name, address, phone	Area served, services provided	Analysis of the Seven A's

Sources of evidence: _____

J. Law Enforcement

Law enforcement service	Area served, services provided (*Size, equipment, response times, types of calls over the past 6 months, neighborhood programs*)	Analysis of the Seven A's
Police force		
Special services (SWAT, bomb squads, emergency response teams)		
Animal enforcement		
Senior watch patrols		
Private security		
Neighborhood watch		
Vigilante groups		

Sources of evidence: _____

K. Fire Department

Fire department stations (*Fire fighters in company, special fire forces*)	Area served, services provided (*Number of companies, equipment, response times, types of calls over the past 6 months, community programs*)	Analysis of the Seven A's

Sources of evidence: _____

L. Communication

Service	Description of services (*Include whether it is community based, state, or national*)	Analysis of the Seven A's
Television (e.g., educational, relaxation, emergency response)		
Radio (e.g., educational, relaxation, emergency response)		
Newsprint (e.g., educational, relaxation, emergency response)		
Internet/Facebook/My Space/text messaging/ Twitter (e.g., educational, relaxation, emergency response)		
Newsletters		
Bulletin Boards		
Telephone Chains		

Sources of evidence: _____

Section 5. Policy and Interventions

"**Policies and interventions** can have a powerful and positive effect on the health of individuals and the community. Examples include health promotion campaigns to prevent smoking; policies mandating child restraints and safety belt use in automobiles; disease prevention services, such as immunization of children, adolescents, and adults; and clinical services, such as enhanced mental health care. Policies and interventions that promote individual and community health may be implemented by a variety of agencies, such as transportation, education, energy, housing, labor, justice, and other venues, or through places of worship, community-based organizations, civic groups, and businesses" (U.S. DHHS, 2000, p.19).

In the table below, include organizational structure of community including political parties of leadership: governor, senators, assemblypersons, mayor, and board members, and others specific to the community under study.

A. Organizational Structure of Community
Once you collect the data below, place the data within an organizational chart that represents a visual model of the hierarchy.

- Titles

- Names

- Method of contact

- Initiatives supported in the past and presently

- Interview one of the above officials or go to a town board meeting

Sources of evidence: _____

B. Political Issues in the Community

Political issues	Action/policy taken

Section 6. Access to Care

"The health of individuals and communities also depends greatly on **access to quality health care**. Expanding access to quality health care is important to eliminate health disparities and to increase the quality and years of healthy life for all people living in the United States. Health care in the broadest sense not only includes services received through health care providers but also health information and services received through other venues in the community" (U.S. DHHS, 2000, p. 20).

A. Assess the Seven A's

	Describe	Identify as a problem statement
Is the individual, family, or population *aware* of their needs and services available in the community?		
Can the individual, family, or population gain *access* to the services they need?		
Are services *available* and convenient for the individual, family, or population in terms of time, location, and place for use?		
How *affordable* is the service for the individual, family, or population?		
Is the service *acceptable* to the individual, family, or population in terms of choice, satisfaction, and congruency with cultural values and beliefs?		
How *appropriate* is the service for the individual, family, or population, or is there a fit?		
Is there *adequacy* of service in terms of quantity or degree for the individual, family, or population?		

Sources of evidence: _____

PART II: ANALYSIS OF HEALTH STATUS

"To understand the health status of a population, it is essential to monitor and evaluate the consequences of the determinants of health. . . .

The health status of the United States is a description of the health of the total population, using information representative of most people living in this country. . . .

Health status can be measured by birth and death rates, life expectancy, quality of life, morbidity from specific diseases, risk factors, use of ambulatory care and inpatient care, accessibility of health personnel and facilities, financing of health care, health insurance coverage, and many other factors. The information used to report health status comes from a variety of sources, including birth and death records; hospital discharge data; and health information collected from health care records, personal interviews, physical examinations, and telephone surveys" (U.S. DHHS, 2000, p. 21).

A. Vital Statistics

	Census track		Community		County		State	
	#	%	#	%	#	%	#	%
Live births								
General deaths								

Source of evidence: _____

B. Communicable Diseases (*Top 10*)

Census track	Community	County	State

Source of evidence: _____

C. Noncommunicable Diseases (*Top 5*)

Census track	Community	County	State

Source of evidence: _____

D. Leading Causes of Death (*Top 10*)

Census track	Community	County	State

Source of evidence: _____

PART III: PRIORITIZE PUBLIC HEALTH ISSUES

A. Issues (*In order of priority***)**

Issues	Targeted population	Short-term goal(s)	Long-term goal(s)

PART IV: PLAN, IMPLEMENT, AND EVALUATE INTERVENTION USING MINNESOTA INTERVENTION STRATEGIES

A. Population-Based Public Health Intervention Strategies and Levels of Practice *(Select the intervention strategy that is most appropriate with the assessment findings.)*

Interventions	Levels of practice			
	Individual, family	Community	System	Outcome evaluation
Surveillance				
Disease and health event investigation				
Outreach				
Screening				
Case-finding				

Interventions	Levels of practice			
	Individual, family	Community	System	Outcome evaluation
Referral/ follow-up				
Case management				
Delegated functions				
Health teaching				
Counseling				
Consultation				
Collaboration				
Coalition building				
Community organizing				
Advocacy				
Social marketing				
Policy development and enforcement				

PART V: REFLECTION

A. Reflect on Information Learned During Public Health Nursing Assessment
(Keep an ongoing journal throughout the assessment process.)

Date	Reflection

FUNDAMENTALS OF EPIDEMIOLOGY AND SOCIAL EPIDEMIOLOGY

SUSAN MOSCOU

Despite my experience in a large metropolitan hospital, and the subsequent knowledge gained through a year's residence in a reformatory and asylum for the waifs of New York, the exposure of that rear tenement in the lower East Side was a most terrible shock, a shock that was at first benumbing. A picture was presented of human creatures, moral, and, in so far as their opportunities allowed them, decent members of society, in rooms reached through a court that held open closets to be used by men and women, from some of which the doors had been torn away; up dirty steps into a sick-room where there was no window, the one opening leading into a small, crowded room where husband, children, and boarders were gathered together, impossible conditions under which to attempt to establish a home and bring up children (Wald, 1902, p. 567).

LEARNING OBJECTIVES

At the completion of this chapter, the reader will be able to

Describe epidemiology and social epidemiology.

Explain how the processes involved in epidemiology and social epidemiology are important within the context of providing for the public's health.

Analyze the different perspectives of epidemiology and social epidemiology in the context of public health nursing.

KEY TERMS

Epidemiology Terms
- Age-specific rates
- Analytical epidemiology
- Attack rates
- Chain of infection
- Crude rates
- Descriptive epidemiology
- Epidemiological triad
  - Agent
  - Environment
  - Host
- Incidence rates
- Prevalence rates
- Rate

Social Epidemiology Terms
- Developmental and life-course perspective
- Life course model
- Multilevel analysis
- Population perspective
- Social context
- Social determinants of health
  - Discrimination
  - Education
  - Income
  - Income inequality
  - Occupation
  - Socioeconomic position
  - Socioeconomic status

This chapter discusses the concepts of epidemiology and social
epidemiology and their use in
public health nursing. Nursing students
should use epidemiological tools when
they want to understand how and why
disease occurs within populations
instead of individuals. Examples of
populations are pregnant adolescents
living in the South Bronx and college-
aged students with sexually transmitted
diseases. Nursing students use social
epidemiological tools when they want
to understand how the effects of
poverty, **income inequality**, and **discrimination** contribute to how and why
disease occurs within specific populations. The purpose of this chapter is to
present the concepts of epidemiology
and social epidemiology to the public
health nurse for application in their
practice.

Florence Nightingale.

EPIDEMIOLOGY

Epidemiology is the scientific discipline
that studies the distribution and determinants of diseases and injuries in human
populations (Tarzian, 2005). The goal of
epidemiology is to limit disease, injury,
and death by specific interventions to prevent or limit outbreaks or epidemics
(U.S. Department of Health and Human
Services [DHHS] & Centers for Disease
Control and Prevention [CDC], 1998,
2006). Epidemiology is concerned with
the health of particular populations,
whereas clinical nursing and medicine
are concerned with individual health
issues. The perspective of epidemiologists is to understand the source of the illness cause or exposure, ascertain who
else has been exposed, if the exposure
has spread beyond the initial point of

contact, and to prevent additional cases
or recurrences (U.S. DHHS & CDC, 1998,
2006). The clinical perspective of medicine and nursing is to obtain information
about the history of the present illness,
conduct a physical, make a diagnosis,
prescribe treatment, and consider this a
single episode. Public health nurses are
more in line with the epidemiology perspective because they are educated to
integrate knowledge about the environment and the community with their
understandings of health and illness as
experienced by the individual, family, and
population. The perspective in medicine
tends to be focused on individual health,
whereas the perspective in epidemiology
tends to be focused on the population.
Box 4-1 illustrates the various ways

BOX **4-1**   Clinical vs. Epidemiology Perspective

Picnic Scenario: Fifty college students attend a picnic. The food is served at noon, and the students eat turkey, cornbread, tuna salad, and ice cream. The students return to campus. One student becomes sick and is taken to the student health center.

Clinical Perspective (Single Episode)

- History/physical finding of present illness
- Diagnosis
- Treatment

The clinician asks about the illness, diagnoses the ailment based on symptoms, and then treats.

Epidemiologist Perspective (Possible Multiple Episodes)

- History of present illness and observation for patterns
- How many students were at the picnic?
- Who else was sick?

- Timing
- What caused the illness?
  - Food
  - Heat
- Is this an epidemic?

The epidemiologist asks about the illness but also wants to know how many students attended the picnic and how many became sick. The epidemiologist also explores with the students what could have caused the illness: Was it the heat or the food? The epidemiologist would also analyze the food and ask if there was mayonnaise in the tuna salad; how long had the tuna salad been sitting in the heat before it was served? Most importantly, after the epidemiologist gathers the information about the illness, the epidemiologist wants to make sure this is not an epidemic and learn how to prevent this illness in the future.

these clinicians, practicing within these two frameworks, would approach a situation in which a college student falls ill and is taken to the student health center.

Florence Nightingale applied this epidemiological framework when attending to soldiers in the Crimean War. Nightingale recognized that addressing environmental problems such as poor nutrition, sanitation, and contaminated blankets contributed to infection and increases in mortality and morbidity. Nightingale's empirical observations of her surroundings enabled her to examine, methodically, the factors that contributed to disease (Pfettscher, 2002). This big pic-

ture allowed Nightingale to deduce how illness occurred and what strategies reduced the spread of disease.

History

Epidemiological tenets have been used to describe and explain disease and the prevalence of these diseases since 400 B.C. A brief history of epidemiological events and well-known persons who used epidemiological thinking is found in **Table 4-1**.

This epidemiological history can be viewed within the context of two revolutions (**Table 4-2**). The first epidemiological revolution focused on infectious

Table 4-1 Epidemiological History and Events

400 BCE	17th Century	18th Century	19th Century	20th Century
Hippocrates (circa 400 BCE) provided an approach to those who wanted to investigate disease. Hippocrates' treatise, *On Airs, Waters, and Places*, noted that these elements affected health. Hippocrates believed that by knowing how these elements were similar and different in specific areas would provide the basis to understand why a disease occurred and the probability of where the disease would occur.	John Graunt (1620–1674) from London. Graunt published *Observations on the Bills of Mortality*, which quantified Britain's mortality data in 1662. Graunt noted birth and death patterns, infant mortality, occurrences of disease, differences in disease by gender, differences in disease in urban and rural areas, and variations in disease by season.	James Lind (1716–1794), studied scurvy (vitamin C deficiency) while sailing on a Navy ship in 1747. In 1753, Lind published *A Treatise on Scurvy in Three Parts*. This publication explained why scurvy occurred and the treatment for scurvy.	William Farr (1807–1883) was responsible for the concept of surveillance data. John Snow (1813–1858), an anesthesiologist, conducted investigations in London during the cholera outbreak.	Joseph Goldberger (1874–1929) discovered why the disease pellagra (niacin deficiency) occurred. The 1964 Surgeon General Report: *Smoking and Health: Report of the Advisory Committee to the Surgeon General* linked tobacco to lung cancer. The Framingham Heart Study was initiated to identify factors contributing to heart disease in the United States. The 1986 Surgeon General's Report: *The AIDS Epidemic.*

Source: Hippocrates (400 B.C.E.); The James Lind Library (n.d.); National Library of Medicine (n.d.a., n.d.b.); Office of History National Institute of Health (2005); Stephan (n.d.); UCLA Department of Epidemiology School of Public Health (n.d.).

Table 4-2 Epidemiological Revolutions

First Epidemiological Revolution (1870–1930)	Second Epidemiological Revolution (1950–Present)

The first epidemiological revolution was largely about infectious diseases. Scientists and public health practitioners discovered the causes of infectious diseases.
 	
Immunizations discovered during this time period:
• Smallpox
• Polio
• Tetanus
 	
Antibiotics discovered:
• Streptomycin: effective against tuberculosis (1947)
• Penicillin
 	
Immunizations and antibiotics accounted for only a 5% drop in mortality rates.
 	
Greatest advances of the first epidemiological revolution:
• Water purification
• Pasteurization
  • Decrease in diarrhea
  • Decrease in gastroenteritis
	The second epidemiological revolution focused on chronic diseases such as asthma, cancer, heart disease, and understanding levels of prevention.
	
	Epidemiologists had little understanding of noninfectious diseases until 1950. During the second revolution epidemiologists began to understand that 38% of deaths were a result of:
	• Tobacco (lung cancer and heart disease)
	• Diet and inactivity (heart disease, diabetes)
	• Alcohol (heart disease, liver disease)
	
	Understanding the factors that contribute to noninfectious diseases paved the way for interventions. Clinicians use the following levels of preventions with their clients:
	• Primary (prevent from the outset)
	  • Immunizations
	  • Health education
	• Secondary (early detection of disease)
	  • Screening tests
	    • PAP
	    • Mammogram
	    • Cholesterol
	    • Colonoscopy
	• Tertiary (reducing mortality and morbidity of the disease)
	  • Cardiac rehabilitation

Source: Adapted from Bodenheimer and Grumbach (2008).

diseases such as influenza, plague, and tuberculosis. These diseases were largely responsible for illnesses and death in previous centuries. It was also during these times that scientists and public health practitioners discovered that the causes of infectious diseases were due to poverty, overcrowding, sanitation, and contaminated food and water supplies (Breslow, 2005). From 1870 to 1930 scientists and public health practitioners began to understand the cause(s) of infectious disease. Once epidemiologists had an understanding of why infectious diseases occurred, public health interventions and some medical advances played a role in the reduction of those diseases.

The **rates** of morbidity and mortality of infectious diseases declined in the 18th and 19th centuries due to food production increases leading to less malnutrition, improvements in nutrition leading to healthier adults and children, and improvements of overall living conditions as a result of improved sanitation and clean water, pasteurization of milk, and less overcrowding. It is important to note that this decrease in infectious disease rates occurred because of public health interventions.

The second epidemiological revolution began in 1950 when epidemiologists started to understand the causes of non-infectious diseases (e.g., heart disease, asthma, diabetes, violence). With this understanding public health practitioners could apply epidemiological principles to shed light on health promotion, disease prevention, and the role of risk factor identification and behavioral change in the promotion of health. Noninfectious diseases are discussed later in this chapter.

To summarize, during the first epidemiological revolution (1870–1930) sci-entists had little understanding about the causes of infectious diseases (e.g., tuberculosis and influenza). Reductions in infectious diseases were largely the result of public health interventions, whereas medical advances (immunizations and antibiotics) contributed about a 5% reduction in mortality rates. During the second epidemiological revolution (beginning in 1950), epidemiologists began to understand causes of noninfectious diseases such as heart disease, asthma, and diabetes, which paved the way for public health and clinical interventions (Bodenheimer & Grumbach, 2008).

Uses of Epidemiology

Why is it important to understand epidemiology and how is epidemiology used? In this section the reader will come to see how epidemiology is applied in public health nursing practice. This process includes the systematic collection of data and how the analysis of these data not only leads to a better understanding of a disease process but the reduction of disease. The reader will also come to understand how the epidemiological process informs the public health nurse's decision making.

The collection and use of epidemiology data for decision making can be viewed in the following ways. Public health nurses engage in an *assessment* process that informs them about the health of the individual, family, population, and community. Chapter 3 is devoted to assessment. The process of assessment provides information so the public health nurse may engage in problem identification and/or potential problem identification along with information that may support program development and, at times, the development of public health policy. For example, the data collected by public health nurses may be presented to policymakers to shed light about the actual and potential problems seen in the population in their targeted home communities. Examples of this information may include data that highlight health, social, or environmental problems in a particular population in a policymaker's constituency; data on risks within their constituency; the history of health problems within a particular population showing trends such as the increase or decrease of a particular disease; and the services available in a community. Knowing this information facilitates these policymakers in their decisions leading to the establishment of law as well as determining resource utilization and allocation.

Epidemiology plays a role in our day-to-day *individual decisions* pertaining to healthy behaviors such as smoking cessation, exercising, weight control, and eating healthy foods. These positive decisions are made because of epidemiological studies. Epidemiology has contributed to the fount of information about associations and causal relationships (we say causal relationships because research can never prove cause and effect) between obesity and diabetes, smoking and lung cancer, and risky sexual practices such as engaging in unprotected sex and sexually transmitted diseases. Without epidemiology we would not know how a disease is transmitted and the strategies to reduce our risks of contracting this disease. Public health nurses use this evidence daily in their practice as they develop educational programs for individuals, families, and populations in an effort to offer information that assists others to make healthy lifestyle choices.

The work of public health practitioners involves public health nurses, epidemiologists, health department officials, clinicians, physicians, scientists, media experts, educators, sanitation officials, and researchers. These individuals all provide particular world views that when joined collectively complete the *clinical picture* needed to understand the disease, the progression and trajectory of that disease, and interventions. Completing the clinical picture is identifying *what* the infectious agent is, *why*/how the disease is transmitted to the host, *where* the disease is most prevalent in terms of the place or location, *when* the disease most makes itself known with regard to time, and *who* the individual is that is affected by the disease. These are known as the 5 W's of **descriptive epidemiology**, discussed below (U.S. DHHS & CDC, 2006, p. 31). Part of this clinical picture is an understanding of the determinants of health, discussed in Chapter 1. One practitioner alone is unable to be a solo artist in this endeavor because effective public health strategies require collaborative and collective efforts between and among many different professions.

HIV is an example of how epidemiologists were able to complete the clinical picture. In the early 1980s a strange pneumonia affected five men who identified themselves as having sex with men. *Pneumocystis carinii* pneumonia was a relatively rare lung disease and appeared to be clustered only within this specific population (Sepkowitz, 2001). Additionally, clinicians were seeing Kaposi's sarcoma (KS), a relatively benign form of cancer, in their younger male patients who had sex with men. KS was also relatively rare in the United States; the skin lesions associated with KS were usually localized to the lower extremities and affected older people in their 70s (Hymes et al., 1981).

Because these cases appeared to be clustered within a specific population and puzzled the medical community, the cases and laboratory results were reported to the CDC for further investigation. In 1981 the CDC provided information about the first cases of *P. carinii* pneumonia and KS among men who have sex with men (CDC referred to this group as homosexuals) to the medical community, and in 1982 the CDC *named* this disease "acquired immune deficiency syndrome" (known as AIDS). It was not until 1986 that the term "human immunodeficiency virus," or HIV, was adopted by the clinical community (Sepkowitz, 2008). Once a particular disease or health event is identified, healthcare professionals make the diagnosis in individual cases, whereas epidemiologists contribute to our understanding of the natural history of the disease. Since this time the work pertaining to HIV has been carried on by a wide and varied group of healthcare professionals. Take a few minutes and just think. Who has contributed to the knowledge of this disease and the treatment of this disease? The list is rather overwhelming, yet at the same time it clearly presents for us the view that in order for the health of the public to be sustained there is a need for the collective wisdom of many working together. Public health nurses are a valued member of this collective group.

Finally, the *search for causes* is epidemiological research. This research is dedicated to the investigation of the causes and individual, societal, and environmental factors that contribute to a person's risk for contracting a disease and/or injury. This research provides evidence for interventions that health professionals can use in their clinical practice, such as counseling about smoking, protective sexual practices, seat belts, car child seats, and immunizations. Public health nurses not only apply this research as evidence in their practice but raise questions for research and conduct research.

Epidemiological Approach

When we see a particular disease in our clinical practice or if we decide to explore a particular disease, we want to know who is affected by this disease, what factors contribute to this disease (environmental, social, or personal factors), are there other cases, when did this disease become known, why are some individuals more prone to this particular disease, and what common factors do diseased individuals have in common? Epidemiologists begin with *case definition* as the standard criteria to guide their practice.

A case definition is that which determines if a person has a particular disease. For example, an individual is diagnosed with diabetes if his or her blood sugar levels are above the cutoff point (above 126 mg/dL) on two separate occasions (U.S. Preventive Services Task Force, 2008). Case definitions standardize the diagnoses of a particular disease, thus ensuring that every case is similarly diagnosed. Additionally, case definitions consist of clinical criteria, including subjective data, which are client complaints, and objective data, which are the clinician's observations inclusive of physical, environmental, and laboratory findings.

NUMBERS AND RATES

Epidemiologists are concerned about numbers and rates because it allows them to measure, describe, and compare the morbidity and mortality of a particular disease and/or injury in populations. Rates are "measures of frequency of health events that put raw numbers into a frame of reference to the size of a population. Rates are determined by statistical adjustments to the raw data, making them useful in making comparisons or examining trends" (Stotts, 2008, p. 91).

In epidemiology the numerator is the actual number of cases or events occurring during a given time period, and the denominator is the total population at risk during the same time period. The denominator is typically converted to a standard base denominator such as 1,000, 10,000, and 100,000 so that comparisons can be made among at-risk populations, communities, and neighborhoods (Tarzian, 2005). Rates are useful to the public health nurse because they can help the nurse identify what populations in the community are at an increased risk for a particular disease and/or injury. For example, City A has a population of 130,000 nursing home residents. City A reported 100 cases of hepatitis A among nursing home residents to the Department of Health (DOH). City B has a population of 120,000 nursing home residents. City B reported 150 cases of hepatitis A among their nursing home residents to the DOH. The DOH determined that the specific rate for hepatitis A was 7.6 cases per 10,000 persons living in a nursing home in City A and was 12.5 cases per 10,000 persons in City B. The DOH specific rate calculations for these cities are found in **Box 4-2**. This type of data helps the public health nurse think about and develop initiatives that target nursing home residents who appear to be a high-risk population for contracting hepatitis A.

In addition to the above specific rates, there are many other rate definitions that measure morbidity (illness rates) or mortality (death rates) for populations at risk for a particular disease, such as asthma, diabetes, or high blood pressure, or death from a particular disease, or cause, such as a motor vehicle accident. Examples of these rates or statistical calculations are **incidence rates, prevalence rates, attack rates, crude rates**, and **age-specific rates** as listed in **Table 4-3**.

DESCRIPTIVE EPIDEMIOLOGY

Descriptive epidemiology describes the extent of an outbreak in terms of *who* gets the disease, *where* the disease occurs, and *when* the disease occurred. These characteristics are described in **Table 4-4**. For example, Lyme disease was classified as a new disease when about 50 children were diagnosed with arthritis in Lyme, Connecticut. This cluster of arthritis in children caused an epidemiologist in Lyme to request that the CDC investigate this outbreak. The epidemiologist was concerned because juvenile rheumatoid arthritis is relatively rare in children (France, 1999). The *who* in this outbreak were children, the *where* in this outbreak was a *wooded hamlet* at the mouth of the Connecticut River, and the *when* for this disease is typically the summer and fall when people tend to spend more time outdoors and thus are more at risk for a tick bite. The collection and analysis of this descriptive information form a critical first step in the epidemiological investigatory process.

This gathering and analyzing of data in descriptive epidemiology is also termed as the gathering of data on *person, time,* and *place*. This information allows the public health nurse to become knowl-

---

BOX **4-2** **Specific Rate Calculations for Hepatitis A Found in City A and City B**

Numbers and rates permit the epidemiologist to measure, describe, and compare the morbidity and mortality of particular diseases. A rate is

$$\frac{\text{Number of cases or events occurring during a given time period}}{\text{Population at risk during the same time period}} \times 10n$$

In epidemiology rates are changed to a common base such as 100,000 because it changes the result of the division into a quantity that permits a standardized comparison.

Example:

City A and City B saw an outbreak of hepatitis A in their nursing home residents. Each city reported these cases to the Department of Health. The Department of Health calculated the specific rates for each city using 10,000 as the standard base number. Hepatitis A specific rate for nursing home residents is calculated as follows:

City A specific rate:

$$\frac{100 \text{ cases of reported Hep A cases}}{130,000 \text{ City A nursing home residents}} \times 10,000$$

City A specific rate: 7.6, which means the rate of hepatitis A in nursing homes for City A is about seven to eight residents in nursing homes contracted hepatitis A.

City B specific rate:

$$\frac{150 \text{ cases of reported Hep A cases}}{120,000 \text{ City B nursing home residents}} \times 10,000$$

City B specific rate = 12.5

By calculating the specific rate, the Department of Health can compare the hepatitis rates in City A and City B. Additionally, the Department of Health knows that nursing home residents are at risk for contracting hepatitis A.

Source: Adapted from U.S. DHHS & CDC (2006).

---

edgeable about the public health problem being studied, thus enabling the public health nurse to provide a comprehensive picture of the health of the population under study and determine who is at risk for acquiring the particular disease. Another part of the epidemiological approach is known as **analytical epi-**demiology, which facilitates the how and why of a particular disease.

ANALYTICAL EPIDEMIOLOGY

Analytical epidemiology illustrates the causal relationship between a risk factor and a specific disease or health condition. In other words, it seeks to answer

Table 4-3 Rate Definitions

Incidence Rate	Prevalence Rate	Attack Rate	Specific Rates	Crude Rate	Age-specific Rate
Applied in the study of acute diseases, a disease outbreak, or in the diagnosis of new cases. Incidence rates are the frequency with which a new condition or event occurs in a population over a period of time.	Applied in the study of chronic disease. Prevalence rate measures the number of people in a given population who have an already existing condition at a given point in time.	Important for the study of a single disease outbreak or epidemic during a short time period. The number is expressed as a percent.	These measure morbidity or mortality for a particular population: • Age specific • Gender specific • Income • Race/ethnicity • Infant mortality • Maternal mortality	A crude rate measures the experience of the entire population in a specific area with regard to the specific disease or condition being investigated.	These rates provide age-specific information for a particular disease.
Example We want to know the number of new cases of flu. In the second week of November the student Health Services diagnosed 3 students with the flu. The total student population is 1,600.	_Example_ We want to know the number of existing cases of flu. There were 3 new cases of the flu in the second week of November and 10 old cases of the flu in the first week of November.	_Example_ 120 people flew from New York to Los Angeles. The meal served was meatloaf. 80 people ate the meal and 40 people chose not to eat meatloaf. 20 of those who ate meatloaf became ill.	_Example_ Age-specific diabetes mortality in 45- to 55-year-olds	The crude mortality rate looks at the entire mortality rate from all causes of death for a population in a particular area during a specific time. _Example_ <u>NYC death rate</u>	Age-specific mortality rate is one limited to a particular age group. The numerator is the number of deaths in that age group and the denominator is the number of persons in that age group in the population. Examples include: Neonatal mortality rate Infant mortality rate
Calculation 3 new flu cases ÷ 1,600 (student population) × 1,000 (comparison denominator)	_Calculation_ 3 + 10 cases ÷ 1,600 (student population) × 1,000	_Calculation_ 20 (ill) ÷ 80 (meatloaf pop) × 100	_Calculation_ Number of diabetes deaths in 45–55-year-olds ÷ Population of individuals 45–55-year-olds × 1,000	_Calculation_ The total number of NYC deaths reported during (1985) ÷ 5 million × 100,000	
Incidence rate is 1.8.	Prevalence rate is 8.1.	Attack rate is 25%.			

Source: Adapted from U.S. DHHS & CDC (2006).

Table 4-4 Descriptive Epidemiological Variables

Person	Place	Time
Person variables are used to understand what makes a person susceptible to a disease or injury. Inherent characteristics include age, race, and sex. Acquired characteristics include marital status, education, occupation, living conditions, socioeconomic status, and access to health care. Inherent characteristics are considered fixed or unchangeable. A person's gender makes him or her at higher risk for some diseases such as breast cancer. However, because age varies the person becomes more susceptible to illness as he or she ages. Acquired characteristics may be modifiable via education. Example A 50-year-old man develops lung cancer. He has smoked for 30 years. The smoking is considered an acquired characteristic because it is potentially modifiable with education. Behavioral changes (quitting or smoking fewer cigarettes) lead to a healthier life and prevention of lung cancer.	Place variables describe the disease event by where the disease occurs such as • Place of residence • School district • Community • Country • State • Hospital unit Place information also provides insight into the geographical location and what factors in that environment facilitate the disease. For example, the temperature and climate may promote a place where a particular agent may grow and multiply. Example Lyme disease was first characterized in Lyme, CT, because the lush wooded environment supported the agent, host, and environment cycle.	Time variables give information about how disease rates change over time. Time information can be reported in • Days • Weeks • Months • Years • Decades • Epidemic period: when the number of cases is greater than normal. Does the disease manifest itself during certain seasons? Is the presentation of the disease predictable? If so why? Can this information be used in the prevention of the disease? Example Seasonality may demonstrate disease occurrences by week or month over the course of a year. For example, flu season typically begins in November and ends in March.

Source: Adapted from U.S. DHHS & CDC (2006).

questions about how and why disease occurs and the effects of a particular disease. Analytical studies use a comparison group to learn why one group has a disease and another does not. These groups are drawn from a healthy population living in the same community in which the disease has occurred. For example, a public health nurse was sent to a community where there was an outbreak of hepatitis A. The nurse interviewed the individuals who were diagnosed with hepatitis A and discovered that they had attended a graduation party at the local high school in the neighborhood. The public health nurse learned about the food that was served at this party and asked each person what he or she had eaten at the party. The public health nurse recognized the need for a comparison group for further investigation of this hepatitis A outbreak. The comparison group in this case would be those individuals at the same party who did not eat those same foods and who were not ill. "When . . . investigators find that persons with a particular characteristic are more likely than those without the characteristic to develop a certain disease, then the characteristic is said to be associated with the disease" (U.S. DHHS & CDC, 2006, p. 32). These characteristics include demographics such as age, race, or sex; constitutional characteristics such as immune state; behavioral characteristics such as smoking; or other characteristics such as living next to a waste site (U.S. DHHS & CDC, 2006).

Analytical epidemiology attempts to search for the causes and effects of the disease under study. Further, epidemiologists discern how or why exposure to a particular agent results in the outcome of disease or no disease. Epidemiologists can study the occurrences of diseases in

two ways: experimental studies and observational studies.

In an experimental study the researcher is the one who determines the exposure status of the individual or population. The researcher does not only observe, but determines and actively initiates what the exposure is, where to deliver the exposure, how to deliver the exposure, when to deliver the exposure, and who will be the recipient of the exposure. The researcher determines recipient characteristics such as age, gender, and **socioeconomic status** (SES). The researcher then carries out the research design to determine the effects of the exposure on the experimental individual or population and compares these outcomes with those not having had the exposure. Those who have not been exposed are the comparison group. This type of study is sometimes referred to as prospective because the research moves forward in time to look at the effects of the exposure. It is also important to note that these studies rarely prove causation but often lead to more research. Experimental studies are generally used to determine the effectiveness of a treatment such as a vaccine or drug. These types of studies are considered the gold standard of clinical trials. Study participants in clinical trials are either given the medication or drug under study or given a placebo such as a sugar pill. Most of the major medications used to treat chronic diseases such as high blood pressure, diabetes, and asthma were subjected to trials in experimental studies.

Observational studies include cohort and case-control studies. In a cohort study a cohort of healthy individuals that share similar experiences or characteristics are identified and classified by their exposures. For example, in a study that wishes to look at tobacco use and lung cancer, the cohort identified may be men 21 years of age who are actively engaged in smoking. This group is studied over a period of years, allowing researchers to compare the disease rates in the exposed group (those who smoked) with the unexposed group (those who did not smoke). In a case-control group the researcher identifies a group of people who have already been diagnosed with a disease (women diagnosed with breast cancer) and a group without the disease. The researcher compares and contrasts the participants' past life experiences, characteristics, and exposures to determine patterns. Again, a comparison group is important in case-control studies. This type of research is sometimes referred to as retrospective because the researcher is looking at a situation in the present and linking it to situations or conditions in the past.

The Framingham Study is an example of a classic cohort study. Since 1949 the National Heart Institute of the U.S. Public Health Service observed men and women living in Framingham, Massachusetts, to identify factors related to developing coronary heart disease (Kannel, Schwartz, & McNamara, 1969). The Nurses' Health Study, another example of a cohort study, was started several decades ago to examine the relationship between oral contraception (birth control pills) and breast cancer (Colditz, Manson, & Hankinson, 1997).

Epidemiological Triad

The **epidemiological triad** (**Figure 4-1**) is the traditional model of infectious disease causation. The three components are agent, host, and environment.

Agent factors refer to an infectious organism such as a virus, bacterium, parasite, or other microbe. **Host** factors that can mediate the effect of a particular

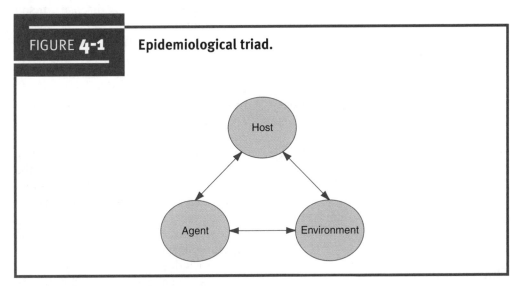

FIGURE **4-1**   **Epidemiological triad.**

Source: Adapted from U.S. DHHS & CDC (2006).

agent are age, sex, SES (**education, income, occupation**), behaviors (smoking, drinking, and exercise), and genetic factors. For example, a 95-year-old man with multiple chronic illnesses who does not get his yearly flu vaccine is more susceptible to influenza than a healthy 20-year-old college student. These host factors are also known as intrinsic factors. **Environmental factors** are known as extrinsic factors. Environmental factors include physical factors such as geography, climate, and physical surroundings (e.g., homeless shelters); biological factors such as insects that transmit the agent (e.g., mosquito transmits malaria); and socioeconomic factors such as sanitation and available health services determine the spread of a particular disease (e.g., tuberculosis increases with overcrowding) (U.S. DHHS & CDC, 2006).

Again, Lyme disease is an excellent example of the epidemiological triad. A particular deer tick infected with the bacterium *B. burgdorferi* (the agent), infects a person (the host). The bacteria enter the skin at the bite site only after the infected tick has been in the host for 36 to 48 hours. The initial symptoms felt by the host are primarily due to the body's response to this invasion. Specific factors such as exposure to heavily wooded areas (environment), the season (infection is most likely during the summer and fall), age (most common in children and young adults), and location (90% of cases occur in the coastal northeast as well as in Wisconsin, Minnesota, California, and Oregon) predispose the host to contracting Lyme disease (Depietropaolo, Powers, & Gill, 2005).

Chain of Infection

Diseases are classified as communicable or noncommunicable. Communicable diseases are considered infectious because they can be transmitted by an infected person to a noninfected person. Viruses that cause colds, HIV, and tuberculosis are examples of communicable diseases. Diseases come about when the body (host) is exposed to an infectious agent (virus or microorganism) and the organism or virus grows within the body. If the organism or virus is able to grow within the host, the host at some point in time might become infectious and then can transmit the particular disease to another susceptible host. Noncommunicable diseases such as diabetes, asthma, and heart disease cannot be transmitted by the person who has that particular diagnosis. The contributing factors of noncommunicable diseases are genetics (e.g., Tay-Sachs disease), environmental factors (e.g., Love Canal), and behaviors such as overeating. These determinants of health are discussed in previous chapters and below.

The **chain of infection** (**Figure 4-2**) shows that infectious diseases result from their interaction with the agent, host, and environment. Transmission, direct or indirect, of an infectious agent takes place after the agent leaves its *reservoir* (host) by a *portal of exit* such as the mouth when coughing. The agent then enters the *susceptible host* via a *portal of entry* such as a skin wound to infect the susceptible host (U.S. DHHS & CDC, 2006).

Direct transmission modes are the immediate transfer of the disease agent between an infected person and susceptible person. Examples of direct transmission modes are direct contact via touching, kissing, and direct projection, which includes large short-range spray of droplets via sneezing or coughing. Indirect transmission takes place as an agent is carried from a reservoir to a host via air

FIGURE **4-2**   **The chain of infection.**

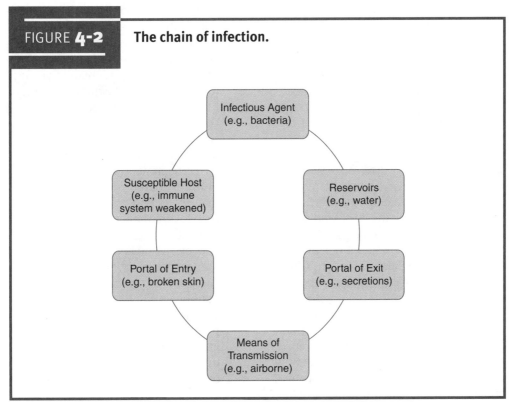

Source: Adapted from U.S. DHHS & CDC (2006).

particles and gains access to the portal of entry via respiratory tract systems (e.g., mouth and nose). Vehicle-borne transmissions are contaminated materials or objects (fomites) in which communicable diseases are transferred (e.g., children's toys in a day care center) and vector-borne transmission methods transfer the disease by a living organism (e.g., mosquito) (U.S. DHHS & CDC, 2006).

Public Health Surveillance Data

Public health surveillance data are used by public health nurses and other health officials to understand disease prevalence and disease patterns. Surveillance data

are critically analyzed and used by these individuals to make decisions about policy, funding, research, and program initiatives. Surveillance is discussed in Chapter 8 as an intervention strategy.

SOCIAL EPIDEMIOLOGY

Social epidemiology is the study of social conditions such as poverty, SES, and discrimination that play a role and influence the health of populations. Social epidemiology goes beyond the analysis of individual risk factors such as age and gender to include the study of the social context or societal implications in which the health–disease phenomenon occurs

(Krieger, 2002). Social epidemiology measures the impact of the social environment on health outcomes, whereas epidemiology is more concerned with the impact of the physical environment on health outcomes (Berkman & Kawachi, 2000).

Social epidemiology attempts to address how social inequality has a role in disease causation. Social epidemiologists investigate social conditions responsible for patterns of health, patterns of disease, and the well-being of populations. Social epidemiology examines how social inequality in the past and social inequality in the present has a role in the health or disease of populations and the well-being of populations (Krieger, 2001a). Social epidemiologists investigate the gradient of income on the health status of lower-income, middle-income, and upper-income classes in society. By looking at the health status at each income level, social epidemiologists can examine how income exerts an influence, either positive or negative, on health outcomes (Krieger, 2001b). For example, people growing up in poorer communities have worse health outcomes than those growing up in wealthier communities. Once a social epidemiologist teases out variations in health status by different income groups, the social epidemiologist then explores the relationship between individual income, which is considered an individual factor, and income inequality, which is considered a contextual factor (Subramanian, Kawachi, & Kennedy, 2001).

The concepts guiding social epidemiology are as follows:

- **Population perspective**, which means that because individuals are rooted in society, their risks for disease or staying healthy are situated with the population in which they belong.
- **Social context** of behavior, which means that certain behaviors such as smoking, drinking, and voter participation are shaped by social influences. For example, children seeing their parents smoke are more likely to smoke when they get older or communities with ample resources such as parks, grocery stores, and health clinics are more likely to shape healthier behavior.
- **Multilevel analysis**, which means that health outcomes are understood within the perspective of individual factors such as income and education and contextual factors that assess environmental exposures at the community, state, national, and global level.
- **Developmental and life-course perspective**, which means the early life experiences of an individual contribute to his or her susceptibility to disease later in life (**Table 4-5**).

Population Perspective

The population perspective is a guiding concept in social epidemiology. As discussed, the population perspective illustrates that an individual's risk for health problems cannot be isolated from the community in which he or she resides or from the population or society in which he or she belongs. An individual's risk for disease must be seen in the context of where he or she lives. For example, breast cancer survival rates of Japanese women are higher than Japanese immigrants living in America and Japanese-Americans. One explanation for the improved survival rate is the low dietary fat intake of Japanese women (Pineda, White, Kristal, & Taylor, 2001). This means that when a Japanese woman

Table 4-5 Guiding Perspectives in Social Epidemiology

Population	Social Context of Behavior	Multilevel Analysis	Developmental and Life Course
This perspective examines an individual's health in the context of the population where the person resides. Example Breast cancer survival rates in women in Japan are higher than Japanese women who become U.S. immigrants.	This perspective makes the case that risky behaviors such as smoking and drinking tend to be clustered in particular communities. The residents in these communities typically have less education, are more socially isolated, and have less access to health-promoting environments. This perspective recognizes that social environments have a large role in positive or negative health behaviors. Example Communities with higher rates of smoking live in areas where smoking is heavily advertised.	This perspective encourages a larger analysis of the problem by assessing all factors that contribute to disease. This analysis assesses the levels of exposures found at the community, state, national, and global level. If we understand the relationship between the individual and the community level, we gain a larger understanding of health outcomes for the individual. Example A person lives in a community that does not have grocery stores with fresh food, but there are several fast food restaurants on every block. Eating fast food almost every day might contribute to becoming overweight and might lead to diabetes in the future.	This perspective examines the cumulative risk of health status based on early life exposures. This perspective recognizes that disadvantages in one's early life may facilitate disease later in life. Example A child grew up in a poor neighborhood next to a medical incinerator. Additionally, several family members smoked cigarettes. The family did not have health insurance until the child was 10 years old. The child, however, was healthy and did not need medical attention. The child went to college and became quite wealthy. The early life experience of deprivation for this child, however, may contribute to developing asthma when older even though the new environment is less conducive to developing asthma.

Source: Adapted from Berkman and Kawachi (2000).

moves from Japan and lives in the United States, her breast cancer survival rate would be less than if she lived in Japan.

Social Context of Behavior

The social context of behavior is a guiding concept of social epidemiology. As discussed, the social context of behavior addresses individual behavioral risk factors such as smoking and drinking and examines these behaviors in a larger social context or by the social influences or conditions that contribute to specific behaviors. For example, the number of green spaces such as parks and supermarkets in a neighborhood often determine how an individual will behave and the choices the person has to make to maintain health and reduce his or her susceptibility to disease. Public health nurses working in the South Bronx, where many of the adults are overweight and at risk for diabetes or high blood pressure, recommend an exercise regimen for these individuals, but because there are few green space areas, no access to walking paths, no gym facilities, and the neighborhood feels less safe in the evening, many of these individuals do not adhere to the exercise recommendations.

Social conditions often determine behavior and play a role in how susceptible a person is to disease or his or her ability to resist disease. Growing up in poverty or wealth determines the type of neighborhoods where people can live (e.g., unsafe vs. safe), the environmental exposures in certain neighborhoods (e.g., lead), how people in these neighborhoods access health care (e.g., emergency room vs. private healthcare office), and the levels of educational attainment (e.g., high-school degree vs. college degree). For example, people living in poorer communities face increased risks of environmental exposures such as living near a medical incinerator, which might cause more asthma; lack of adequate housing that might lead to overcrowding, which can increase the prevalence of tuberculosis; reduced availability of medical resources that might lead to the increased use of the emergency room versus seeing a primary care clinician; and lower educational attainment that creates the context for detrimental behaviors such as smoking and drinking, which contribute to disease later in life such as lung cancer, cirrhosis of the liver, or emphysema.

Social conditions do not create disease but generate a susceptibility to disease. Social epidemiology takes into account that the continued exposure to adverse social conditions has a role in how well the host can resist disease and that these exposures often lay the groundwork for poorer health in the future (Berkman & Kawachi, 2000).

Multilevel Analysis

Multilevel analysis is a guiding concept of social epidemiology. As discussed, multilevel analysis is necessary to understand all factors that contribute to disease. These factors are examined on an individual level and on an environmental level such as a neighborhood, community, city, state, and so forth. The individual level is a *contextual* effect and the environmental level is a *compositional* effect (Berkman & Kawachi, 2000). A contextual effect on the individual level would be the relationship between the individual's income and income inequality. A compositional effect on the environmental level would be the proportion of people living in poverty.

Before we can examine the relationship of income and income inequality, we need to look at the data collected on household income in the United States.

The U.S. Census collects data on household incomes and then ranks the level of income into five quintiles; quintile one represents those households with the lowest income and quintile five represents those households that have the highest level of income. For example, a family lives in a lower middle-income neighborhood; their median income is $60,000, and the median income for the neighborhood is $40,000. The median income in 2007 for all households in the United States was $50,233. Based on this income, 3.4% of households were in the first (lowest) quintile, 8.7% were in the second quintile, 14.8% were in the third quintile, 23.4% were in the fourth quintile, and 49.7% were in the fifth (highest) quintile. The Gini index measures income inequality. The Gini index range is 0 to 1. Perfect equality is 0 and perfect inequality is 1. In 2007 the U.S. Gini index was 0.470. The 2007 federal poverty threshold for a family of four (two adults and two children) was $21,027. The proportion of households in 2007 living at 50% below the poverty level ($19,975) represented 5.2%, households living at 100% below the poverty level ($18,924) represented 12.5%, and households living at 125% below the poverty level ($18,398) represented 17% of all households (DeNavas-Walt, Proctor, & Smith, 2008).

The median income for this family ($60,000) was above the U.S. median income ($50,233), and the neighborhood income ($40,000) was below the U.S. median income. Knowing the income distribution for this family, the income distribution for the neighborhood, and the proportion of households in the neighborhood living in poverty would be of interest to the public health nurse because he or she would have an idea about the differences in health outcomes and health behaviors for the different income groups and have an understanding of the neighborhood's access to resources.

Life Course Model or Perspective

The life course perspective is a guiding concept in social epidemiology. The **life course model** puts forward that the **socioeconomic position** of the family during childhood affects the child's health status, educational choices, and occupation choices in the future. Children growing up in families with less economic means or a lower socioeconomic position might have more health problems than children growing up in families with more economic means or a higher socioeconomic position. For example, children growing up in poverty might have more health problems such as asthma, which then might contribute to a lower level of education because frequent asthma episodes result in more school absences, which in turn leads to less occupational choices because they did not do well enough in school to attend college, and less education results in lower income levels that can precipitate downward mobility (Dike van de Mheen, Stronks, & Mackenbach, 1998). Children, however, growing up in more prosperous neighborhoods tend to have better health outcomes than children in economically disadvantaged communities because they attend better schools, have access to health care, and their parents are better educated and therefore have better jobs (Acevedo-Garcia, Lochner, Osypuk, & Subramanian, 2003). Economic disadvantages in early life can set in motion negative consequences that build up over time to produce disease after 20, 30, 40, or 50 years of being disadvantaged (Berkman & Kawachi, 2000).

Multilevel Approaches to Understanding Social Determinants of Health

Social determinants of health refer to the interaction of environmental and social processes that can affect an individual's biological processes that make him or her susceptible to a disease. For example, a child is exposed to secondhand smoke and develops asthma when he or she is 6 years old. Additionally, this child might even develop lung cancer later in life because of the continued exposure to secondhand smoke and the early development of lung disease. We know that early life experiences can contribute to subsequent health outcomes, good or bad. Solving the direct effects of material conditions such as pollution, malnutrition, and housing are important, but the person might still be at risk for health problems depending on how long he or she was exposed to the offending agent or experienced economic or social deprivation.

Socioeconomic factors such as income, education, occupation, medical care, healthcare barriers, language, environmental exposures, discrimination, and so forth are all correlated with health outcomes in one context or another. The public health nurse considers the above variables to bring about a better understanding of health disparities noted in individuals, families, populations, and communities. Additionally, analyzing the interaction between socioeconomic factors, health, and discrimination gives the public health nurse a framework to

develop interventions for specific individuals, families, or populations in specific areas. What follows is a discrete and detailed discussion of these social determinants of health.

SOCIOECONOMIC STATUS
AND SOCIOECONOMIC POSITION

The relationship of SES and health status has been documented for centuries (Lynch & Kaplan, 2000; Mirowsky, Ross, & Reynolds, 2000). SES consists of family income, educational level, and occupation. Additionally, SES determines an individual's socioeconomic position within society. How much money a person has, educational attainment, and occupation have a bearing on and reflects his or her socioeconomic position or standing in society. Additionally, populations have a socioeconomic position, and this is based on the economic resources available to the community. Like SES, the relationship between the socioeconomic position of a person or population and health status has been well established (Lynch & Kaplan, 2000). The effects of SES and socioeconomic position on health have been consistent with regard to health outcome disparities across different time periods, different geographical areas, and in nearly all measurements used to assess health and disease (Lantz et al., 2001).

An individual's SES and socioeconomic position in society are based on his or her educational level, annual income, occupation, and level of assets such as stocks, bonds, and home ownership. A person's SES and socioeconomic position matter to health status because living in a relatively poor community can be bad for one's health, whereas living in a relatively affluent community can be good for one's health. The SES or socioeconomic positions of an individual or population contribute to positive or negative health behaviors. For example, individuals growing up in lower socioeconomic circumstances are more likely to live in an area where there may be *health-damaging exposures,* such as living near a sewage treatment plant, as opposed to individuals in upper socioeconomic circumstances who are more likely to grow up in communities with *health-enhancing resources,* such as supermarkets containing fresh fruits and vegetables (Lynch & Kaplan, 2000). The SES and socioeconomic position of an individual or group reflect the social and economic risks (e.g., living in unsafe neighborhoods) or rewards (e.g., living in safe neighborhoods) of that particular class in society (Mirowsky et al., 2000).

INCOME

One of the most significant determinants of good health is income; therefore many have suggested that economic policy is a powerful form of health policy. By increasing a person's income, you increase the health status for everyone in society (Kaplan, 2001). Income matters in society because income gives a person access to resources that are necessary to maintain health (Kawachi, 2000; Wilkinson, 1999). For example, stress has been shown to have a negative impact on one's health. Being able to relieve stress is an important resource. A 55-year-old executive is able to relieve stress during the day because she has access to a gym in her office, whereas a 55-year-old bus driver does not have that resource available. The bus driver's inability to relieve stress makes him more susceptible to health problems.

Public health nurses work with individuals, families, and populations daily who experience stressors. How one responds to a particular stressor sets in motion physiological, behavioral, and psychological responses in the person. Additionally, how one handles a particular stressor depends on his or her coping mechanisms, support systems, and personality (Marmot, 2000). Sister Callista Roy, although not a social epidemiologist but a nursing theorist, recognized that adaptation to a particular stimuli is shaped by perceptions of the event and interpretation of the event. How the person interprets an event brings about a particular adaptive response. This response could have been formed by earlier life experiences. The Roy Adaptation Model puts forth that adaptation mechanisms used by a person have health consequences in the present and possibly in the future (Phillips, 2002). This example is presented for the reader in an attempt to demonstrate that public health nurses must also bring into their practice nursing's own unique body of knowledge.

INCOME INEQUALITY

Income inequality describes where wealth is concentrated and who controls the wealth in society. Income inequality measures the degree of income variation in a population. Income inequality on a community level contributes to the loss of social capital. Social capital refers to social resources such as parks, medical facilities, schools, and economic investments that are needed to ensure that communities have the resources to maintain health (Kawachi, 1999). Hence, communities with higher income are more likely to have higher social capital or resources such as parks for their population to enjoy and enhance health as opposed to communities with lower income and lower social capital. Income inequality also influences the average life expectancy for citizens in society.

Income inequality is either relative or absolute. Relative income inequality (growing up poor in a rich society vs. growing up poor where everybody is poor) has health consequences because individuals' perceptions of the social and material world can trigger biological processes (e.g., stress), which can lead to a current illness such as a headache or a future illness such as heart disease. For example, a child whose family is lower-income attends an expensive preparatory school on scholarship. This child is surrounded by students who have money and privilege. Further, the child's classmates vacation in Europe, wear the latest fashions, and see a movie every weekend. The child often feels sad because he or she does not have the money to buy new clothes, go to the movies, or travel. Had this child, however, gone to the local school with children of similar economic means, he or she might have better health outcomes in the present and the future. This model posits that socioeconomic inequalities as experienced by this child may activate psychosocial factors that contribute to health and illness (Wilkinson, 1999).

EDUCATION

Education is positively associated with employment and an important variable in understanding the social determinants of health. For example, an individual with a college degree is more likely to have employment that is more secure, higher paying, with health benefits, and limited environmental exposures to hazards than an individual with a high-school diploma.

The *New York Times* reported that staying in school for a long period of time and not smoking resulted in the best outcomes; thus extreme education has a role in longevity (Kolata, 2007). Adults with more years of education are less likely to engage in risky health behaviors such as smoking and drinking. Additionally, more education leads to a greater sense of personal efficacy. Of note, educational attainment and income returns vary over time and often differ by gender, race, and ethnicity. What this means is even though women may have the same educational degree and same occupation, they may make less money over time because they leave work to have children.

OCCUPATION

Occupation is studied less by researchers in the United States but is an important indicator in health outcomes. Great Britain uses occupation in its analysis of health outcomes. A person's occupation tells us about his or her educational opportunities, economic independence, environmental exposures, and likely health stressors. For example, a coal miner in West Virginia has limited educational opportunities and less economic independence because he or she has skills that are unique to coal mining. These same individuals are exposed to coal dust, which affects their lungs and can lead to illnesses such as asthma, emphysema, and chronic respiratory infections. Further, coal minors experience a multitude of on-the-job stressors. Existing health problems may be worsened by stress because coal miners have less autonomy in their job and are unable to control or relieve their stress levels. A white-collar worker or executive has more education; thus his or her job is considered more prestigious. The more prestigious jobs are more likely to be held by individuals who are healthier, wealthier, and have more autonomy, which contributes to feelings of control. Further, autonomy or how well one controls his or her life can improve social status and social supports and lead to better health status (Marmot & Wilkinson, 2006).

DISCRIMINATION, DISPARITY, AND HEALTH

Studies of racial and ethnic disparities find that being a member of a minority group is a risk factor for less intensive and lower quality of healthcare services (Institute of Medicine, 2002). Racial and ethnic disparities have been consistently noted in cardiovascular procedures (LaVeist, Arthur, Plantholt, & Rubinstein, 2003), cancer diagnosis and treatment (Shavers & Brown, 2002), and colorectal cancer (Cooper, Yuan, & Rimm, 1997). Thinking about how discrimination harms health requires the public health nurse to consider the different experiences of those considered a dominant group, such as white men, and those considered a suborbinate group, such as women. Social epidemiology considers that discrimination has an adverse effect on health, and some social epidemiologists hypothesize that discrimination actually creates a biological pathway for disease to occur in the body.

Social epidemiologists posit "inequality hurts and discrimination harms health" (Krieger, 2000, p. 36). How discrimination affects one's health status necessitates a conceptual framework that provides measurements and methods that permit an analysis of how discrimination can affect health in the present and in the future. Discrimination is the process by which people are treated differently because they are members in a particular group. Particular "isms" such as racism (bias against racial and ethnic groups), sexism (bias against women), ageism (bias against elders), heterosexism (bias against gays and lesbians), ableism (bias against disabled), and classism (bias against class) are forms of discrimination. How these "isms" become pathways for poor health is called the ecosocial theory of disease distribution. Ecosocial theory seeks to *integrate* the biological and social mechanisms of discrimination within a historical and multilayered analytical perspective. Ecosocial theory leads social epidemiologists to develop knowledge about (1) how a person *embodies* disease or how disease grows within the body, (2) the social and biological pathways that contribute to this embodiment, and (3) the cumulative interaction between exposure, susceptibility, and resistance to disease (Krieger, 2001c). Additionally, ecosocial theory examines the biological and social mechanisms of discrimination and how they become expressions for disease or poor health.

The public health nurse assesses discrimination on an individual level and a population level. The individual level examines indirect or *unobserved* forms of discrimination (how clinicians treat their clients differently based on race or gender) and direct forms of discrimination as reported by the client and then linking these to an *observable* outcome measure such as uncontrolled high blood pressure, as noted in **Figure 4-3**.

On the population level, institutional discrimination is examined. Institutional discrimination refers to policies that are

FIGURE 4-3   **Conceptual model to understanding discrimination.**

Individual Level		Population Level
Indirect discrimination by clinician (unobserved)	Direct discrimination self-reported by the client	Institutional discrimination (unobserved)
Clinical implications Treats clients differently resulting in difference in treatment. Example A 55-year-old gay man presented to the ER complaining of chest pains. The man was discharged and was not scheduled for a cardiac catheterization. Possible explanations for treatment difference: • Comorbidity • Illness severity • Age • Insurance status • Economic resources • Patient preference	*Clinical implications* Experiencing discrimination brings about emotional responses. Example The 55-year-old gay man leaves the ER distressed, fearful, and angry. Physiological responses: • Cardiovascular—heart disease • Endocrine—diabetes • Neurological—headache	*Policy Implications* Racial steering practices by real estate brokers. Example Residential segregation is observed in many poor and lower-income communities. Residential segregation might facilitate: • Concentration of poverty • Poor housing stock • Population density and overcrowding • Lack of economic and medical resources
Differences in observed health outcome: increase in morbidity and mortality.	Differences in observed health outcome: increase in morbidity and mortality.	Differences in observed health outcome: increase in morbidity and mortality.

Source: Adapted from Krieger (2000).

part of the standard working relationships of institutions. An example is corporate policies that often make it difficult for women or people of color to advance into upper management even though they are qualified. The public health nurse should always consider how the individual level and population level of discrimination contribute to poorer health outcomes as evidenced by increases in morbidity and mortality rates.

Discrimination can tell the public health nurse how groups are treated differently. Racism is a subset of discrimina-

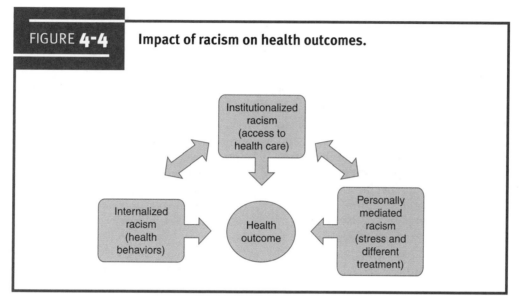

Source: Adapted from Jones (2001).

tion. Jones (2001) developed a framework for understanding racism on three levels: institutionalized, personally mediated, and internalized.

- Institutionalized racism describes resources that are available to certain groups in society and their ability to access them. For example, the wait times in the emergency room in a private hospital are less than the wait times in a public hospital. Additionally, a wealthy community will have more grocery stores with fresh food than a poorer community.
- Personally mediated racism describes prejudice and discrimination as experienced by particular groups of people because of their race. This type of racism can be intentional and unintentional. For example, a black student attending Yale might experience feelings of racism when a classmate asks if he or she was accepted into Yale because of the affirmative action program. This action may be intentional and/or unintentional.
- Internalized racism describes how members of a stigmatized race accept or internalize the negative messages about their abilities. Manifestations of internalized racism might be hopelessness, self-devaluation, and other behaviors that reflect loss of self-esteem. For example, a child of color may play only with a white doll.

Understanding how racism exemplifies itself on all three levels gives the public health nurse an understanding of the resulting health outcomes for individuals, families, populations, and communities. **Figure 4-4** illustrates the relationship between and among the three.

CONCLUSION

A historical review of epidemiology looked at special events in history that facilitated the need for epidemiological practices. Further, epidemiological practices evolved after each significant revolution (infectious disease control vs. noninfectious disease control). Today, public health nurses and other public health practitioners apply epidemiological principles and tools to systematically collect health-related data, analyze these data, interpret these data, and recommend public health actions in terms of policy initiatives that address preventing and controlling disease(s) in particular populations and communities. Descriptive and analytical epidemiology was described and explored as well as the epidemiological triad and the chain of infection. Examples were offered throughout the reading to bring this material to life for the readers.

Social epidemiology makes the case that social determinants of health, which consists of SES (income, occupation, and education), socioeconomic position, and discrimination can influence health outcomes in the future. Additionally, it is the economic and educational advantages of an individual that facilitate better health outcomes. Social epidemiologists study how social equality and inequalities contribute to the biological expression of disease and positive or negative health outcomes.

References

Acevedo-Garcia, D., Lochner, K. A., Osypuk, T. L., & Subramanian, S. V. (2003). Future directions in residential segregation and health research: A multilevel approach. *American Journal of Public Health, 93*(2), 215–221.

Berkman, L. F., & Kawachi, I. (2000). A historical framework for social epidemiology. In L. F. Berkman & I. Kawachi (Eds.), *Social epidemiology* (pp. 3–12). New York: Oxford University Press.

Bodenheimer, T. S., & Grumbach, K. (2008). *Understanding health policy: A clinical approach* (5th ed.). New York: McGraw-Hill Lange Medical Books.

Breslow, L. (2005). Origins and development of the International Epidemiological Association. *International Journal of Epidemiology, 34,* 725–729.

Colditz, G. A., Manson, J. E., & Hankinson, S. E. (1997). The Nurses' Health Study: 20-year contribution to the understanding of health among women. *Journal of Women's Health, 6*(1), 49–62.

Cooper, G. S., Yuan, Z., & Rimm, A. A. (1997). Racial disparity in the incidence and case-fatality of colorectal cancer: Analysis of 329 United States counties. *Cancer, Epidemiology, Biomarkers, & Prevention, 6,* 283–285.

DeNavas-Walt, C., Proctor, D. B., & Smith, J. C. (2008). *Income, poverty, and health insurance coverage in the United States: 2007.* U.S. Census Bureau, Current Population Reports, P60-235. Washington, DC: U.S. Government Printing Office.

Depietropaolo, D. L., Powers, J. H., & Gill, J. M. (2005). Diagnosis of Lyme disease. *American Family Physician, 72*(2), 297–303.

Dike van de Mheen, H., Stronks, K., & Mackenbach, J. P. (1998). A lifecourse perspective on socioeconomic inequalities: The influences of childhood socioeconomic conditions and selection processes. In M. Bartley, D. Blane, & G. D. Smith (Eds.), *The sociology of health inequalities* (pp. 193–216). Oxford: Blackwell Publishers.

France, D. (1999, May 4). Scientists at work: Allen C. Steere; Lyme disease expert developed the big picture of tiny tick. *The New York Times.*

Retrieved December 7, 2008, from http://query.nytimes.com/gst/fullpage.html?sec=health&res=9C00EED8173CF937A35756C0A96F958260

Hippocrates. (400 B.C.E.). Translated by Francis Adams. *On airs, waters, and places.* Retrieved November 5, 2009, from http://classics.mit.edu//Hippocrates/airwatpl.html

Hymes, K. B., Greene, J. B., Marcus, A., William, D. C., Cheung, T., Prose, N. S., et al. (1981). Kaposi's sarcoma in homosexual men—A report of eight cases. *Lancet, 318*(8247), 598–600.

Institute of Medicine. (2002). *Unequal treatment: Confronting racial and ethnic disparities in health care.* Washington, DC: Author.

The James Lind Library. (n.d.). *Treatise of scurvy.* Retrieved November 5, 2009, from http://www.jameslindlibrary.org/trial_records/17th_18th_Century/lind/lind_tp.html

Jones, C. P. (2001). Race, racism, and the practice of epidemiology. *American Journal of Epidemiology, 154*(4), 299–304.

Kannel, W. B., Schwartz, M. J., & McNamara, P. M. (1969). Blood pressure and risk of coronary heart disease: A Framingham study. *Chest, 56*(1), 43–52.

Kaplan, G. A. (2001). Economic policy is health policy: Findings from the study of income, socioeconomic status, and health. In J. A. Auerbach & B. K. Krimgold (Eds.), *Income, socioeconomic status, and health: Exploring the relationships* (pp. 137–149). Washington, DC: National Policy Association.

Kawachi, I. (1999). Social capital and community effects on population and individual health. *Annals of New York Academy of Sciences, 896,* 120–130.

Kawachi, I. (2000). Income inequality and health. In L. F. Berkman & I. Kawachi (Eds.), *Social epidemiology* (pp. 76–94). New York: Oxford University Press.

Kolata, G. (2007, January 3). A surprising secret to long life: Stay in school. *The New York Times.* Retrieved September 1, 2009, from http://www.nytimes.com/2007/01/03/health/03aging.html

Krieger, N. (2000). Discrimination and health. In L. F. Berkman & I. Kawachi (Eds.), *Social epidemiology* (pp. 36–75). New York: Oxford University Press.

Krieger, N. (2001a). Theories for social epidemiology in the 21st century: An ecosocial perspective. *International Journal of Epidemiology, 30,* 668–677.

Krieger, N. (2001b). Historical roots of social epidemiology: Socioeconomic gradients in health and contextual analysis. *International Journal of Epidemiology, 30,* 899–900.

Krieger, N. (2001c). A glossary for social epidemiology. *Journal of Epidemiology and Community Health, 55,* 693–700.

Krieger, N. (2002). A glossary for social epidemiology. *Epidemiological Bulletin, 23*(1). Retrieved October 26, 2008, from http://www.paho.org/English/SHA/be_v23nl-glossary.htm

Lantz, P. M., Lynch, J. W., House, J. S., Lepkowski, J. M., Mero, R. P., Musick, M. A., & Williams, D. R. (2001). Socioeconomic disparities in health change in a longitudinal study of US adults: The role of health-risk behaviors. *Social Science and Medicine, 53,* 29–40.

LaVeist, T. A., Arthur, M., Plantholt, S., & Rubinstein, M. (2003). Explaining racial differences in receipt of coronary angiography: The role of physician referral and physician specialty. *Medical Care Research and Review, 60*(4), 453–467.

Lynch, J., & Kaplan, G. (2000). Socioeconomic position. In L. F. Berkman & I. Kawachi (Eds.), *Social epidemiology* (pp. 13–35). New York: Oxford University Press.

Marmot, M. (2000). Multilevel approaches to understanding social determinants. In L. F. Berkman & I. Kawachi (Eds.), *Social epidemiology* (pp. 349–367). New York: Oxford University Press.

Marmot, M., & Wilkinson, R. (2006). *Social determinants of health* (2nd ed.). Oxford: Oxford University Press.

Mirowsky, J., Ross, C. E., & Reynolds, J. (2000). Links between social status and health. In C. E. Bird, P. Conrad, & A. M. Fremont (Eds.), *Handbook of medical sociology* (pp. 47–78). Upper Saddle River, NJ: Prentice Hall.

National Library of Medicine (n.d.a.). *The reports of the surgeon general: The AIDS epidemic.* Retrieved November 5, 2009, from http://profiles.nlm.nih.gov/NN/Views/Exhibit/narrative/aids.html

National Library of Medicine. (n.d.b.). *The reports of the surgeon general: The 1964 report on smoking and health.* Retrieved November 5, 2009, from http://profiles.nlm.nih.gov/NN/Views/Exhibit/narrative/smoking.html

Office of History National Institute of Health. (2005). *Dr. Joseph Golberg & the war on pellagra.* Retrieved November 5, 2009, from http://history.nih.gov/exhibits/goldberger/index.html

Pfettscher, S. A. (2002). Florence Nightingale: Modern nursing. In A. M. Tomey & M. R. Alligood (Eds.), *Nursing theorists and their work* (5th ed., pp. 65–83). Philadelphia: Mosby.

Phillips, K. D. (2002). Sister Callista Roy: Adaptation model. In A. M. Tomey & M. R. Alligood (Eds.), *Nursing theorists and their work* (5th ed., pp. 269–298). Philadelphia: Mosby.

Pineda, M. D., White, E., Kristal, A. R., & Taylor, V. (2001). Asian breast cancer survival in the US: A comparison between Asian immigrants, US-born Asian Americans, and Caucasians. *International Journal of Epidemiology, 30,* 976–982.

Sepkowitz, K. A. (2001). AIDS—The first 20 years. *New England Journal of Medicine, 344*(23), 1764–1772.

Sepkowitz, K. A. (2008). One disease, two epidemics—AIDS at 25. *New England Journal of Medicine, 354*(23), 2411–2414.

Shavers, V. L., & Brown, M. L. (2002). Racial and ethnic disparities in the receipt of cancer treatment. *Journal of the National Cancer Institute, 94*(5), 334–357.

Stephan, E. (n.d.). *John Graunt.* Retrieved from http://www.edstephan.org/Graunt/graunt.html

Stotts, R. C. (2008). *Epidemiology and public health nursing.* Clifton Park, NJ: Delmar Cengage Learning.

Subramanian, S. V., Kawachi, I., & Kennedy, B. P. (2001). Does the state you live in make a difference? Multilevel analysis of self-rated health in the US. *Social Science & Medicine, 53,* 9–19.

Tarzian, A. J. (2005). Epidemiology: Unraveling the mysteries of disease and health. In F. A. Maurer & C. M. Smith (Eds), *Community/public health nursing practice: Health for families and populations* (3rd ed., pp. 150–174). St. Louis, MO: Elsevier Saunders.

UCLA Department of Epidemiology School of Public Health. (n.d.). *John Snow.* Retrieved November 5, 2009, from http://www.ph.ucla.edu/epi/snow.html

U.S. Department of Health and Human Services [DHHS] & Centers for Disease Control and Prevention [CDC]. (1998). *Principles of epidemiology: An introduction to applied epidemiology and biostatistics* (2nd ed.). Atlanta, GA: Author.

U.S. Department of Health and Human Services [DHHS] & Centers for Disease Control and Prevention [CDC]. (2006). *Principles of epidemiology: An introduction to applied epidemiology and biostatistics* (3rd ed.). Atlanta, GA: Author.

U.S. Preventive Services Task Force. (2008). *Guide to clinical preventive services: Recommendations of the U.S. Preventive Services Task Force.* Rockville, MD: Agency for Healthcare and Research Quality.

Wald, L. (1902). The nurses' settlement in New York. *American Journal of Nursing, 2*(8), 567–575.

Wilkinson, R. (1999). Income distribution and life expectancy. In I. Kawachi, B. Kennedy, & R. Wilkinson (Eds.), *The society and population health reader: Income inequality and health* (pp. 28–35). New York: The New Press.

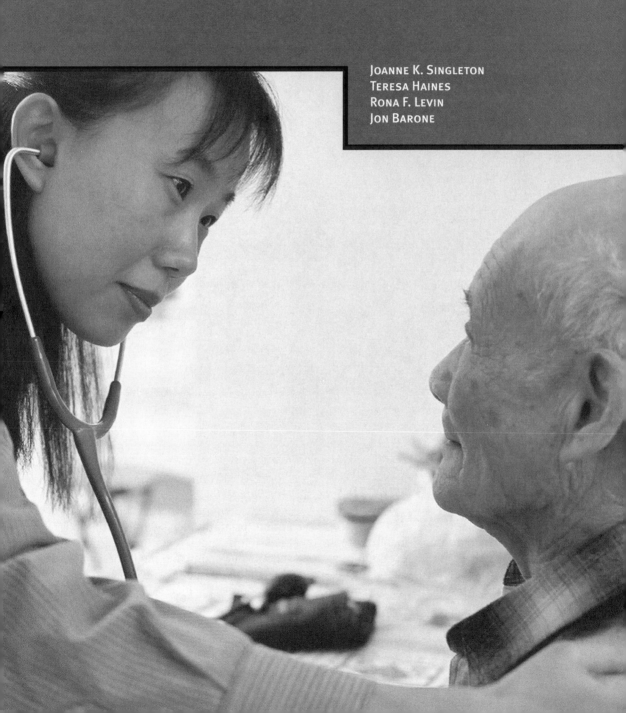

CHAPTER 5

EVIDENCE-BASED PRACTICE FROM A PUBLIC HEALTH PERSPECTIVE

JOANNE K. SINGLETON
TERESA HAINES
RONA F. LEVIN
JON BARONE

An uneducated woman may become a good nurse, but never an intelligent one; she can obey orders conscientiously and understand thoroughly a sick person's need, but should an emergency arise, where is she? She works through her feelings, and therefore lacks judgment . . . theory fortifies the practical, practice strengthens and retains the theoretical (Brennan, 1897/1991, p. 25).

LEARNING OBJECTIVES

At the completion of this chapter, the reader will be able to

- Define evidence-based practice.
- Describe the systematic approach to finding best available evidence.

- Explore the application of evidence-based practice to public health issues of health literacy and tobacco use.

KEY TERMS

- Evidence-based medicine
- Evidence-based practice
- Health literacy
- Morbidity

- Mortality
- Prevalence
- Tobacco use

INTRODUCTION TO EVIDENCE-BASED PRACTICE AND PUBLIC HEALTH

"In a world where public health threats range from AIDS and bioterrorism to an epidemic of obesity, the need for an effective public health system is as urgent as it has ever been" (Gebbie, Rosenstock, & Hernandez, 2003, p. 1). This quote comes from an Institute of Medicine (IOM) report, *Who Will Keep the Public Healthy? Educating Public Health Professionals for the 21st Century.* Although this report is aimed primarily at schools of public health, it includes recommendations for schools of nursing and medicine as well. For schools of nursing the recommendations address the inclusion of an ecological perspective of health in nursing curricula, collaboration among all public health professionals from a variety of disciplines, and the provision of clinical experiences in the public health arena. Also included in the report's recommendations is the need to include "**health literacy**" as a public health goal.

On the heels of this report, the IOM published *Health Professions Education: A Bridge to Quality* (Griener & Knebel, 2003), which included the following new vision for all health professions education: "All health professionals should be educated to deliver patient centered care as members of an interdisciplinary team, emphasizing evidence-based practice, quality improvement approaches, and informatics" (p. 3).

Healthy People 2010 is a federal government initiative that contains health objectives for the citizens of our nation (U.S. Department of Health and Human Services [DHHS], 2000). This document is built on past government initiatives intended to guide action that would improve people's health. Healthy People 2010 addresses two very important health issues—**tobacco use** and health literacy. Among the leading health indicators, which reflect the major health concerns in the United States, is tobacco use. The objective included in Healthy People regarding this health problem is

> Reduce illness, disability, and death related to tobacco use and exposure to secondhand smoke.

Although health literacy was not included as a leading health indicator in Healthy People 2010, the need for improved consumer health literacy is addressed in Objective 11-2. This objective highlighted the importance of health literacy in relation to health communication, medical product safety, and oral health.

The focus of this chapter is on an evidence-based approach to these two very important public health challenges: health literacy and tobacco use. Before discussing these two public health challenges and introducing the **evidence-based practice** (EBP) approach to understanding them, an overview of population-based concepts will help you to put the subsequent discussions about specific public health issues in context.

What Are "Need to Know" Population-Based Concepts to Inform Our Understanding?

The three major population-based or epidemiological concepts we discuss in relation to these major public health challenges are **prevalence**, **morbidity**, and **mortality**. For clarity, we provide the definitions of these terms here.

Prevalence is ". . . the number of affected persons present in the population at a specific time, divided by the number of persons in the population at that time" (Gordis, 2009, p. 43). This is a simple concept that tells us how many people in a specific population have the health problem. So, for example, in terms of health literacy this indicates how many people are not considered health literate among the Hispanic population who are receiving home care services.

Morbidity includes prevalence of a health problem but goes beyond prevalence to include the concept of incidence. The incidence rate of a health problem may be defined according to Gordis (2009) as ". . . the number of new cases of a disease that occur during a specified time period in a population at risk for developing the . . . [health problem]" (p. 38).

Clearly, *mortality* has to do with the rate of death from disease. There are, however, different ways of calculating mortality rates, and each way may give us a different perspective on a health problem. Suffice it to say for our purposes that mortality is defined as the death rate.

WHAT IS AN EBP LENS FOR VIEWING POPULATION-BASED HEALTH ISSUES?

The term "evidence based" was first used by medicine in 1992 by Gordon Guyatt, a Canadian physician from McMaster University, and the Evidence-Based Medicine Working Group. Although the term **"evidence-based medicine"** originated within the medical profession as a new paradigm for medical practice (Oxman, Sackett, & Guyatt, 1992), the essence of this paradigm, using research evidence as the best evidence to guide professional decision making, has recently spread to other professions both within and outside the healthcare arena. Singleton, Levin, and Keefer (2007) discussed several examples from the disciplines of law, education, and management. In addition, Cullum, Ciliska, Haynes, and Marks (2008) cite the use of the term "evidence based" in professions such as physiotherapy and police science.

Regardless of the field or discipline in which this paradigm or model is applied, EBP has several conceptual and process components that cross disciplinary boundaries. EBP is a framework for decision making that uses the *best available evidence* in conjunction with the *professional's expertise* and the client's, customer's, or consumer's *values and preferences* to guide problem solving and judgments about how to best approach a situation to achieve desired outcomes (Levin, 2006; Melnyk & Fineout-Overholt, 2005; Straus, Richardson, Glasziou, & Haynes, 2005). The key to the EBP model is the systematic approach to finding the best available evidence to answer a focused question and to implementation of the answer in practice as follows:

1. *Ask* and frame a *clinical question*.
2. *Find* the *evidence* to answer the question.
3. *Appraise* the *evidence* for validity, source reliability, and applicability to practice.
4. *Select* and *synthesize* the best evidence for use.
5. *Implement* the evidence-based *intervention* in practice.
6. *Evaluate* the intervention and *results*.

The search for and retrieval of this evidence is not always approached in the systematic way advocated in the EBP paradigm, which is to try to find the highest level of evidence first and then proceed methodically through the hierarchy of evidence that exists to answer the focused question. Thus a major principle from EBP that informs the practice improvement paradigm is, "Not all evidence is created equal" (Levin, 2008, p. 30). That is, some types of evidence carry more weight than other types of evidence. For example, a single study carries less weight than a systematic review. A systematic review combines the results of several studies on the same clinical question or questions. We always want to use the highest level of evidence available to guide our clinical practice. Health professionals, therefore, have developed schema that rank evidence according to levels. The higher the level of evidence, the more confidence we are able to have in a study's validity (Levin, 2008). There are many different schemata for ranking the level of a piece of evidence. **Box 5-1** presents the one we use.

Although it is important to determine the levels of evidence upon which a recommendation for practice is based, it is also important to assess the quality of that evidence, whether it is a study or expert opinion. The quality of evidence depends on the critical appraisal of the study or the background of and resources used by an expert panel.

The schema shown in **Box 5-2** provides one approach for assigning a quality rating to a piece of evidence. Using this approach, a rating for any level of evidence may range from A to D and reflects the basic scientific credibility of the overall study/project or other type of evidence.

Leveling schemes and quality ratings may differ according to agency or organization or author. Under any circumstances, however, the leveling and determination of the quality of evidence are essential components of this model. Some evidence-based guidelines, such as

---

BOX **5-1**   **Levels of Evidence**

- Level I: Systematic reviews (integrative/meta-analyses/CPG's based on systematic reviews)
- Level II: Single experimental study (randomized controlled trials)
- Level III: Quasi-experimental studies
- Level IV: Nonexperimental studies
- Level V: Case report/program evaluation/narrative literature reviews
- Level VI: Opinions of respected authorities

Source: From Levin (2008).

BOX **5-2**   **Quality Ratings**

A: A very well-designed study/project (Stetler et al., 1998)

B: A well-designed meta-analysis with at least 5 studies but less than 12; well-designed meta-analysis with large sample but some flawed studies*; individual studies in level IV, which may have a large sample size, but are secondary analyses of previously conducted randomized clinical trials (Singleton et al., 2005)

C: Well-designed individual studies with small sample sizes (Singleton et al., 2005)

D: Study/project has a major flaw that raises serious questions about the validity of the findings (Stetler et al., 1998)

*For example, use of nonrandomized trials in a meta-analysis seeking to answer questions of treatment effectiveness.

Source: From Singleton et al. (2005); Stetler et al. (1998).

the tobacco-dependence guidelines introduced below, identify and define "strength" of evidence for the specific guideline. When reading EBP guidelines, therefore, it is important to identify the criteria used to assess the level, quality, or strength of evidence. This is the approach we have taken in providing readers with the best available evidence on two very important public health challenges: helping people to stop smoking and increasing the health literacy of our population.

PUBLIC HEALTH CONDITIONS: AN EVIDENCE-BASED PERSPECTIVE

This chapter focuses on two health conditions from a public health perspective: health literacy and tobacco addiction. We discuss the national incidence and prevalence and morbidity and mortality of these health conditions, the evidence to guide or develop population-focused interventions for these conditions, and specific public health interventions in action for health literacy and tobacco addiction.

Health Literacy as a Public Health Condition: Overview and Definition

Before the 1990s the impact of literacy on population health in the United States was either unappreciated by health professionals or was generally thought of as a problem of an individual; literacy was not considered to be a public health condition. Today, it is known that literacy and its healthcare counterpart, "health literacy," has far-reaching effects on both the individual with low health literacy

and the U.S. population as a whole (Shohet & Renaud, 2006). As an indication of this new significance, Healthy People 2010, the U.S. national health promotion and disease prevention program, has formally included health literacy as a defined objective for study and intervention during the current decade (U.S. DHHS, 2000).

The definition of health literacy is continually being refined. The current most widely accepted definition states that health literacy is "the degree to which individuals have the capacity to obtain, process, and understand basic health information and services needed to make appropriate health decisions" (IOM, 2004, p. 32). This definition has been expanded more recently to reflect the even broader impact that health literacy has on individual lives. "Literacy facilitates access to information, and enables individuals to make informed health decisions, to influence events and to exert greater control over their lives" (Shohet & Renaud, 2006, p. 10). In more concrete terms, health literacy impacts an individual's ability to access health care, to make choices in obtaining appropriate health insurance coverage, and to seek out high-quality facilities to obtain evidence-based health screening and illness care as well as comprehend written health information about disease prevention or self-care of chronic disease. In addition, if an individual has responsibility for the care of children or elderly family members, the individual needs to advocate and make decisions for those in his or her care. Clearly, health literacy has far-reaching effects on individuals, families, communities, and the U.S. population as a whole.

INCIDENCE, PREVALENCE,
MORBIDITY, AND MORTALITY

Incidence and Prevalence. Although low health literacy is now widely recognized to have a significant negative impact on both the individual and public health, tools to measure health literacy and strategies to improve care of the low literacy population have only recently been developed. For the third time in as many decades, the National Center for Education Statistics (2006) measured the English literacy of the U.S. population in the 2003 National Assessment of Adult Literacy. This survey was the first to include measurement of health literacy in addition to overall U.S. English literacy. The National Assessment of Adult Literacy surveyed a representative sample of 18,000 U.S. households as well as 1,200 persons in prisons. For the purpose of this study, health literacy was defined using the previously quoted IOM definition (National Center for Education Statistics, 2006).

Health literacy was measured using the three literacy measures used in the overall English literacy assessments by the 2003 National Assessment of Adult Literacy survey: prose, document, and quantitative measures. Prose literacy is defined as the ability to search, comprehend, and use information from continuous text. Document literacy is defined as the ability to search, comprehend, and use information from noncontinuous text (e.g., application forms or maps). Quantitative literacy is defined as the ability to identify and perform computation using numbers embedded in print materials (e.g., balancing a checkbook). In addition, three domains specific to health literacy were identified and measured: clinical, prevention, and navigation of the health

system. The clinical domain was defined as the activities involved in the provider–patient interaction, such as completing forms and understanding medication dosages. The prevention domain was defined as activities related to disease prevention and self-management of illness. Navigation of the health system included activities such as understanding health insurance plans and consent forms.

Results of the 2003 adult health literacy survey showed that 36% of the U.S. population, or approximately 87 million adults, had either below basic (14%) or basic (22%) health literacy levels, defined as

- Below basic: No more than the most basic and concrete literacy skills
- Basic: Skills necessary to perform simple and basic everyday activities

Disparities among particular subpopulations were also noted. Hispanic populations had the lowest percentage of health literacy among ethnic groups. More men (16%) than women (12%) had below basic health literacy levels. Persons who did not speak English before attending primary school had lower health literacy than those who spoke English at early ages. Adults over age 65 had lower health literacy than other age groups. Educational attainment was significantly associated with below basic health literacy. Forty-nine percent of individuals who did not complete either high school or a General Educational Development program had below basic health literacy scores. Adults living in poverty had lower health literacy levels than other socioeconomic groups. Persons who had self-perceived overall health at lower ratings also had lower health literacy levels. Persons who had no health insurance or had Medicaid/Medicare had lower health literacy levels. Those who obtained their basic health information from television or radio had lower health literacy than those who obtained information from print media (National Center for Education Statistics, 2006).

Low health literacy may contribute significantly to the notable health disparities across specific populations in the United States. One of the overarching goals of Healthy People 2010 is to reduce these health disparities, which lead to increased morbidity and mortality as well as inefficient and ineffective use of public resources. Estimates of the cost of low health literacy to U.S. society range from $106 to $236 billion dollars annually (Vernon, Trujillo, Rosenbaum, & DeBuono, 2007). Clearly, low health literacy is a public health condition of great consequence.

Morbidity and Mortality and Level of Evidence. Many studies have documented how low health literacy impacts a person's ability to obtain preventive screening services and to manage one's chronic diseases. Based on the level of evidence ratings in Box 5-1, the following evidence is reported. In a systematic review of the literature, DeWalt, Berkman, Sheridan, Lohr, and Pignone (2004) found that patients with low health literacy used health resources less frequently than their higher literacy counterparts (level 1). Maniaci, Heckman, and Dawson (2008) found that patients with lower levels of health literacy were found to have less medication knowledge after hospital discharge (level IV). In addition, patients with type 2 diabetes mellitus and low health literacy were found to have higher HgA_{1C} levels and higher rates of retinopathy than those with higher health literacy levels

(Schillinger et al., 2002) (level IV). Patients with low health literacy were less likely to use preventive services (IOM, 2004) (level V). Also, higher mortality rates were associated with lower health literacy scores (Baker et al., 2007) (level IV). Patients with low health literacy have higher rates of hospitalizations and complications and higher emergency room use (Baker, Parker, Williams, & Clark, 1998; Baker et al., 2002) (level IV). Moreover, patients with low health literacy were two to three times more likely to experience poor outcomes (DeWalt et al., 2004) (level I).

EVIDENCE TO GUIDE POPULATION-FOCUSED INTERVENTIONS

Evidence on the morbidity and mortality related to health literacy provides guidance on population-focused interventions. The cost to society as a whole mandates that action is taken to remedy the low health literacy problem. Paasche-Orlow and Wolf (2007) identified three areas for intervention "access points" across the U.S. healthcare system: systemic, interactional, and self-care.

A systemic intervention to improve care of low literacy patients is the three-pronged strategy adopted by The Joint Commission (Murphy-Knoll, 2007). The first strategy makes clear communication an organizational priority. The second strategy mandates that clear communication needs to be addressed across the continuum of care, from the acute care to the primary care setting. The third strategy states that policy changes must be pursued to improve provider–patient communication.

Another systemic intervention involves increasing access to healthcare coverage for the entire population. During 2008, 46.3 million persons in the United States under the age of 65 were uninsured

(National Center for Health Statistics, 2008). Persons with low health literacy are more likely to be uninsured than those with intermediate or proficient levels of health literacy.

An important point to note, however, is that the uninsured are not the only persons with low health literacy. Seventy-five million persons with low health literacy are currently insured. Simplification of the existing system may also have a significant impact on those with low health literacy who are currently insured. Currently, physicians frequently drop out of insurance plans and formularies change, requiring a change of primary care provider or a change in medication. In addition, a single individual may have three different plan requirements for his or her medical, dental, and pharmacy coverage. Reducing insurance barriers for all persons may mean taking steps such as minimizing confusing health insurance requirements and documents. Systemic interventions include improved access to care as well as streamlining existing healthcare plans.

The second access point for intervention is interaction between individuals and healthcare professionals. This interaction could be improved by increasing basic health literacy education of primary care providers. Institutions educating healthcare professionals need to include clear communication techniques as part of their basic curriculum. Methods such as "teach back" (Pfizer Clear Health Communication Initiative, 2008) and "ask me three" (National Patient Safety Foundation, 2008) have been shown to improve patient comprehension and ability for self-care. Healthcare providers need to understand that health education materials should be written in easy-to-use formats, with large font, short sentences, and action-oriented content to improve

readability and patient comprehension (Doak, Doak, & Root, 1998). Providers need to be aware that certain populations respond to different educational techniques. In a study by Volandes and colleagues (2008), specific teaching techniques were shown to enhance decision-making ability regarding end-of-life care preferences.

Healthcare providers need to understand the negative impact of health literacy on their individual clients. The literature suggests that individuals do not access health care due to the "shame" related to their literacy problems. Organizations and healthcare providers can make changes to reduce this negative impact by creating "shame-free environments." Providing written materials at low literacy levels and offering assistance for those completing intake forms are suggested methods to remove barriers to care for those with low health literacy. If healthcare providers wish to measure their individual client's health literacy, the "newest vital sign" tool has been developed. This tool is a 3-minute, face-to-face individual measurement available in both English and Spanish (Weiss et al., 2005). If time and/or personnel constraints do not permit specific measurement, there is a proxy measure for health literacy, the Demographic Assessment for Health Literacy (Hanchate, Ash, Gasmararian, Wolf, & Paasche-Orlow, 2008). This measure uses the demographic data of age, educational attainment, gender, and race/ethnicity to estimate health literacy levels.

Interactional intervention access points can also be found in the person's community. People with low health literacy cannot distinguish different medications and the appropriate dosing schedules (Jacobson et al., 2007). The

Agency for Health Research and Quality developed a tool for community pharmacies to improve outcomes in medication safety with improved prescription drug labeling and health education materials. Community adult literacy initiatives need to be integrated with the healthcare community to foster improved health literacy. The Literary Information and Communication System system in the United States is a web-based organization dedicated to connecting resources from both the adult education and healthcare communities (National Institute for Literacy, 2008).

HEALTH LITERACY AND TOBACCO USE: SPECIFIC PUBLIC HEALTH INTERVENTIONS (CASE STUDY)
An organization reviews the current tobacco use health education materials it provides to nonsmoking adolescent clients (e.g., Did you know that tobacco addiction is one of the hardest habits to break?). These education materials could be evaluated for both reading level, using the Simplified Measure of Gobbledygook, or SMOG (McLaughlin, 2008), or Fry formula (Doak et al., 1998), and readability, using the Suitability of Assessment Materials, or SAM, tool (Doak et al., 1998). When designing materials for adolescents, in particular, it is important that patients "see themselves" in the illustrations on the material. The SAM tool gives very valuable guidelines that improve design for health education materials that are targeted to a specific audience. Revision of an organization's existing tobacco use materials to reduce reading level, improve readability, and clearly target a specific population is one example of a low cost and effective means to begin a system-wide movement toward clear communication.

FUTURE PROJECTIONS
Unfortunately, the problem of low health literacy may worsen in the United States. Projections for population English literacy levels are projected to decrease in the United States (Sum, Kirsch, & Yamamoto, 2004). If healthcare systems and individual providers do not make health literacy and clear communication a priority, public health outcomes can be expected to decline over the next decade.

Tobacco Dependence as a Public Health Condition: Overview

Tobacco, a green leafy plant that grows in warm climates, has a long history in America. Dating back to the first American settlers in 1621 in Jamestown, Virginia, tobacco was the first crop grown for money in North America. Tobacco is dried and can be smoked or chewed. There are over 4,800 chemicals in tobacco and its smoke; nicotine is the chemical that makes tobacco addictive. Although, starting with the first settlers, tobacco was used in small amounts, the invention of the cigarette-making machine in 1881 resulted in widespread cigarette smoking. Nevertheless, it was not until 1964 that the Surgeon General of the United States reported on the dangers of cigarette smoking, identifying that the nicotine and tar in cigarettes may cause lung cancer. The U.S. Congress in 1965 passed the Cigarette Labeling and Advertising Act that required every cigarette pack to carry on its side the warning "Cigarettes may be hazardous to your health." This was followed by later legislation in 1971 banning radio and television advertising of cigarettes. Cigarette companies responded to the government warnings about the hazards of smoking related to tar. By the 1980s cigarette companies made, sold, and promoted low and ultra low tar ciga-rettes. Congress passed another law in 1984, the Comprehensive Smoking Edu-cation Act, that created four different warning labels (**Figure 5-1**) and required cigarette companies to rotate among these warnings every 3 months.

Federal, state, and local governments as well as private companies have been taking action since the 1980s to restrict and ban smoking in public places. The American Lung Association tracks and reports tobacco control trends in the United States (see http://stateoftobacco control.org). As of 2009 the Lung Associa-tion's smoke-free map reveals that still a little over half of the 50 states have yet to enact comprehensive smoke-free laws to protect their citizens. Although the U.S. House of Representatives passed the Fam-ily Smoking Prevention and Tobacco Con-trol Act in July 2008 to regulate tobacco products, the Senate did not act on this. This means this legislation will have to start over again, leaving tobacco products unregulated by the federal government.

INCIDENCE, PREVALENCE, MORBIDITY, AND MORTALITY

In the United States cigarette smoking continues to be identified as the most avoidable cause of death and disability (Centers for Disease Control and Preven-tion [CDC], 2007a). Tobacco use begins in adolescence, with first use almost always occurring before 18 years of age.

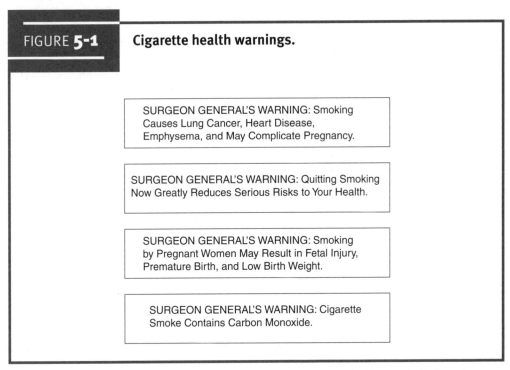

FIGURE **5-1**   **Cigarette health warnings.**

SURGEON GENERAL'S WARNING: Smoking Causes Lung Cancer, Heart Disease, Emphysema, and May Complicate Pregnancy.

SURGEON GENERAL'S WARNING: Quitting Smoking Now Greatly Reduces Serious Risks to Your Health.

SURGEON GENERAL'S WARNING: Smoking by Pregnant Women May Result in Fetal Injury, Premature Birth, and Low Birth Weight.

SURGEON GENERAL'S WARNING: Cigarette Smoke Contains Carbon Monoxide.

Source: From Public Law 98-474, Comprehensive Smoking Education Act, 1984. Smoking Tobacco & Health, Centers for Disease Control and Prevention.

Cigarette smoking carries a significant disease burden for the primary smoker that may result in respiratory diseases, lung cancer, and/or cardiovascular disease and may have harmful reproductive effects and results in more than 438,000 deaths per year in the United States (CDC, 2007b). Exposure to secondhand smoke for the nonsmoker creates a significant health risk, especially for individuals with respiratory or cardiac conditions, resulting in premature death and disease. According to a CDC report, direct medical costs in the United States from tobacco dependence are more than $96 billion per year and an additional $97 billion resulting from lost productivity (CDC, 2007b).

Although most smokers report a desire to quit, most quit attempts fail. New smokers from adults to children are continually recruited. Not only are interventions critical to help those who already smoke to quit, interventions to prevent people, especially children, from starting to smoke are essential to eliminating smoking-related illnesses.

About 45 million adults (21%) in the United States smoke (CDC, 2007a), and each day about 4,000 children ages 12 to 17 smoke their first cigarette, with about 1,200 becoming addicted to tobacco and smoking daily (Substance Abuse and Mental Health Services Administration, 2005, 2007). In 2006 it was reported that 3.3 million adolescents ages 12 to 17 years were tobacco users, with 2.6 million of this population cigarette smokers. About 82% of adolescent smokers are interested in quitting, but only about 4% of the 77% who attempt to quit are successful (Engels, Knibbe, de Vries, & Drop, 1998; Zhu, Sun, Billings, Choi, & Malarcher, 1999). Quit attempts in ado-

lescents are usually unassisted and unplanned, yet those who enroll in quit programs are twice as likely to succeed as those who are not enrolled (McCuller, Sussman, Wapner, Dent, & Weiss, 2006).

Over the past 50 years the prevalence of smoking in the United States has decreased by about 50% to about one-fifth of the population. Men smoke more than women (23% vs. 19%). Native American/Native Alaskans smoke more (33%) than blacks and whites (both at 21%), Hispanics (15%), and Asians/Pacific Islanders (11.3%). In 2005, 19 million adults attempted to quit, but only 4% to 7% are estimated to have been successful (Hughes, 2003). Although there is now "a robust evidence base about effective interventions . . . the United States has not yet achieved the goal of making tobacco use a rare behavior" (CDC, 2007c, p. 7).

EVIDENCE TO GUIDE POPULATION-FOCUSED INTERVENTIONS

Decreasing smoking in public places not only protects nonsmokers from the effects of secondhand smoke, but it may also promote smoking cessation by restricting smoking behavior. Comprehensive multicomponent strategies to enforce no-smoking policies within organizations were found to be the most effective strategies to decrease smoking in public places. A moderate effect was found with the use of educational material and posted warnings to enforce no-smoking policies (Serra, Bonfill, Pladevall, & Cabezas, 2008). From 2002 to 2004 smoking prevalence in New York City decreased from 21.5% to 17.5%. This has been attributed to increased taxes that increased the price of cigarettes as well as the law that made all indoor workplaces smoke free. This percentage decrease equates with approximately 240,000 fewer smokers (CDC, 2007a).

Mass media interventions, such as those delivered by leaflets, booklets, posters, billboards, newspapers, radio and television, are used to promote smoking cessation in adults. One example of this type of intervention is the media campaign initiated by the New York City Department of Mental Health and Hygiene. In 2006 the Department launched a television advertising blitz with disturbing images and graphic descriptions of the health consequences of smoking. One vignette showed a man speaking with a robotic voice after a laryngectomy due to throat cancer. This campaign reduced smoking rates overall among men and Hispanic New Yorkers (CDC, 2007a). It is difficult, however, to specifically identify the contribution of mass media interventions. What the evidence does indicate is that when mass media interventions are used as part of a comprehensive tobacco cessation program, they can be effective for adults (Bala, Strzeszynski, & Cahill, 2008).

Healthcare financing systems may also be effective in increasing the use of tobacco dependence treatment. The evidence to date shows that health insurance coverage or reducing the direct cost of smoking cessation treatment may increase the number of successful quit attempts as well as the number of smokers who are successful with smoking cessation. This evidence must be looked at cautiously because the studies in the meta-analysis that produced this evidence had methodological problems (Kaper, Wagena, Severns, & van Schayck, 2005).

In May 2008 the U.S. Public Health Service released the updated the guidelines on tobacco use treatment and dependence (Fiore et al., 2008). These evidence-based guidelines recommend treatment for individuals who are tobacco dependent. Recommendations from the guidelines represent strength of evidence with A through C ratings. The strongest recommendations, A, are based on multiple, well-designed, randomized trials that are directly relevant to the recommendation. Level B ratings indicate that some evidence from randomized clinical trials supported the recommendation but the scientific support was not optimal. Level C ratings are "reserved for important clinical situations in which the Panel achieved consensus on the recommendation in the absence of relevant randomized controlled trials" (Fiore et al., 2008, p. 15). According to the guidelines, "It is difficult to identify any other condition [than tobacco dependence] that presents such a mix of lethality, prevalence, and neglect, despite effective and readily available interventions" (Fiore et al., 2008, p. 2).

The guidelines strongly recommend that clinicians screen and document patients' tobacco use status and deliver evidence-based tobacco dependence treatment (strength of evidence A) (Fiore et al., 2008). Simple reminders, like chart stickers or electronic prompts, can be instituted within an organization to remind clinicians to "ask" about smoking status. For smokers who are not currently interested in quitting, motivational techniques can be used to encourage a future quit attempt (strength of evidence B). Clinicians and clinicians-in-training should be taught effective smoking cessation strategies to assist individuals who want to make a quit attempt and those who are not yet motivated to do so (strength of evidence B). Further, because the tobacco dependence treatments identified in the guidelines are cost effective, they should be offered to all smokers (strength of evidence A). Counseling for tobacco dependent adolescents has been found to be effective and therefore is recommended for adolescents (strength of evidence B). Cessation counseling has been found to be effective with parents to help protect children from secondhand smoke (strength of evidence B).

What Does Additional Evidence Tell Us About Adolescents?

The evidence indicates that tobacco advertising and promotion increases the likelihood that nonsmoking adolescents will become smokers at a later time (Lovato, Linn, Stead, & Best, 2003). "Joe the Camel" was an example of an advertising strategy that was specifically directed to promote adolescent smoking. Community interventions, specifically coordinated multicomponent programs, can help to reduce smoking behavior in people under age 25 years. Multicomponent programs might include mass media interventions, age restrictions on tobacco purchase, and school programs (Sowden, 1998).

Overall, there is weak evidence that mass media can be effective in preventing young adults from starting to smoke. Mass media campaigns that developed and focused their message based on their target audience were more effective than those that did not use this strategy. Campaigns of greater intensity and duration were more successful than those that were not (Sowden, 1998). An example of a media campaign targeting young adults was the billboard advertising in New York City featuring star athletes from various local sports teams. The slogan, "I don't smoke, do you?" was prominently displayed along major highways throughout the city. It is believed that if young people are unable to purchase cigarettes this may reduce the number who start to smoke. Although during compliance checks interventions with retailers to discourage the illegal sale of cigarettes, such as warnings and fines, were shown to be effective in decreasing sales, the outcome of this intervention on young adults' smoking behavior has not shown a clear effect (Stead & Lancaster, 2005). Further, it is believed that the behavior of a child's/adolescent's family may influence the likelihood of the child/adolescent starting to smoke. Although there is evidence that family interventions may prevent adolescents from smoking, other evidence showed neutral or negative outcomes (Thomas, Baker, & Lorenzetti, 2007).

Do school-based programs prevent children who are nonsmokers from becoming smokers? Thomas and Perera (2006) reviewed 23 high-quality, randomized controlled trials. The interventions in these studies included information giving, social influence approaches, social skills training, and community interventions. Information giving alone was not supported by the evidence as an effective intervention, and there was limited evidence for the effects of the other interventions.

Through increased implementation of evidence-based interventions, tobacco dependence in adolescents declined 40% from 1997 to 2003. Progress has stalled, however, and may be attributed to decreased state funding for tobacco dependence prevention programs, increased tobacco industry marketing, and decreased effectiveness of mass media campaigns (CDC, 2007a).

The tobacco epidemic in the United States is an example of how putting evidence into practice can stop this epidemic and accelerate declines in the related morbidity and mortality associated with tobacco dependence.

PUTTING EVIDENCE INTO PRACTICE
Because of the accomplishments of modern public health, the United States has seen a 30-year increase in life expectancy in the 20th century. Still, many public health challenges remain. To achieve the goals as outlined in Healthy People 2010 and meet the expectations for continued public health improvement, a drive toward more widespread use of evidence-based strategies for effectively addressing current challenges in public health is needed (Brownson, Baker, Leet, & Gillespie, 2003).

The concerns related to smoking and secondhand smoke have become the focus of a public health issue that has for years gone without intervention. Lawmakers are now recognizing the detrimental effects of smoking to a community at large. Not only is smoking the number one preventable cause of death in the United States today with over 430,000 deaths each year from tobacco-related causes, but another 53,000 non-smoking Americans die annually from inhaling secondhand tobacco smoke.

Breathing tobacco smoke can be harmful to anyone, but it is especially harmful to the elderly, the very young, and those with existing respiratory problems. The Surgeon General's 2006 report stated "there is no risk-free level of second hand smoke exposure. Even brief exposures can be harmful to children" (U.S. DHHS, 2006).

Many believe that children are the forgotten victims in the secondhand smoke debate and should be protected as much, if not more, than adults who are exposed to secondhand smoke. It is questionable whether or not many children are able to avoid cigarette smoke at home, but there should be no doubt that they cannot escape if they are in a car with someone smoking. Can you imagine how much damage is done to the health of a young child, sitting in a car for hours, while his or her parents chain smoke? A no-smoking advocate stated that it would be like "being locked up in a mobile gas chamber." To me, the example is a bit drastic, but the point is well taken.

ADVERSE HEALTH EFFECTS OF SECONDHAND SMOKE ON CHILDREN
Secondhand smoke is a major, preventable contributor to acute and chronic adverse health outcomes that affect children. Another quote from the Surgeon General's report states that "Secondhand smoke contains more than 250 chemicals known to be toxic or carcinogenic, including formaldehyde, benzene, vinyl chloride, arsenic, ammonia, and hydrogen cyanide. Children who are exposed to secondhand smoke are inhaling many of the same cancer-causing substances and poisons as smokers" (U.S. DHHS, 2006).

- Babies born to mothers who smoked during pregnancy, or who are exposed after birth, have weaker lungs, which increases the risk of other health issues (U.S. DHHS, 2006).
- Because the lungs of infants and young children are still developing, exposure results in decreased lung function (U.S. DHHS, 2006).
- Secondhand smoke causes an estimated 430 deaths from sudden infant death syndrome annually (California Environmental Protection Agency [EPA], 2005).

- Infants and children are more likely to suffer from cough, wheezing, phlegm, and breathlessness (U.S. DHHS, 2006).
- Secondhand smoke exacerbates 400,000 to 1,000,000 cases of asthma in the United States and is a risk factor for induction of new cases of asthma among children and adolescents (California EPA, 2005).
- Sixty percent of middle and high schoolers combined are exposed to secondhand smoke in their own homes (National Youth Tobacco Survey, 2004).
- Based on levels of cotinine (a biological marker of secondhand smoke exposure), an estimated 40 million children aged 3 to 19 were exposed to secondhand smoke in the United States in 2000 (U.S. DHHS, 2006).
- Secondhand smoke causes 150,000 to 300,000 acute lower respiratory tract infections (pneumonia and bronchitis) annually in children 18 months and younger, which results in 7,500 to 15,000 hospitalizations each year (California EPA, 2005).
- Secondhand smoke causes otitis media, resulting in 790,000 to 1.6 million physician office visits (California EPA, 2005).
- It is the most common cause of childhood hearing loss (California EPA, 2005).

Need for Change: One Nurse's Voice

Jon Barone is a voting member of the Keyport, New Jersey, Board of Health and also a commissioner and voting member of the Monmouth County Regional Health Commission, which oversees the boards of health of 24 townships in New Jersey.

He became involved in the local political scene because a newly elected Councilman remembered him from the Councilman's door-to-door campaign. The Councilman had expressed Barone's views on how to improve the health of the community. After his election the Councilman knocked on Barone's door again, this time to ask him to become a member of the Board of Health. Barone accepted an appointment by the Mayor and joined the Board of Health. The Board of Health then appointed Barone to represent them on the Monmouth County Regional Health Commission.

One day after reading the Surgeon General's Report and reviewing the evidence-based data, it was clear to Barone that there was a need for change in existing laws to enhance EBP in the community at large. The idea for an ordinance to prohibit adults from smoking in vehicles when children are present in late 2006 to early 2007 seemed appropriate.

Are We Going Too Far? Some members of the community may say that this is overstepping bounds and infringing on the constitutional rights of the individual and question whether this dictates what may be considered as poor parenting skills. Additionally, others might believe that because it is becoming harder and harder to smoke in public, violating the privacy and sanctity of their personal space is just too much to bear. However, this is not so much about infringing on the rights of the individual as it is about preserving the rights of our children and protecting those who do not have the ability or are unable to choose for themselves (Barone, 2007).

Public Health Education. After researching the idea further, drafting an ordinance, and getting advice from a nonsmoking organization, Barone presented the legislation to the Keyport Town Council. Before the vote Barone spoke to the Mayor and Council in support of the law, presenting the evidence-based data. It passed by an overwhelming margin, making Keyport the first township in New Jersey, and only one of a select number of places in the country, to pass legislation that protects children against secondhand smoke in a confined space. As a result of this new law, Keyport, New Jersey, received national attention and was all over the news and Internet the rest of that week. As a result of the publicity received related to the passage of this public health–related law, many people in communities nationwide were thinking more about the detrimental effects of secondhand smoke.

Influence Through Action. After these events Barone was contacted by New Jersey State Senator Raymond Lesniak's office, who wanted to use this precedent as a catalyst for a state law in New Jersey and hopefully influence surrounding states as well. To assist in that effort, Barone drafted a resolution to the Monmouth County Regional Health Commission supporting a state law prohibiting adults from smoking in vehicles when children are present. Additionally, in June 2007 Barone was invited to speak and testify before the New Jersey State Senate Health & Human Services Committee in Trenton, New Jersey, in support of a state law. He was also invited to speak at a press conference in support of a similar law in New York City at City Hall.

A Time of Empowerment. Whether you are a registered nurse or an advanced practice nurse, you can analyze the health status data to identify a public health issue and affect change in the community. We all know that if you wait for the other person to initiate change, it may not happen. Empowerment is the key. If you are passionate about the issues, don't be afraid to get involved. Participate in organized lobbying efforts to help effect change in your profession and community. It is important to help promote more effective public health prevention strategies through legislative interventions. Allow your voice to be heard. It takes only one person to become a catalyst for a health promotion idea. One nurse can make a difference.

Reflecting on the case above, it is evident that whereas public health nurses use data as evidence to inform policymakers, the other public health strategies are intertwined. Once policy is established, it does not end there; other public health strategies, such as advocacy and the use of media for educating the population, to name a few, must take shape and form.

TOBACCO DEPENDENCE: FUTURE DIRECTIONS THROUGH BEST PRACTICES

According to the CDC (2007a) the most effective evidence-based, population-based approaches result from the synergistic effect produced from putting into the place the following program components: state and community interventions, health communication interventions, cessation interventions, surveillance and evaluation, and administration and management. The IOM (2007) put forth the goal of reducing smoking so that it is no longer a significant health problem for our nation. The IOM believes, based on substantial evidence, that this can be achieved through state tobacco control programs that are comprehensive, integrated, and maintained

over time. In fact, it has been shown that the more spent by states for sustained comprehensive tobacco control programs, the greater and faster the impact (CDC, 2007a). Putting into practice evidence-based interventions is an example of how to curtail a public health condition such as the tobacco epidemic in the United States.

References

Baker, D. W., Parker, R. M., Williams, M. V., and Clark, W. S. (1998). Health literacy and the risk of hospital admission. *Journal of General Internal Medicine, 13*(12), 791–798.

Baker, D. W., Gamazian, J. A., Williams, M. V., Scott, T., Parker, R. M., Green, D., et al. (2002). Functional health literacy and the risk of hospital admission among Medicare managed care enrollees. *American Journal of Public Health, 92*(8), 1278–1283.

Baker, D. W., Wolf, M., Feinglass, J., Thompson, J. A., Gasmaranian, J. A., and Huang, J. (2007). Health literacy and mortality among elderly persons. *Archives of Internal Medicine, 167*(14), 1503–1509.

Bala, M., Strzeszynski, L., & Cahill, K., (2008). Mass media interventions for smoking cessation in adults. *Cochrane Database of Systematic Reviews* (Issue 1), Art. No.: CD004704. DOI: 10.1002/14651858.CD004704.pub2.

Barone, J. (2007, June 4). The second hand smoke issue lights up in New Jersey. *The Nursing Spectrum, 19A*(12).

Brennan, A. S. (1897/1991). Comparative value of theory and practice in training nurses. In N. Birnbach & S. B. Lewenson (Eds.), *First words: Selected addresses from the National League for Nursing 1894–1933* (pp. 358–369). New York: National League for Nursing Press.

Brownson, R. C., Baker, E. A., Leet, T. L., & Gillespie, K. N. (2003). *Evidence based public health.* London: Oxford University Press.

California Environmental Protection Agency [EPA]. (2005, June). *Health effects of exposure to ETS.* Retrieved September 6, 2009, from http://www.oehha.ca.gov/air/environmental_tobacco/2005etsfinal.html

Centers for Disease Control and Prevention [CDC]. (2007a). *Best practices for comprehensive tobacco control programs—2007.* Atlanta, GA: U.S. Department of Health and Human Services, Centers for Disease Control and Prevention, National Center for Chronic Disease Prevention and Health Promotion, Office on Smoking and Health.

Centers for Disease Control and Prevention [CDC]. (2007b). Cigarette smoking among adults—United States, 2006. *Morbidity and Mortality Weekly Report, 56,* 1157–1161.

Centers for Disease Control and Prevention [CDC[. (2007c). MMWR synopsis for June 21, 2007. Retrieved February 12, 2007 from http://www.cdc.gov/media/mmwrnews/2007/n070621.htm#3

Cullum, N., Ciliska, D., Haynes, R. B., & Marks, S. (2008). *Evidence-based nursing: an introduction.* Hong Kong and Singapore: Blackwell.

DeWalt, D. A., Berkman, N. D., Sheridan, S., Lohr, K. N., & Pignone, M. P. (2004). Literacy and health outcomes: A systematic review of the literature. *Journal of General Internal Medicine, 19*(12), 1228–1239.

Doak, L., Doak, C., & Root, J. (1998). *Teaching patients with low literacy skills.* Philadelphia: Lippincott.

Engels, R. C., Knibbe, R. A., de Vries, H., & Drop, M. J. (1998). Antecedents of smoking cessation among adolescents: Who is motivated to change? *Preventive Medicine, 27*, 348–357.

Fiore, M. C., Jaén, C. R., Baker, T. B., Bailey, W. C., Benowitz, N. L., Curry, S. J., et al. (2008). *Treating tobacco use and dependence: 2008 update.* Rockville, MD: U.S. Dept. of Health and Human Services.

Gebbie, K., Rosenstock, L., & Hernandez, L. M. (Eds.), Committee on Educating Health Professionals for the 21st Century, Board on Health Promotion and Disease Prevention, Institute of Medicine of the National Academies. (2003). *Who will keep the public healthy? Educating public health professionals for the 21st century.* Washington, DC: National Academies Press.

Gordis, L. (2009). *Epidemiology* (4th ed.). Philadelphia: Saunders.

Griener, A. C., & Knebel, E. (Eds.). Committee on the Health Professions Summit, Institute of Medicine of the National Academies. (2003). *Health professions education: A bridge to quality.* Washington, DC: National Academies Press.

Hanchate, A. D., Ash, A. S., Gasmararian, J. A., Wolf, M. A., & Paasche-Orlow, M. K. (2008). The Demographic Assessment for Health Literacy (DAHL): A new tool for estimating associations between health literacy and outcomes in national surveys. *Journal of General Internal Medicine, 23*(10), 1561–1566.

Hughes, J. R. (2003). Motivating and helping smokers to stop smoking. *Journal of General Internal Medicine, 18*, 1053–1057.

Institute of Medicine. (2007). *Ending the tobacco problem: A blueprint for the nation.* Washington, DC: The National Academies Press.

Institute of Medicine [IOM]. (2004). *Health literacy: A prescription to end confusion.* Washington, DC: National Academies Press.

Jacobson, K. L., Gazmararian, J. A., Kripalani, S., McMorris, K. J., Blake, S. C., & Brach, C. (2007). *Is our pharmacy meeting patients' needs? A pharmacy health literacy assessment tool users guide.* Retrieved November 30, 2008, from http://www.cdc.gov/nchs/data/hus/hus07.pdf#fig30

Kaper, J., Wagena, E., Severns, J. L., & van Schayck, O. P. (2005). Healthcare financing systems for increasing the use of tobacco dependence treatment. *Cochrane Database of Systematic Reviews,* (1), CD004305.

Levin, R. (2006). Evidence-based practice in nursing: What is it? In R. F. Levin & H. R. Feldman (Eds.), *Teaching evidence-based practice in nursing: A guide for educators.* New York: Springer.

Levin, R. F. (2008). Translating research evidence for WOCN practice. Evidence levels and quality ratings: What do they mean? *WCET Journal, 28*(1), 30–31.

Lovato, C., Linn, G., Stead, L. F., & Best, A. (2003). Impact of tobacco advertising and promotion on increasing adolescent smoking behaviors. *Cochrane Database of Systematic Reviews,* (4) CD003439.

Maniaci, M., Heckman, M., & Dawson, N. (2008). Functional health literacy and understanding of medicines at discharge. *Mayo Clinic Proceedings, 83*(5), 554–558.

McCuller, W. J., Sussman, S., Wapner, M., Dent, C., & Weiss, D. J. (2006). Motivation to quit as a mediator of tobacco cessation among at-risk youth. *Addictive Behaviors, 31*, 880–888.

McLaughlin, G. H. (2008). *Simplified measure of gobbledygook.* Retrieved November 30, 2008, from http://www.harrymclaughlin.com/SMOG.htm

Melnyk, B. M., & Fineout-Overholt, E. (2005). *Evidence-based practice in healthcare.* Philadelphia: Lippincott.

Murphy-Knoll, L. (2007). Low health literacy puts patients at risk. *Journal of Nursing Care Quality, 22*(3), 205–209.

National Center for Education Statistics. (2006). The health literacy of America's adults: Results from the 2003 National Assessment of Adult Literacy. Retrieved November 15, 2008, from http://nces.ed.gov/pubs2006/2006483.pdf

National Center for Health Statistics. (2008). *Fast Stats.* Retrieved September 8, 2009, from http://www.cdc.gov/nchs/fastats/uinsure.htm

National Institute for Literacy. (2008). Literary Information and Communication System [LINCS]. Retrieved November 30, 2008, from http://www.nifl.gov/lincs/

National Patient Safety Foundation. (2008). Ask me three. Retrieved November 30, 2008, from http://www.npsf.org/askme3/PCHC/

National Youth Tobacco Survey. (2004). Retrieved September 6, 2009, from http://www.cdc.gov/mmwr/preview/mmwrhtml/mm5412a1.htm

Oxman, A., Sackett, D., & Guyatt, G. (1992). Evidence-based medicine workgroup. *Journal of the American Medical Association, 268*(9), 1135–1136.

Paasche-Orlow, M. S., & Wolf, M. (2007). The causal pathways linking health literacy to health outcomes. *American Journal of Health Behavior, 31*(Suppl 1), S19–S26.

Pfizer Clear Health Communication Initiative. (2008). Help your patients succeed: Tips for improving communication with your patients. Retrieved November 30, 2008, from http://clearhealthcommunication.com/public-health-professionals/tips-for-providers.html

Schillinger, D., Grumbach, K., Piette, J., Wang, F., Osmond, D., Daher, C., et al. (2002). Association of health literacy with diabetes outcomes. *Journal of the American Medical Association, 288*(4), 475–482.

Serra, C., Bonfill, X., Pladevall-Vila, M., & Cabezas Pena, C. (2008). Interventions for preventing tobacco smoking in public places. *Cochrane Database of Systematic Reviews* (3), CD001294.

Shohet, L., & Renaud, L. (2006). Critical analysis on best practices in health literacy. *Canadian Journal of Public Health, 97*, S10.

Singleton, J., Levin, R. F., Feldman, H. R., & Truglio-Londrigan, M. (2005). Evidence for smoking cessation: Implications for gender-specific strategies. *Worldviews on Evidence-Based Nursing, 2*(2), 1–12.

Singleton, J. K., Levin, R. F., & Keefer, J. (2007). Evidence-based practice. Disciplinary perspectives on evidence-based practice: The more the merrier. *Research and Theory in Nursing Practice, 21*(4), 213–216.

Sowden, A. J. (1998). Mass media interventions for preventing smoking in young people. *Cochrane Database of Systematic Reviews,* (4), CD001006.

Stead, L. F., & Lancaster, T., (2005). Interventions for preventing tobacco sales to minors. *Cochrane Database of Systematic Reviews,* (1), CD001497.

Stetler, C. B., Morsi, D., Rucki, S., Broughton, S., Corrigan, B., Fitzgerald, J., et al. (1998). Utilization-focused integrative reviews in a nursing service. *Applied Nursing Research, 11*(4), 195–205.

Straus, S. E., Richardson, W. S., Glasziou, P., & Haynes, R. B. (2005). *Evidence-based medicine: How to practice and teach EBM* (3rd ed.). Edinburgh: Elsevier.

Substance Abuse and Mental Health Services Administration. (2005). *Results from the 2005 National Survey on Drug Use and Health.* Rockville, MD: Office of Applied Studies.

Substance Abuse and Mental Health Services Administration. (2007). *Results from the 2006 National Survey on Drug Use and Health: National findings.* Rockville, MD: Office of Applied Studies.

Sum, A., Kirsch, I., & Yamamoto, K. (2004). *A human capital concern: The literacy proficiency of U.S. immigrants.* Princeton, NJ: Education Testing Service.

Thomas, R. E., Baker, P. R. A., & Lorenzetti, D. (2007). Family-based programmes for preventing smoking by children and adolescents. *Cochrane Database of Systematic Reviews,* (1), CD004493.

Thomas, R., & Perera, R. (2006). School-based programmes for preventing smoking. *Cochrane Database of Systematic Reviews, 19,* 3.

U.S. Department of Health and Human Services, Centers for Disease Control and Prevention, National Center for Chronic Disease Prevention and Health Promotion, Office on Smoking and Health. (2000). *Healthy People 2010.* Conference Edition, in two volumes. Washington, DC: U.S. Government Printing Office.

U.S. Department of Health and Human Services. (2006). *The health consequences of involuntary exposure to tobacco smoke: A report of the Surgeon General.* Atlanta, GA: U.S. Department of Health and Human Services, Centers for Disease Control and Prevention, Coordinating Center for Health Promotion, National Center for Chronic Disease Prevention and Health Promotion, Office on Smoking and Health.

Vernon, J. A., Trujillo, A., Rosenbaum, S., & DeBuono, B. (2007). Low health literacy: Implications for national health policy. Partnership for Clear Health Communication. Retrieved November 24, 2008, from http://npsf.org/askme3/pdfs/Case_Report_10_07.pdf

Volandes, A., Paasche-Orlow, M., Gillick, M. R., Cook, E. F., Shaykevich, S., Abbo, E. D., et al. (2008). Health literacy not race predicts end-of-life care preferences. *Palliative Medicine, 11*(5), 754–762.

Weiss, B. D., Mays, M. Z., Martz, W., Castro, K. M., DeWalt, D. A., Pignone, M. P., et al. (2005). Quick assessment of literacy in primary care: The newest vital sign. *Annals of Family Medicine, 3,* 514–522.

Zhu, S. H., Sun, J., Billings, S. C., Choi, W. S., & Malarcher, A. (1999). Predictors of smoking cessation in U.S. adolescents. *American Journal of Preventive Medicine, 16,* 202–207.

CHAPTER 6

APPLYING TECHNOLOGY IN PUBLIC HEALTH NURSING

MARTHA KELLY

SANDRA B. LEWENSON

MARIE TRUGLIO-LONDRIGAN

How impossible to portray with any justice to the subject the superb panorama of the progress of human betterment under the leadership of science through successive generations of ardent devotees blazing ever new trails, evolving ever new methods, achieving ever more outstanding results, facing ever new problems . . . (Goodrich, 1931, p. 1385).

LEARNING OBJECTIVES

At the completion of this chapter, the reader will be able to

- Define the terms used in informatics.

- Describe the application of information technology in public health nursing practice.
- Discuss the use of nursing informatics in public health nursing.

KEY TERMS

- Data
- Database
- Data mining
- Informatics
- Information

- Information technology
- Knowledge
- Nursing informatics
- Public health informatics
- Wisdom

Using technology is essential to public health and, specifically, to public health nursing. Information systems play an important role in the public health arena where accurate and up-to-date information is needed. Historically, data collection has always been one of the hallmarks of public health. Florence Nightingale spoke to the need for accurate statistics about morbidity and mortality using pie graphs and the like to demonstrate the necessity for quality nursing care (Agnew, 1958). Ozbolt and Saba (2008) recognized Nightingale's quest for this kind of data, saying,

"Nightingale called for standardized clinical records that could be analyzed to assess and improve care processes and patient outcomes. Nursing informatics thus springs from the roots of modern nursing" (p. 199). Lillian Wald, the noted public health nursing pioneer and founder of Henry Street, compared and contrasted the data collected by the Henry Street Settlement House visiting nurses with data from four New York City hospitals. Using these data Wald (1915) showed that care provided in the home improved patient outcomes. Nightingale and Wald valued statistical data. They collected and analyzed the data from their clinical experiences, all without the use and speed that information technology and other forms of technology can now provide public health nurses.

This chapter highlights the use of technology as a competency that must be achieved by all practitioners (U.S. Department of Health and Human Services [DHHS], 2004). Like all nursing professionals, public health nurses need to have a basic understanding of technology and how to put that technology to use. Skiba (2008) wrote that "informatics tools can help mitigate error, provide interdisciplinary communication, promote quality, support clinical decision making, and provide the necessary infrastructure for evidenced-based practice" (p. 301). Although not specifically focused on public health nursing curricular activities, Skiba supports the case that students need to understand and use **informatics** in all healthcare settings. Skiba echoes the American Nurses Association (ANA, 2008) statement that "the evolving mandate for electronic information systems and increasing complexity of health care services and practice have raised the bar for the nursing professional. Select informatics competencies will soon be required in all undergraduate and graduate nursing curricula" (p. 17). Public health nurses must know how to use computers and information technology as well as incorporate newer online learning technology (U.S. DHHS, 2004) into their practice.

This chapter examines the various aspects of technology and its use in public health nursing. Throughout the chapter vignettes from nurses who work with the public's health in mind reveal how information technology is being used, or not, in the practice setting. Their stories show the advances that have been made as well as the issues related to the diffusion of new ideas into practice (Rogers, 1983). These vignettes serve as a conduit where the true experts, those individuals working with populations in a variety of settings, tell us how they integrate information technology in the care they render. The future directions of nursing information technology for public health nursing provide the reader with additional reflections on the current status and strategies to move into the future.

ROLE OF TECHNOLOGY IN PUBLIC HEALTH NURSING PRACTICE

The need for information systems and the technology to support that need is transforming public health nursing practice. Public health nurses work in health departments, clinics, visiting nurse services, ambulatory care settings, and anywhere that nursing takes place in the community. Their work emphasizes "population-focused services" (ANA, 2007, p. 11). Technology affords these nurses and society a better way of systematically collecting data, analyzing those data, and then applying the data analysis in a way that informs practice and improves the health of the individual, family, population, and community.

Public health nurses have always collected data on their patients, like Lillian Wald at the Henry Street Settlement in New York City. These nurses collected data to assess the health of the patients and families they served in the community (Buhler-Wilkerson, 2001). In 1914, two years after the formation of the National Organization for Public Health Nursing, the Executive Secretary, Ella

Phillips Crandall (1914), wrote a letter to the philanthropist, John D. Rockefeller, explaining the success that the organization had accomplished by developing a "standardization of record cards" (n.p.). With the adoption of these record cards nationally, Crandall believed public health nurses could collect data in a way that would make previously "incoherent statistics" more "homogenous or at least comparable" (n.p.).

Public health nurses knew that records needed to be kept and somehow the statistical data needed to be collected in a way that made them useful and comparable. In 1950 Freeman wrote that "nursing will be carried on within the framework of a comprehensive program for public health" and this included maintaining "vital statistics, or the recording, tabulation, interpretation, and publication of the essential facts of births, deaths, and reportable diseases" (Freeman, 1950, p. 20). In today's world information technology assists the public health nurse to systematically collect, organize, and analyze data as well as share it with stakeholders as they have done in the past. Now technology allows the collection and analysis to occur at a faster and more comprehensive level than ever before. Furthermore, technology affords us a way to save data and analyze large data sets that provide the needed evidence to support changes in practice. The transformative nature of technology continues this year and into the future.

In today's healthcare arena public health nurses must ask how technology can be used to

- Provide care
- Access information to monitor the health of the public

- Identify best evidence for practice
- Enhance education for the individual, family, population, and community
- Improve public health nursing
- Communicate to others in health care
- Support research

The answers to these questions will serve to enhance the public health nurses' practice in education, research, and the delivery of care.

INFORMATION TECHNOLOGY

It is important for the reader to understand the concepts and terms used in **information technology** as they are applied to public health practice and public health nursing. This understanding is critical as public health nurses work toward better communication, integration, and application of information technology. Vignettes throughout this section and the chapter illustrate the technology that nurses use in their practice and how it informs practice, provides solutions, and creates challenges.

Data

Data are considered the "essential element of information" containing the "measurements and facts" (Institute of Medicine [IOM], 2003a, p. 126) that public health nurses need to make decisions in practice. According to Thede (2003), data are defined as "discrete elements that have not been interpreted . . ." (p. 11). The ANA (2008) uses similar language explaining that "data are discrete entities that are described objectively without interpretation" (p. 3). For example, a newly diagnosed case of tuberculosis in a small town is considered data and is reported to the local county department of health, which then reports this case to the state department of health. This newly diagnosed case of tuberculosis singularly is considered data and is entered into a database. Certain other diseases may also be reported to the Centers for Disease Control and Prevention (CDC) and to the World Health Organization. These data once reported are also entered into a database.

There are many sources of data, some of which include mortality reports, vital statistics, morbidity data, and hospital data such as falls, length of stay, wounds, injuries, and occupational illnesses. Once data are reported and located in a database, analysis may be carried out. Often, the amount of data may be so overwhelming that the message the data would ordinarily convey is overlooked. It is only when the data are reported and placed into a database that patterns emerge to inform the practitioner as to what the best practice interventions may be.

Databases

Databases are systems or structures that allow for data to be stored in an organized way and support access and retrieval (Hebda, Czar, & Mascara, 2005). For example, in a database that maintains surveillance data, such as epidemic reporting, the database holds those data for use by public health nurses. The ANA (2008) explains that data become information after they are "interpreted, organized, or structured" (p. 3). The various database systems help to organize data so they can become information and eventually knowledge. The data may be accessed and shared but may be different for each user depending on who retrieves

the information and how they interpret it. Public health nurses who note an increase in mumps, a nationally reportable disease, may see the need to develop a health education program for young families if an outbreak were to occur in their community. Immunization programs may be another intervention to consider, and yet who interprets the data, such as a private practitioner or an outpatient clinic, may direct the kind of immunization program developed. It is therefore important that the public health nurse know the different types of databases available to them, how to find databases, and how to use the statistics and other vital information for their practice at the local, state, and national level. **Box 6-1** provides some examples of the types of databases that are available for the public health nurse.

Creating a Database

Public health nurses need to be comfortable enough with information technology to develop appropriate databases for their nursing practice when needed. In the vignette on page 143, the nurse recognizes a need to collect and organize data to better assess and serve the population of interest. The nurse recognizes an opportunity to use technology from a nursing informatics perspective. Marisa Cortese-Peske, a nurse researcher, noted that the Hispanic population in the community was being overlooked in a clinical trial. Based on a concern for culturally competent and congruent care, Cortese-Peske collected data on the population of interest and initiated a database to understand patterns and trends within this population.

Using Databases for Tracking

The process of monitoring or tracking the data is critical for public health nurses to

BOX **6-1** Examples of Databases

Federal Government and Health Statistics Agencies

These are federal agencies that gather, analyze, and report statistical data:

Agency for Healthcare Research and Quality (AHRQ): http://www.ahrq.gov

AHRQ is the lead scientific research federal agency charged with supporting research to improve quality of health care, reduce cost, improve patient safety, decrease medical errors, and broaden access to services.

Centers for Disease Control and Prevention (CDC)

Behavioral Risk Factor Surveillance System (BRFSS): http://www.cdc.gov/brfss/

BRFSS tracks health risks of adults in the United States.

National Notifiable Disease Surveillance System (NNDSS): http://www.cdc.gov/epo/dphsi/nndsshis.htm

State health departments report notifiable infectious diseases to the CDC.

National Vital Statistics System: http://www.cdc.gov/nchs/nvss.htm

Information from states on vital events such as births, deaths, marriages, divorces, and fetal deaths

State and Local Data Sources

Many states have their own systems for reporting data; the following are some examples:

Arizona Public Health Services: http://www.hs.state.az.us/plan/index.htm

California Department of Health Services: http://www.dhs.ca.gov/

International Data

United Nations Statistics Division: http://unstats.un.org/unsd/

World Health Organization-Statistical Information Systems (WHOSIS): http://www3.who.int/whois/menu.cfm

Hospital and Healthcare Records

National Hospital Discharge and Ambulatory Surgery Data: http://cdc.gov/nchs/about/major/hdasd/listpubs.htm

Mortality and Morbidity Data

Mortality Data from the National Vital Statistics System: http://www.cdc.gov/nchs/about/major/dvs/mortdata.htm

Pubic Health Preparedness

Bioterrorism and Emerging Infections Site: http://www.bioterrorism-uab.ahrq.gov/

Source: Adapted from National Network of Libraries of Medicine and National Library of Medicine (2005).

Case Study

Vignette From a Nurse Researcher
Marisa A. Cortese-Peske, RN, MS, PNP

As per Healthy People 2010 the cancer rates among Hispanics and African Americans are much higher than those of the non-Hispanic white population. This disparity may be due to many factors such as access to care, education, and genetic make-up. Healthy People 2010 describes three steps in decreasing cancer death rates. The first step is providing culturally and linguistically appropriate information for prevention, early detection, and treatment of cancer. The second step is to provide state-of-the-art services such as radiological scans and cutting edge treatments for detecting and treating cancer. The third step is encouraging clients to participate in clinical research. Clinical research is necessary to obtain important information on preventing and effectively treating cancer (U.S. DHHS, 2000).

I serve as the director of the cancer clinical trials office at a metropolitan teaching hospital in New York City. Our office offers a variety of clinical trials in both solid tumor and hematological malignancies. In the past most clinical trials were chosen by an investigator's disease interest. Many times the investigator would not look into the population of clients that were seen or the eligibility criteria needed to enroll a patient into a study. Most clients enrolled into a clinical trial were from white, middle class backgrounds. In the past year, however, there has been a dramatic movement to enroll more clients from different cultures. This may be due in part to the fact that this hospital is applying for a National Cancer Institute designation that requires more clinical trials on populations with health disparities.

During my practice at this hospital, I have noticed many barriers in conducting clinical research properly to represent all client populations. The first barrier is actually finding clients who are eligible to participate in a clinical trial. Many of the lower socioeconomic clients are seen in a separate Medicaid clinic. Most investigators do not see the clients in this clinic because the clients are followed by the fellows. Even though the fellows do have intentions of enrolling these clients in the clinical trial, there seems to be a disconnect. I have met with clients in the clinic, and it is difficult to convince them to enroll in a clinical trial when I am not the primary provider for their care. Another problem is the language barrier. Not only am I not fluent in Spanish, but many of the investigators are not fluent in Spanish either. This creates a problem to properly explain the risks and benefits of a clinical trial. In addition, the informed consent forms are available only in English. Based on this failure to properly communicate, I believe that clients have a sense of distrust and decline to participate in a clinical trial.

At this hospital I have begun my own health initiative in expanding the number of Hispanic clients currently enrolled in clinical trials. My first step was to create a client database to capture all cancer clients that are seen at this hospital, including a diagnosis, age, ethnicity, and prior treatments. This database went into use in January 2008, and it has already helped to identify groups of clients by disease or ethnicity.

With this database it was identified that many clients at this hospital are diagnosed with HIV-related lymphoma. In the past, however, it was never recognized exactly how many of these clients are seen at this hospital with this diagnosis.

I also realized there are numerous clients diagnosed with hepatocellular carcinoma due to hepatitis C. However, we do not have a clinical investigator at this hospital who specializes in this disease. I have expressed my concern with the director of the cancer institute, and we are currently conducting a search for a hepatocellular carcinoma specialist.

After a complete analysis of my client database, I realized that only 13% of the clients enrolled in an oncology clinical trial in 2007 were Hispanic. Hispanics account, however, for 49% of the population in the catchment area of this hospital. Whereas this disparity seems shocking, I previously recognized that many Hispanic clients who I have tried to enroll did not feel comfortable signing up for a study when they did not understand the risks and benefits of participation. I discussed this issue with the director of the cancer institute. I explained that one reason why Hispanic clients were refusing participation in a clinical trial was because they could not understand the informed consent form because it is available only in English. After months of debate I finally received the funding to translate all informed consents into Spanish. So far I have currently translated three consent forms. As a direct result accrual numbers in the Hispanic population have increased.

With an increase in the number of Hispanic clients enrolling in clinical trials, I believe it will help to understand the physiological and/or genetic factors that cause the higher incidence of certain cancers in the Hispanic population. This information hopefully will lead to finding better treatments and preventive medicine for this population. The development of a database enabled our hospital to be more successful in this attempt.

---

be able to see trends and at the same time note the implication of these trends. The tracking of data provides important evidence for the public health nurse to support decision making and effective planning. For example, public health nurses track Lyme disease and may note an increase in a particular county. The data initially alert the public health nurse to ask critical questions. Once the proper assessment is conducted to answer these questions and the cause of the increase in the diagnosis of Lyme disease made, appropriate interventions are planned and implemented followed by evaluation. The public health nurse continues to track and monitor the Lyme disease in the county to determine if their planned intervention was effective.

The vignette on the next page describes one nurse's experience in a home care setting that uses technology to track clients' healthcare information. In addition, the vignette shows how data tracking can be used in billing, communication, and education.

Data Mining

Another important application of technology and nursing informatics for practice is **data mining**. In 1849 the gold rush in California brought people from all over the world to small towns in northern California, like Grass Valley. The gold mine established in Grass Valley is open to visitors today. Tourists can see how the various veins of gold were identified and then extracted from the earth to create wealth and improve lives. Likewise, the rich veins of data stored in databases can be extracted to show relationships and patterns to help us develop new information and knowledge. The data collected

Case Study

Vignette of a Home Care Nurse
Irene S. Rempel, BS, RN, LMSW

Home care is using computers and informatics more and more. Our intake department is able to obtain patient referral via direct telephone referrals, faxes, and two computerized systems, "Eason" and "E-discharge." Both systems are expensive but frequently used as a referral source in home care.

Patient referrals are initiated at local hospitals. Patients in need of home care are identified on either system, including their admitting diagnosis, chief complaint, demographics, insurance, medications, diagnosis, any type of procedure the patient might have had while in the hospital, physician's name, license number, National Provider Information number, and a physician's order for home care. Those orders differ from patient to patient. Some may require specific wound care. Others need diabetic teaching and intervention.

Home care companies interested in servicing a particular client make a check mark next to the patient's name and wait for confirmation from the social worker staff. Meanwhile, social workers review all companies interested in taking care of a particular patient and then make their decision which company they believe would take the best care of the patient. Once the decision is made, the social worker confirms electronically and provides a patient discharge date for a particular healthcare agency that has been authorized to provide care.

Once the company is approved to provide specific patient care, a registered nurse is sent out to assess the patient, his or her environment, and provide care authorized by the primary medical doctor. When making the initial assessment, the nurse always has his or her laptop provided by the agency. The company I work for uses a system called "McKesson." It is a detailed software application that covers all aspects of certified home health agency services. It generates patient information, plan of care, doctors' orders, and specific instructions for each discipline professionally involved in patient care. Our computer system provides medical and billing codes for different diagnoses and serves as a communication tool among providers. When our patients are prescribed more than one medication at the same time, McKesson identifies whether these medications are compatible or not. Frequently, our software identifies adverse effects and provides educational information for our patients regarding food and drug interactions as well.

Once the nurse assesses the patient in his or her own home, information is logged into our software that is specific to initial assessment, revisit forms, and discharge. If the nurse finds the information originally transmitted from the hospital differs in any way from his or her assessment, the doctor is contacted and a change of order is completed on a separate form and transmitted to the doctor and the agency for approval. Every revisit made by the nurse is recorded and transmitted to the doctor and the agency. Our system is able to generate a patient's plan of care, addendum to plan of care, and change of care. Those forms are required by the department of health and patients' insurance providers for review of medical necessity for home care, services provided, and payment to the home care agency.

Computers assist communications among all team members involved in patient care. If my patient is receiving the services of a registered nurse, physical therapist, occupational therapist, social worker, dietitian, and home health aide services, the patient's progress can be analyzed and inter-disciplinary conferences made without members of the team physically being in the office. Computer access has made patient information, treatment, and follow-up considerably easier than in the past. Members are communicating with each other and the doctor without leaving their offices.

---

through surveillance processes and then collected and stored can be "mined," just as the veins of gold were mined, for any number of purposes to enhance and enrich lives in the public sphere. Data mining looks for patterns and relationships from large aggregate data sources. Data, however, have to be considered "clean" enough to be mined. Gold, when it was extracted, went through a chemical process to obtain the pure gold. The process used to clean data in preparation for effective data mining consists of "scrubbing" the data for errors that have the potential to skew any relationships or patterns. Cleansing the data, as it is called, means looking at the data for inconsistencies such as typographical errors, misspelled words, and multiple names for similar terms (e.g., "SOB" could mean "short of breath" or some other term). Abbreviations vary from institution to institution, and this can skew the data, making them difficult to use. Software packages exist to help scrub the data and remove the inconsistencies (Hebda et al., 2005).

McGonigle and Mastrian (2009) state that data mining "helps to identify patterns in aggregate data, gain insights, and ultimately discover and generate knowledge applicable to nursing science" (p. 148). Thede (2003) explains data mining as "the automated processes that permit the conversion of data to information and knowledge by finding hidden relationships within data" (p. 277). The use of data min-

ing is a key concept in nursing informatics that has relevance to public health nursing. The challenge for nursing is to continue to refine and develop a standardized language that will enable data to be coded in like formats. The data then may be later mined for patterns and relationships.

Information, Knowledge, and Wisdom

The practice of public health nursing can be viewed from the nursing informatics perspective of data, information, knowledge, and wisdom (ANA, 2008). Three areas of information science that IOM (2003a) identify include "data, information, and knowledge" (p. 126). Data become information as they are organized and "placed in context" in information systems (IOM, 2003a, p. 126). The IOM (2003a) explains that information and information systems are essential tools that public health agencies need to monitor a population's health status and identify health hazards and risks. The information gained from these systems helps the public health nurse provide evidenced-based care to the individual, family, population, or community they serve.

Information is defined as "data that are interpreted, organized, or structured" (ANA, 2008, p. 3). **Knowledge** is information that has been "synthesized so that relationships are identified and formalized" (ANA, 2008, p. 3). Information enhances knowledge and guides decision making. The ANA (2008) further explains that **wisdom** is the "appropriate use of knowledge to manage and solve human problems" (p. 5). Understanding how and when to apply knowledge to make appropriate decisions is relevant to the work of public health nurses. Information technology affords public health nurses a way of making informed decisions and evaluating them to support the work they do in the community. The vignette by Cortes-Peske, above, provides an example of how information technology creates opportunities to use data that are more inclusive of populations in the community. By using the data and knowledge to gain wisdom, public health nurses are able to understand the important influence technology plays in providing culturally competent, evidenced-based health care.

Figure 6-1 provides a visual depiction of the transformation of data, information, knowledge, wisdom, and evaluations leading to the potential for new knowledge formation. Data, information, and knowledge lead to wisdom. This data collection takes place within a context, such as a system, and can then be reviewed, organized, and synthesized to support the work of public health nurses.

For public health nurses to practice effectively and efficiently, the public health infrastructure must be designed so that the system seamlessly facilitates information input, storage, access, and management. The public health care system in the United States is a complex one, and the amount and types of information necessary for practice are staggering. The types of information systems necessary

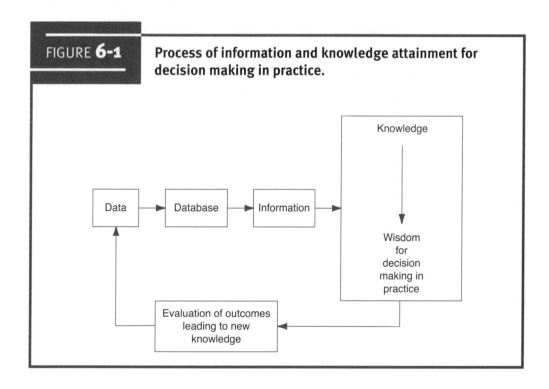

FIGURE **6-1**   **Process of information and knowledge attainment for decision making in practice.**

to facilitate the health of the public, therefore, are numerous, and each of these systems must "speak to each other." According to Thede (2003), "in a well designed system, there is an interface or an exchange of information, between systems to support the sharing of data so that the data do not have to be reentered" (p. 224).

An example of such a system is the National Environmental Public Health Tracking Program. According to the CDC (2008), a lack of information needed to document links between environmental hazards and chronic disease exists. Air and water pollution are considered by the CDC (2008) as the two "most common environmental hazards" (p. 4) and "asthma, cancer, and lead poisoning . . . the most frequent adverse health effects" (p. 4). A tracking system that links these environmental hazards and chronic diseases provides a valuable tool for all public health workers and specifically for public health nurses. This facilitates an easier identification of the environmental causes of chronic illness. The National Environmental Public Health Tracking Program, developed by the CDC, is an attempt to address this issue with the start of this system. The national system tracks environmental hazards and the diseases they cause, updating traditional medical detective work with "computers, satellites, and geographic information systems" (CDC, 2008, p. 10). This system connects data sources, provides the tools to make sense of them, and makes that crucial information available to those who need it. In addition, the CDC has been working to develop the National Environmental

Public Health Tracking Network. The CDC hopes this network

> [W]ill promote information system standards to integrate local, state, and national databases of environmental hazards, environmental exposures, and health effects, will be a crucial component of the National Environmental Public Health Tracking Program. With the help of the National Environmental Public Health Tracking Network, scientists, communities, policymakers, and the public soon will have access to the information they need to make good decisions about preventing disease, keeping the American public healthy, and saving lives. (2008, p. 5)

INFORMATION TECHNOLOGY IN PUBLIC HEALTH NURSING

In 2001, as a result of a national crisis, it became known to the public and those responsible for policy that the public health infrastructure was lacking in a number of areas. One of those areas was the country's public health infrastructure with regard to technology and information systems (IOM, 2003a, 2003b). Since that time public health technology and information systems have been an evolving area. Three core functions of public health, assessment, policy development, and assurance, depend on information and access to that information (IOM, 1988). Public health informatics supports this goal (IOM, 2003b).

Public health informatics is defined as the "systematic application of information, computer science, and technology to public health practice and learning" (IOM, 2003b, p. 63). The IOM (2003b) document builds on the work of Yasnoff, O'Carroll, Koo, Linkins, and Kilbourne (2000) where the scope of public health informatics "includes the conceptualization, design, development, deployment, refinement, maintenance and evaluation of communication, surveillance, and information systems relevant to public health" (p. 68). Friede, Blum, and McDonald (1995) define public health informatics as follows:

[A]pplication of information science and technology to public health practice and research. Specifically, this means developing innovative ways to use inexpensive and powerful computers, online databases, the capacity for universal connection of people and computers, and multimedia communications to support the mission of disease prevention and health promotion. (p. 240)

The Association of Community Health Nursing Educators also defines public health informatics as the "systematic application of information, computer science, and technology to public practice" (Levin et al., 2007, p. 13).

In 2008 the ANA revised its standards and practice for **nursing informatics**, building on its earlier definition of nursing informatics to include the term "wisdom." The ANA (2008) defines nursing informatics as the "integration of nursing science, computer science, and information science to manage and communicate data, information, knowledge, and wisdom in nursing practice" (p. 1). The goal of nursing informatics is to "improve the health of populations, communities,

families, and individuals by optimizing information management and communication" (ANA, 2008, p. 1). Informatics in public health nursing includes "the conceptualization, design, development, refinement, maintenance, and evaluation of communication, surveillance and information systems relevant to public health" (Levin et al., 2007, p. 13).

Public health nursing practice uses technology to do more than just outreach and screening. It now encompasses areas such as consumer health, tele-health, cyberhealth, and e-health. The use of Internet blogs and podcasts also impacts the practice of public health nursing. Technology enhances the design, conduct, and dissemination of research studies (Bakken, Stone, & Larson, 2008). It also plays a critical role in developing sustainable public health infrastructures (IOM, 2003b). For example, in the area of surveillance systems, one of the intervention strategies of the Minnesota Department of Health Population-Based Public Health Nursing Practice Intervention Wheel, the need for technology, is noted in the following citation:

Improved surveillance systems are likely to tax the public health system's capacity to process the growing quantity of health data required for public health improvement. Progressively, state and local governments are collecting and disseminating health status data at greater levels of detail, the number of reportable diseases is enlarging, and new developments in electronic laboratory reporting systems and electronic medical records systems will also increase the volume of data available to the public health system. Informatics methods and applications, such as decision supports and expert systems, modeling and simulation techniques, can help public health face this challenge by providing increased capacity to handle, analyze, and act on data that is likely to increase during the coming years. (IOM, 2003b, pp. 63–64)

Other areas such as health promotion, disease prevention, and consumer health informatics are noted as having potential beneficial effects with the infusion of public health informatics (IOM, 2003b). In addition, evidence-based practice and the development of online educational programs for the public and public health nurses serve to promote an effective and efficient public health system.

Access and Adaptability

Not only is the use of technology critical for public health nurses, but the population's ability to access information via technology is equally important. The possibility of a "digital disparity" is an issue that must be addressed. Digital disparity refers to whether or not an individual has access to information technology. This means that people who do not have access to technology for any number of social, political, or economic reasons may experience greater healthcare risks than those who do have access (Cronin, 2002). Access to technology by the public health nurse as well as the public becomes an essential part of the quality health care that can be provided. Later vignettes in this chapter demonstrate the importance of access to technology.

People, however, are not always ready to accept new technology, even if the technology is available to them. Rogers (1983) describes how innovations are accepted at varying speeds based on how people perceive the innovation. Some people embrace change and technology in nursing practice resonates with them, whereas others take a longer time to accept change (Thede, 2003). Five perceived attributes influence the speed in which an idea, like the use of computers in home care or a new information system that requires training, is accepted. Rogers (1983) identifies these five attributes as relative advantage of service, compatibility, complexity, trialability, and observability. The first attribute, relative advantage, refers to the idea that the adopter (in this instance, the public health nurse) perceives that the proposed innovation, such as using a computerized scheduling system, is better than the way previous scheduling was done. The greater the understanding of the relative advantage of the innovation, the more likely the public health nurse will quickly adopt the innovative method proposed. Second, how the public health nurse connects with or values the new system, defined as compatibility, also influences the rate of acceptance of an innovative measure. Third, If public health nurses do not understand the use of technology in the work they do (i.e., complexity), they are less likely to accept the new innovation. Fourth, the ability to test a new product (i.e., trialability), like the use of laptops in the home or a personal digital assistant (PDA) in the field, will aid in the acceptability. And, fifth, observability occurs when, for example, the public health nurse can easily recognize how the technology adds value to his or her work and thus the innovation is more likely to be adopted and adopted earlier rather than later.

The public health workforce, of which nursing is a critical member, must be educated to ensure the healthcare needs of the population. Knowledge of informatics along with epidemiology, biostatistics, environmental health, health services administration, social and behavioral sciences, informatics, genomics, communication, cultural competence, community-based participatory research, global health, policy and law, and public health ethics, are essential for all public healthcare workers (IOM, 2003b). Although all these areas are important, informatics and its use in public health nursing stands out. Informatics initiatives that will redesign the public health system are critical, and public health nurses must be ready and competent not only in their understanding of these systems but in their early adaptation and application to ensure the health of the public.

The next two vignettes presented below provide two examples of how innovative information technology has the potential to improve practice. Both show how some people more readily accept innovations in practice than others.

Case Study

Adapting a Computerized Scheduling System
Martha Kelly, EdD, RN

My introduction into the world of nursing informatics started with the implementation of a computerized scheduling system in a large medical center in 1980. Very few hospitals had a computerized scheduling system at that time. From an informatics standpoint, the software package purchased allowed us to use our current staffing patterns; however, the concept of taking the control away from the role of the head nurse was a major paradigm shift. Until that time nurses did not typically have control of their unit's budget and subsequently used the time sheets as part of their reward system. The real issue was how to show nurses they still retained the decision-making portion of the schedule. The computerized system generated the first draft of the schedule, but the final decision was made by the head nurse who knew the staff and what the staffing mix should be for the unit to run well.

During this period I attended what was the first national nursing conference engaged in computer technology, entitled "Computer Technology and Nursing," that was hosted by the Clinical Center at the National Institutes of Health and held in Bethesda, Maryland. Many of the speakers at that conference addressed what we see today. Computerized patient records and computerized care plans were discussed at the conference. To my chagrin some of those in attendance seemed quite resistant to these new computer applications for nursing. For example, some were not supportive and others were critical of the concept of computerized care plans. Although the speakers were innovative, there was reluctance for early adaption on the part of some in the audience. Their reluctance was most likely reflective of this new field and the role of nursing informatics that was still being carved out. It was a time when there were mainframes but few desktop computers in a clinical setting. Even as a novice informatics nurse, it was clear that a merger of computer technology and nursing would soon come together.

In the next vignette, Carole Baraldi explains some of the challenges nurses face in home care settings. Technological equipment can be cumbersome, as is the collection of data. For technology to be supported by the very people who use it and benefit from it, adaptation to various settings may be required. Rural settings versus urban environments create different challenges for nurses using technology.

Connections

Information technology is used in a variety of settings, including hospitals, private practices, voluntary visiting nurse services, and municipal health departments. Currently, many institutions have their own data systems; however, many of the systems do not talk to each other within or between institutions. The lack of inter-

Case Study

Making Technology Work in Home Care
Carole A. Baraldi, MS, RN

I left home care more than 10 years ago, in part because of the implementation of the OASIS Tool, which created additional time on the already laborious paperwork required in home care because computers were not widely used. Furthermore, I was working fee for service for two agencies in New York City, and this additional work greatly impacted my financial profitability.

I decided to make a "career change" and began working in clinical trials for an international pharmaceutical company, which enhanced my computer skills. This year I reentered the home care arena and was introduced to the "tablet." My first impression was the weight of the laptop, which was necessary to ensure an extended life of the battery.

After the orientation I began making home visits with the computer and supplies stored in a luggage bag with wheels. Negotiating the New York City subways with this bag was quite challenging, because the turnstiles and stairs are antiquated and not conducive to travel.

Once in the member's home, the computer was placed on a barrier and secure table, which at times was difficult to locate. The computer frequently would crash, necessitating rebooting, which was frustrating to both me and the member. The focus of the visit was the computer and not the member and his or her environment.

Overall, I was dissatisfied with this experience and subsequently resigned after 3 months of employment. In addition, one of the nurses I met in orientation was asked to leave the agency after 6 months because her computer skills were not up to par. Several months earlier this same nurse had been mentored in the field and praised for her excellent clinical skills.

I am presently working as a consultant for a home care agency, which allows the nurses to decide how information is obtained. They can use the computer in the field or pen and paper, which is later entered into the database by administrative assistants. Information technology is vital to the healthcare industry, but I believe that in home care a certain amount of flexibility in the procurement of same should be offered, particularly with the paucity of experience.

faces and compatibility is related to the inability to share information. The integration of systems is costly but critical for a comprehensive model of care. This is an area where focused attention will be directed to in the coming years. How to develop systems that do interface with each other will be a question to consider.

Through the Internet both the public and public health nurses gain access to a wide range of information, research, and Web sites. This form of communication is "reshaping how information is accessed and shared" (IOM, 2003a, p. 329). The Internet connects individuals to information that was not easily available to them before, if at all. Networking opportunities for both healthcare providers and consumers of health care abound, and the ability to disseminate information at a lower cost than more traditional means adds to the many advantages the Internet presents (IOM, 2003a).

One of the concerns when using the Internet is how one can judge the quality, accuracy, and reliability of the infor-

mation that can be found on the World Wide Web (Thede, 2003). Public health nurses who work with populations must teach individuals to ask critical questions to determine the validity of the information. Thede (2003) suggests three possible ways to help the public determine the quality of a site: look for the Health on the Net Foundation logo, an organization that accredits health-related Web sites, check for the organizational domain (.org), and check for a copyright symbol. The use of the Internet, however, opens up many avenues that will serve public health nurses well. For example, today many home care nurses use the Internet in their practice as they apply home healthcare monitoring or seek out information and knowledge to support their clinical decisions.

In the next vignette, Teresa Haines writes about her work in student health services where Internet access is crucial to her successful decision making. The importance of using accurate and reliable sites for information is demonstrated.

Case Study

Information Technology in Student Health Services
Teresa M. Haines, DNP, RN, FNP-BC

I am a family nurse practitioner and have worked at the Student Health Service at a college in New York City for 11 years. During that time I have seen dramatic change in the use of information technology at my clinical setting.

Ten years ago I purchased my first computer and started down the road toward becoming computer literate. At that time there were no computers in use at the Student Health Service. Gradually, computers were installed for use by the clerical staff to check student status and electronically convey student compliance with New York State vaccination requirements to the Registrar's office. Nurse practitioners were still using textbooks when they needed reference materials for patient care decision making. Next, computers were installed at many clerical workstations around the clinic and could be used by providers to look for online resources in lieu of potentially outdated textbook resources. Most recently, there is a computer installed in the conference room explicitly for provider resource and reference searches.

After a recent typical workday, I thought about how technology was now an integral part of my clinical practice. I saw a patient with hypothyroidism. She had blood tests on a prior visit and was returning for test results and ongoing care. Her thyroid function studies were atypical. After a brief consultation with colleagues, I went immediately to the computer to find references to aid in decision making about a treatment plan for this patient. Access to information gave a speedy resolution to an uncommon problem.

Later in the day I saw a patient who had an upper respiratory tract infection. She was taking an over-the-counter medication with which I was unfamiliar, and I needed to know the active ingredients. Again, consultation with colleagues did not provide the answer I needed to make an appropriate treatment plan for this patient. I looked in an over-the-counter drug reference on the shelf and could not find this particular product information because the product was only recently put on the market. Back at the computer terminal I searched and found, very quickly, the active ingredients of this product. Again, access equaled expedience and an accurate treatment plan.

In addition to my personal utilization of information technology during the workday, the Health Service has plans to grow the information technology at the clinic. A Health Service Web site is available for students to make electronic appointments and access health information. Educational podcasts are being developed and will soon be linked to the Web site to enhance patient education. Computers are planned for each examination room, and electronic medical records are also in the planning stage. Information technology in the community healthcare setting provides an invaluable resource for providers and enhances both quality and efficiency of patient care.

Using Technology to Communicate

Communication for public health is imperative. Information technology, online systems, and Internet opportunities, as well as other electronic information systems, continue to expand the volume and accessibility of information (U.S. DHHS, 2000). The use of the PDA enables one to organize information. Along with the PDA, other wireless devices, like laptop computers, allow the nurse more flexibility and greater access to computers or the network. In addition, the legislative requirements for the Health Insurance Portability and Accountability Act of 1996 (HIPAA) includes a privacy rule to protect patient information. Many HIPAA requirements are designed to allow for the transmissions of electronic health information, including transactions of providers, health insurance plans, and for the safeguarding and security of health data (Thede, 2003).

In any process of communication, evaluative feedback is required so that adjustments may be made. McBride and Detmar (2008) consider the need for nurses to take on a leadership role in transforming care in the community using information systems and communication. They question, however, why informatics is viewed as important for a few rather than for the entire profession. They also question why the building of feedback loops in practice is so slow when it is these feedback loops that are essential for promotion of safety and the advancement of the profession. McBride and Detmar (2008) ask, "Are we afraid that we will be regarded as less professional if we pay more attention to the context of care than to individual care plans?" (p. 195). In other words, if we are looking at individual care and the nursing process, we feel more legitimate. But when we look at nursing informatics, we are looking beyond the individual care and focusing on the environment where that care takes place; therefore this may be perceived as not legitimate.

McBride and Detmar (2008) speak about the need for feedback loops, and technology supports the communication of the data within these loops. Online systems, for example in a health department, organize and collect data about births, deaths, and communicable diseases and then transmit these data to a regional repository and CDC, where other public health nurses or professionals can access these data and use them to support their practice.

A method of communication is demonstrated in the next vignette. Madeline R. Cafiero describes her experiences in home care when pagers were first being introduced as a way of communication. She evaluates the use of pagers, providing the rationale for moving toward this, at the time, innovative use of technology and some of the problems it created.

Case Study

From Coronary Care to Pagers in Home Care
Madeline R. Cafiero, MS, RN, FNP, CWOCN

Transferring to the home care department from the coronary care unit in 1986 was a culture shock. There were no cardiac monitors or automated blood pressure cuffs or arterial lines in home care; just me and my stethoscope. I soon became accustomed to this reliance on my senses and clinical judgment. It took a while to adjust to staying connected to the office while being out all day on the road.

Before each nurse left the home care office each day, the supervisors secured a list of each nurse's scheduled patients numbered in the order they were to be visited. Patients' names were listed in the large block calendars on each nurse's desk and copied onto the supervisor's master schedule for the day. The calendar was the only way the supervisor could contact the nurse if necessary during the day. If something came up, the supervisor or office secretary would call the patient's home and ask for the nurse or leave a message for the nurse to call the office when he or she arrived. With this method, much relied on the patient's memory of the call, the patient's willingness to let the nurse use the phone, and the skill of the office staff to predict what patient to call and when to actually catch the nurse in the minimum number of phone calls.

This system was abandoned when all the nurses received pagers in 1988. No longer dependent on the patients to find the nurse, the office would page the nurse and expect the nurse to call the office back within 15 minutes of the page. This was a lofty goal in our precellular phone days. Once a page was received on the beeper, the nurse might be 20 or 30 miles between patients. In rural areas this meant no return call until the nurse arrived at the patient's home. In urban areas if a pay phone was accessible, the nurse needed to have enough change and be in a safe enough area to park and call the office back. In the early 1990s nurses often avoided pay phones in certain neighborhoods because they were the "property" of the area drug dealers. Sometimes pages were not even received in the hill towns of our area. This caused a return to the old call-and-catch method of locating the nurse.

Pagers were known to go off multiple times during the day and usually after the nurse had gloved for a procedure. The pager would beep incessantly until a button could be pushed to silence it. Although the pager had a very wide clip to secure it, it often fell off onto the patient's driveway or stairwell, necessitating a search and rescue effort of calling the pager to locate it. Some days the pager would beep so often the nurse would place it on silent just to be able to concentrate on the patient. Of course, this meant remembering to check on the beeper afterward and return the pages received.

This system was used until I left the home care agency in 1998. Cell phones were being carried by individual nurses who chose to obtain them on their own, but most nurses continued to carry the pager. It became an essential part of their equipment, much as the cell phone and computer are today.

Applying Technology in Public Health

The next three vignettes are told by nurses who work in home care and research initiatives where a variety of tools, databases, tracking systems, cameras, and computers are used in their work. Each vignette provides a glimpse into how technology can add value to their work and offer a means to communicate and shows an increasing comfort level with the use of technology in practice.

A common tool used to collect data over the past 10 years is the Outcome and Assessment Information Set (OASIS). OASIS "is a group of data elements that: Represent core items of a comprehensive assessment for an adult home care patient; and Form the basis for measuring patient outcomes for purposes of outcome-based quality improvement (OBQI)" (U.S. DHHS, n.d., n.p.).

The collection of outcome data on all home care patients using OASIS is required by the Centers for Medicare & Medicaid Services (Schneider, Barkauskas, & Keenan, 2008). Visiting nurses collect outcome data using computers loaded with OASIS and other systems. They also use various technological tools, like digital photography and the telephone to support their work. They gather data, place them into databases, and gain information, knowledge, and wisdom to make decisions in their practice and then evaluate the outcomes. This continuous process occurs while public health nurses care for the individual, family, community, and population. Although a systematic way of connecting all data that nurses collect may not yet exist, in the next vignette Doreen Gallagher Wall shows how visiting nurses have been using systems like OASIS designed to record data sets in conjunction with other technology such as digital photography to support the work they do.

The vignette on page 158 shows how the use of information technology

Case Study

Using Technology as a Visiting Nurse
Doreen Gallagher Wall, MS, RN, BC

The use of technology in the public health, home care setting has clearly been established in the Visiting Nurse Service setting where I work. Visiting nurses use technology in the provision of care and as a support for decision making. Visiting nurses carry laptop computers where they may document and have access to important data for information and hence be connected in a wireless way. For example, Mr. J. Gomez was admitted to the Visiting Nurse Service in the summer of 2008. Part of the intake process is the gathering of information commonly referred to as OASIS. This intake process can take up to 2 hours. Today, OASIS is fully loaded onto all laptop computers, thereby freeing nurses from being tied to paperwork. In addition, these nurses can now extract data and look for patterns and trends. Other data that are collected include care plans, finger sticks, vital signs, blood pressures, and weights.

Digital photography has also improved management of care. Visiting nurses may take a digital photo of a wound that is then sent to the primary care provider who may view the wound and make decisions about options for treatment. This is also helpful for risk management. For example, if a nurse is conducting an intake assessment and notes an area of impaired skin integrity, he or she may take a digital photograph as evidence that this break in integrity was present before admission.

The TeleHealth program is another form of technology that supports clients to remain in their home. With the use of this technology, the visiting nurse can facilitate the management of a client's care supporting promotion of health and identify problems early, thus preventing acute care admissions or readmissions. For example, Mr. Gomez has a diagnosis of chronic obstructive pulmonary disease and his past history is marked by multiple emergency department visits and admissions. Since Mr. Gomez has been enrolled in the TeleHealth program, these emergency department admissions have declined. The reason for this outcome is that the nurse coordinator is able to monitor critical information on an ongoing basis without making daily home visits. The client is taught how to operate the needed technology and to transmit the objective information, such as vital signs, to the home office where the nurse coordinator monitors the data. In this way the nurse coordinator notes changes quickly in physiological functioning, thus identifying those at risk. When a client is at risk, the nurse and other primary care providers can take charge quickly, alter treatment options, and avert emergencies.

and informatics supports a clinical research initiative where the nurse works. Whether a common language exists, public health nurses and all nurses work in collaborative roles requiring understanding of how technology supports the research process. Lois O. Carnochan provides a look at the use of large data sets, protocols generated by computer, and the need to communicate with other healthcare providers. Public health nurses work with others and need to be able to communicate and collaborate effectively.

Case Study

Using Information Technology in Research
Lois O. Carnochan, MS, RN

I worked on a complex clinical trial/investigation in which the strategies and interventions for participants were hypothesis driven and protocol based. The interventions were for the prevention and control of some of the most common causes of morbidity and mortality among older women. The study was a multicentered, nationwide, clinical trial. It was designed to allow for double-blind, placebo-controlled evaluation of distinct interventions. The central focus in each of the interventions was the overall risk-to-benefit assessment of the participants.

Computerized data-based resources were essential to the conduction of the study and to the ongoing analysis of data, which continues. Strict adherence to the protocol was essential to the validity and reliability of the research. Custom data extracts and user-defined fields were used. Participants were carefully screened according to the protocol standards to be enrolled. The user-defined fields were designed to reject any participant who did not meet the criteria. Similarly, participants were randomized into the study by the computer, allowing for and ensuring that the correct interventions were assigned and that the assignments remained consistent and double blind. Also, all visit-specific tasks were determined when the participant started in the study and the visit tasks were computer generated.

Very careful participant monitoring via custom data extracts were essential to participant safety and protocol adherence. The participant-specific data were easily determined via computer-generated reports. This information further guided nursing assessments and interventions within protocol adherence. For example, nurses were able to assess and use the following clinical information for individuals and participant groups:

- All radiographic and laboratory results requiring follow-up.
- Dispensation of all medication by computerized number was participant specific and ensured that the medication given remained double blind.
- Clinical tasks specific to a particular visit type were computer determined as well as nonroutine visits generated by untoward effects and needing immediate clinical attention.
- User-defined fields were flagged if medications were inconsistent.
- Medication-taking compliance was determined by participant adherence percentage, again computer determined.

This helped to assess if the individual could be enrolled in a medication intervention arm and also if the participant could remain in that arm.

The large database of healthcare information generated had to be protected for privacy and confidentiality. Some examples defined by HIPPA as health information that must be protected are name, Social Security number, medical record number, health plan beneficiary number, vehicle identifiers, and biometric identifiers, including finger and voice prints. Under HIPAA's "safe harbor" standard, a participant is de-identified if all identifiers have been removed and there is no reasonable basis to believe that remaining information could identify a given person. Information released by a clinical trial is done by cohort groups and never given on individuals except to the participant directly and under protocol standards.

All individuals were unblinded at the end of the study and informed of the intervention in which they participated. The unblinding process could be done only by computer query. Again, user-defined fields and custom extracts yielded this information, and it was given to each participant individually to ensure confidentiality and privacy.

In the final vignette Lisa Seiff speaks about the need to introduce technology into practice and shows how she has made a change in the home care agency where she works.

Challenges

Several challenges are before us as we consider the role of technology and public health nursing practice. A few of the most urgent challenges that warrant consideration are as follows:

- Standard language to include nursing as a member of the team and to begin to code it in some way so that there is understanding between and among all professionals.
- Funding on federal, state, and local levels to provide financial support.
- Communication between various information systems and between clinicians and the experts in informatics to help build systems that incorporate and interface systems.
- Education of Public Health Work Force Competencies developed to help educate the workforce. Categories are computer science and electronic communication, online access, data system protection, and so on. The second group of competencies is the development and

maintenance of information systems to improve the effectiveness.
- Readiness of public health nurses to accept innovation and be comfortable with applying and adapting changing technology in practice.

Although all the challenges listed above are important for consideration, the development and use of a standardized language are two of the most pressing needs for the best utilization of technology resources and practice. Standardized language and the power of its potential allow for the ability to aggregate and analyze data so that feedback will happen in a timely manner. Aggregate data can also be used for research, quality improvement, and decision-making support. Vendors need to incorporate the use of standardized language (Ozbolt & Saba, 2008). Ozbolt and Saba (2008) believed in the importance of standardized language. Although not specifically directed to public health nursing practice, their implications for standardized language and practice are clear:

Clinical experts must work with terminology experts to develop computable, semantically interoperable standard language for those practice domains not adequately covered by existing standard languages. Researchers and

Case Study

Introducing Technology as a Home Care Nurse
Lisa Seiff, RN, BSN

I began working for a relatively small home care agency in New York City 6 years ago as an assistant to the Director of Nursing at a time when I was just beginning my baccalaureate nursing education. I realized immediately that the agency remained in the technological stone age, which I knew would be a challenge for a 21-year-old who grew up with computers and technology. Five people staffed the office that ran all operations for the agency, which provided RNs, LPNs, home health aides, personal care aides, and live-ins to people requiring various levels of health care in their homes. Of the five people working in the office, only the receptionist had a computer. The minimal technology used in the office reflected the lack of technology used in the field. The nurses and aides working in patients' homes used only one type of technology—cell phones. All documentation was completed with pen and paper.

Most of my coworkers were older, which I believed at least partially explained the minimal technology being used. I soon began to question the lack of technology, specifically the lack of computers in the office. I was surprised by the receptiveness and openness that my superiors expressed in response to my suggestions. Two additional computers with Internet were quickly added to the office, but I then realized that availability of technology would not solve the problem alone. The office staff in general was averse to dedicating the time necessary to make often time-consuming changes. The agency had been in business for about 20 years, and the Director of Nursing had been there for almost 15 of those years; therefore the attitude was "why change a model that works even if it is outdated?" I worked hard to computerize many of the forms and spreadsheets that were previously in paper format, but I often found it difficult to convince the other workers to use the technology because they had so little time to dedicate to learning the new way. They were all so proficient at doing things the old way on paper that convincing them to take the time to complete a task on the computer that could be completed without it in half or a quarter of the time was challenging.

Once I became a registered nurse and began working for the agency in that capacity, I realized quickly that I needed a way to carry with me patient information and medical reference material. I made the mistake of initially packing my nursing bag not only with the nursing items that I needed but with reference books as well. I soon realized the impracticality of my endeavor after carrying such a heavy bag for only a short period of time. I then understood the need for technology in the field. The Agency agreed to purchase for me a PDA that I could use to store all necessary patient information in addition to medical reference software. I use this PDA every day and during every nursing visit. I use it to access all necessary patient information, including diagnoses, physician information, and medication. The medical software provides me with reference information regarding medications, symptoms, diagnoses, and lab work.

Readiness and motivation to change remain a barrier, but cost is an especially difficult challenge. I sit on the agency's Performance Improvement Committee and thus am privy to conversation and debate about spending for technology. Improved patient quality of care is always a strong argument for improved technology, but where quality of care is not obviously improved by technology, the argument against investing the money remains strong. Home care nurses practice in unfamiliar and unpredictable settings every day, and technology can certainly help nurses working in the community to document faster and to share ideas and information in seconds rather than hours or days, but this comes at a large cost, especially for smaller agencies. Hopefully, with the right motivation and increasing availability of affordable technology, my agency and others can continue to expand on and improve the technology used.

---

developers must discover ways to use computable language and data to support nursing clinical and management decision at the point of need. Nursing records must be integrated with other records to support communication and retrieval of critical information. (Ozbolt, & Saba, 2008, p. 204)

The need to refine the languages for nursing classification systems, such as North American Nursing Diagnosis Association, Nursing Intervention Classifications, Nursing Outcome Classifications, or the Omaha Classification System, runs a parallel course with the need for standardized language and data mining as noted earlier in this chapter. Although beyond the scope of this chapter, the discussion about the need to standardize nursing data through minimum data sets, standardized language, and nursing classification systems is essential for the reader to explore further. Since the late 1950s, nursing leaders began to classify nursing problems. In 1973 the North American Nursing Diagnosis Association began to explore the idea of establishing nursing diagnoses. This led to a movement to examine more closely nursing's need to standardize the terminology that described the work that nurses do. As public health nursing informatics gains momentum, the issues of these standard-

izing features will be crucial to the success of public health nursing interventions.

CONCLUSION

As the reader considers the public health interventions suggested in the intervention wheel, the potential for the use of technology to enhance the process becomes important. Technology, information systems, and the applications for nursing informatics play a significant role in public health nursing to enhance practice and address quality of care issues. Throughout nursing's history data are needed, not just as a repository of information but as a driver for knowledge generation and decision making and as a basis for evidence-based practice.

The vignettes from nurses in the field show how nurses working in home care, visiting nurse associations, research initiatives, and schools already use nursing informatics and technology in their practice. Knowledge of how nursing informatics and technology can inform and transform practice is essential for success. The rate of acceptance of the various tools and instruments may vary. The evolutionary nature of using nursing informatics and technology in practice is woven throughout the vignettes. They show how the use of the electronic medical records, pagers, cell phones, laptops, digital cameras, PDAs, systems that support clinical decision making, bar coding for medications, Internet connections, and the use of TeleHealth activities provide better access and services to their clients. Information technology has the potential to transform education and practice so that nursing care, in whatever public health setting, is delivered effectively, safely, and with the best outcomes (Ozbolt & Saba, 2008). If one considers technology as an essential part of today's social fabric, then the words of the former Dean of the Vanderbilt University's School of Nursing, Shirley C. Titus (1933/1991), resonate with us still:

> Nursing, like every form of life activity, is a part of the warp and woof of the whole social fabric. Nursing cannot be an isolated, separated thing-in-itself; the flow, the interplay of social forces inevitable as day follows the night exerts an effect on nursing and nursing education. (p. 345)

References

Agnew, L. R. C. (1958). Florence Nightingale: Statistician. *American Journal of Nursing, 5*(58), 664–665.

American Nurses Association [ANA]. (2007). *Public health nursing: Scope and standards of practice.* Silver Springs, MD: American Nurses Association.

American Nurses Association [ANA]. (2008). *Nursing informatics: Scope and standards of practice.* Washington, DC: American Nurses Publishing.

Bakken, S., Stone, P. W., & Larson, E. (2008). A nursing informatics research agenda for 2008–18: Contextual influences and key components. *Nursing Outlook, 56*(5), 206–214.

Buhler-Wilkerson, K. (2001). *No place like home: A history of nursing and home care in the United States.* Baltimore: Johns Hopkins University Press.

Centers for Disease Control and Prevention [CDC]. (2008). National Environmental Tracking Program. Retrieved January 3, 2009, from http://www.cdc.gov/nceh/tracking/keepingtrack.htm

Crandall, E. (1914). Letter dated October 13, 1914, from Ella Crandall, Executive Secretary, National Organization for Public Health Nursing, to John D. Rockefeller requesting funding for the organization. Collect RC, Record Group 1.1, Series 200, Box 121, Folder 1498, Rockefeller Archives, Pocantico, NY.

Cronin, B. (2002). The digital divide. *Library Journal, 127*(3), 48.

Freeman, R. B. (1950). *Public health nursing practice.* Philadelphia: Saunders.

Friede, A., Blum, H., & McDonald, M. (1995). Public health informatics: How information age technology can strengthen public health. *Annual Review of Public Health, 16,* 239–252.

Goodrich, A. W. (1931). The past, present, and future of nursing. *American Journal of Nursing, 31*(12), 1385–1394.

Hebda, T., Czar, P., & Mascara, C. (2005). *Handbook of informatics for nurses and health care professionals* (3rd ed.). Upper Saddle River, NJ: Pearson-Prentice Hall.

Institute of Medicine [IOM]. (1988). *The future of public health.* Washington, DC: National Academy Press.

Institute of Medicine [IOM]. (2003a). *The future of the public's health in the 21st century.* Washington, DC: National Academy Press.

Institute of Medicine [IOM]. (2003b). *Who will keep the public healthy? Educating public health professionals for the 21st century.* Washington, DC: National Academy Press.

Levin, P., Cary, A., Kulbok, P., Leffers, J., Molle, M., & Polivka, B. (2007). Graduate education for advanced practice public health nursing: At the crossroads. Association of Community Health Nursing Educators (ACHNE), 1–24. Retrieved July 14, 2009, from http://www.achne.org/files/public/GraduateEducationDocument.pdf

McBride, A. B., & Detmar, D. E. (2008). Guest editorial: Using informatics to go beyond technology thinking. *Nursing Outlook, 57*(5), 195–196.

McGonigle, D., & Mastrian, K. (2009). *Nursing informatics and the foundation of knowledge.* Sudbury, MA: Jones and Bartlett.

National Network of Libraries of Medicine and National Library of Medicine. (2005). Public health information and data: A training manual. Retrieved January 28, 2009, from http://phpartners.org/pdf/phmanual.pdf

Ozbolt, J., & Saba, V. (2008). A brief history of nursing informatics in the United States of America. *Nursing Outlook, 56*(5), 199–205.

Rogers, E. (1983). *Diffusion of innovation* (3rd ed., rev. ed.). London: The Free Press.

Schneider, J. S., Barkauskas, V., & Keenan, G. (2008). Evaluating home health care nursing outcomes with OASIS and NOC. *Journal of Nursing Scholarship, 40*(1), 76–82.

Skiba, D. J. (2008). Moving forward: The informatics agenda. *Nursing Education Perspectives, 29*(5), 300–301.

Thede, L. Q. (2003). *Informatics and nursing: Opportunities and challenges* (2nd ed.). Philadelphia: Williams & Wilkins.

Titus, S. C. (1933/1991). The new Scutari. In N. Birnbach & S. B. Lewenson (Eds.), *First words: Selected addresses from the National League for Nursing, 1894–1933* (pp. 344–353). New York: National League for Nursing Press.

U.S. Department of Health and Human Services [DHHS], Centers for Medicare & Medicaid Services. (n.d.). OASIS. Retrieved January 30, 2009, from http://www.cms.hhs.gov/OASIS/046_DataSet.asp#TopOfPage

U.S. Department of Health and Human Services [DHSS]. (2000). *Healthy people 2010* (Vol. 1). Washington, DC: U.S. Government Printing Office.

U.S. Department of Health and Human Services [DHSS], Public Health Service. (2004). The public health workforce: An agenda for the 21st century. Retrieved January 23, 2009, from http://74.125.47.132/search?q=cache:r3T4ANrDgb4J:www.health.gov/phfunctions/pubhlth.pdf+The+Public+Health+Workforce+21st+century+agenda&hl=en&ct=clnk&cd=1&gl=us

Wald, L. (1915). *The house on Henry Street.* New York: Henry Holt & Company.

Yasnoff, W. A., O'Carroll, P. W., Koo, D., Linkins, R. W., & Kilbourne, E. M. (2000). Public health informatics: Improving and transforming public health in the information age. *Journal of Public Health Management Practice, 6*(6), 67–75.

CHAPTER 7

CONSIDERATIONS OF CULTURE IN THE HEALTH OF THE PUBLIC

ASTRID HELLIER WILSON
MARY DE CHESNAY

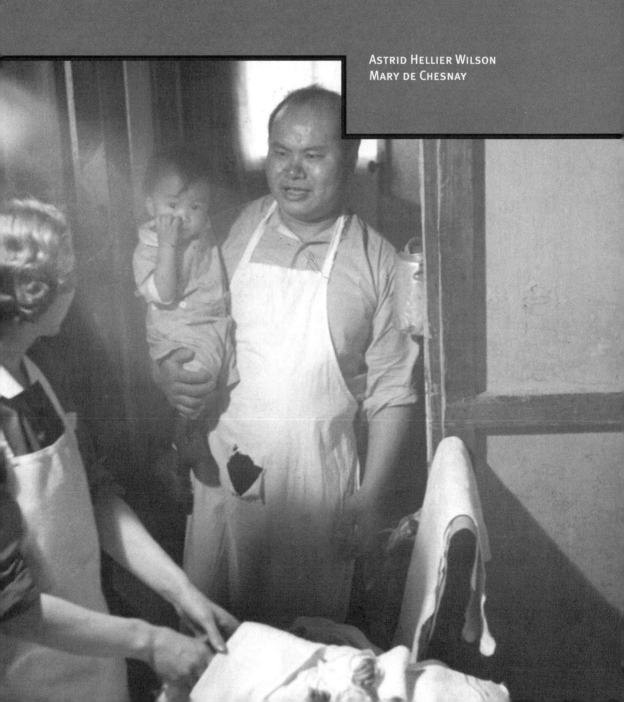

These opportunities that I have so slightly touched upon bear the closest relationship to the immigrants because they are the most helpless of our population and the most exploited; the least information and instructed in the very matters that are essential to their happiness. The country needs them and uses them and it is obviously an obligation due them as well as a safe guarding of the country itself to give them intelligent conception and education of what is important to their and to our interest (Wald, 1908, p. 467).

LEARNING OBJECTIVES

At the completion of this chapter, the reader will be able to

- Define subconcepts associated with culture as a concept.
- Compare and contrast two public health issues in terms of cultural influences.
- Analyze public health nursing interventions for selected cases in terms of cultural competence.

KEY TERMS

- Culture
- Culturally competent care
- Ethnocentrism
- Participant observation
- Ritual
- Xenophobia

The purpose of this chapter is to provide a culturally based framework for public health nursing interventions. Although community health nurses certainly provide care to individuals and families, public health nursing is generally aggregate service, and there is heavy reliance on prevention strategies directed toward populations. The chapter provides a cultural context for health care that maximizes respect for cultural diversity while accomplishing the objectives of best practices. In the first part of this chapter, basic concepts of **culture** are defined and related to important aspects of public health. In the second part of the chapter model programs are presented that are examples of providing **culturally competent care** to populations.

CULTURE

Anthropologists specialize in the study of culture: the lifeways, folkways, **rituals**, taboos, and practices of a group of people who share symbols, values, and patterns of behavior. These shared aspects of living are socially determined and taken for granted by members of the culture. Cultural practices are learned and become ingrained in the subconscious to the extent that they become automatic. A common example is how members of the culture greet each other. In Russia men might kiss each other on both cheeks. In corporate America executives shake hands with a firm grip. In Mediterranean countries women hug each other.

There are, however, many variations within cultural groups, particularly racial subcultural groups, and it is inappropriate to assume that all members of a group react the same in all situations. To generalize to all members of a group is considered stereotyping. For example, low-income, inner-city African Americans probably have more in common with low-income, inner-city whites and Hispanics than they do with upper-class African Americans regardless of where they live. In this case the culture of poverty dominates over the concept of race.

Cultural beliefs are learned and shared without conscious thought or analysis of the logic behind them. Studies that demonstrate the power of cultural beliefs are easily found in the literature (Kwong & Lam, 2008), and although some highlight the differences (Koffman, Morgan, Edmonds, Speck, & Higginson, 2008), there are examples of similarities among cultural groups that might seem to be at odds with each other. For example, Cassar (2006) studied cultural expectations about pregnancy with groups of orthodox

Jews and Muslims living in the United States and found similarities in need for modesty, special diet, limited spousal role in delivery, and beliefs specific to the newborn. The two groups differed on same-sex provider, period of postpartum confinement, consulting with religious leaders, and observing the Sabbath.

Interpretation of the world according to the norms of one's own culture is called *ethnocentrism* and involves the belief that the way things are done within one's own culture is the right way. Ethnocentrism is neither good nor bad but rather a shared perception by members of a group who have in common a set of values and mores. Ethnocentrism, however, can interfere with the ability of a person to respect different ways of doing things. For example, dogmatic assertions that prescribed rituals must be followed to maintain social control can interfere with a person's empathy for individuals who do not share one's cultural beliefs.

Ethnocentrism carried to the extreme of racism has resulted in oppression throughout modern history and the violence associated with racism justified on the basis of false conclusions about the actions and intentions of others. For example, stereotypes of African Americans as a high-crime population might lead one to fear and avoid all African Americans on the basis that some might be dangerous. A few years ago one of the authors had a young research assistant who was African American. This young man was careful to dress up for interviews (coat and tie) and to carry a briefcase to convey an image of respectability, yet he was repeatedly stopped by the police while traveling to interviews in predominantly white neighborhoods. Because he gave no signals that he might be dangerous, and because he took pains to blend in with the white middle class neighbors, the police actions can most reasonably be interpreted as racism.

Carried to an extreme, ethnocentrism can result in violence against those who simply do not share the cultural beliefs of the ones in power. An example in some modern-day communities is mixed marriage. Imagine a black man and white woman trying to raise a family in a rural area of the Deep South. At the other end of the continuum of ethnocentrism is behavior that might be construed simply as rude. For example, simple greeting rituals, if not followed precisely, can be interpreted as insulting to the host. Imagine an acquaintance arriving at your home for dinner and you say "hello" but in return the person starts complaining about a problem.

Strict rules about gender-appropriate behavior apply in many countries. Women who break these rules or who are perceived by the abuser to break the rules are subjected to sanctions that often include beatings and torture. In a study of spousal abuse of pregnant women in Bangladesh, it was found that most women abused during pregnancy had a long history of prior abuse (Naved & Persson, 2008). In families in which women are regularly beaten by their male partners and relatives, the women are perceived to break rules that involve the honor of the family or the man and therefore "deserve" the beatings. This process is an internalization of blame that destroys the women's self-esteem and transcends culture or country.

Closely related to the concept of ethnocentrism is *xenophobia*, a term that describes conscious fear of foreigners. Foreigners can be interpreted as anyone of a different ethnic or racial group than one's own and can reside in close prox-imity to the group that is xenophobic. Xenophobia is distinguished from racism in that the phenomenon does not necessarily apply to people of minority groups. Indeed, it can be the minority group that is xenophobic about others in the community. For example, Tsai (2006) reported an ethnographic study of Taiwanese immigrant youth who settled in a Mandarin-speaking neighborhood of Seattle and who experienced xenophobia in relation to their American neighbors, excluding them from their play groups.

Critical to the study of culture is to understand the *rituals* associated with the culture. A ritual is a type of action that might be as simple as shaking hands when greeting a newcomer or as complex as those found in religious ceremonies. Rituals and traditions associated with key life events can enhance joy in the case of celebratory traditions such as weddings and holidays, provide a sense of comfort in the case of death and dying, and promote a gracious lifestyle as noted in table manners and the offering of food to guests.

Rituals also protect health and are especially important in public health nursing. Consider what would happen if aseptic techniques are not practiced when providing care in homes with varying degrees of cleanliness. What would happen if the sterile techniques used to package medications were not followed? Contamination of foods and drugs has been responsible for many deaths that might have been prevented if the rituals and rules about mass production were followed.

An example of a set of complex rituals is how to care for patients after death (Pattison, 2008). There are prescribed procedures, such as how to wash the body, and prescribed actions that are contraindicated. Often, prescribed actions are related to religious rituals. An example is performing a routine autopsy on a member of certain religious groups. Although sometimes autopsies must be legally mandated as in the case of murder, the process can be extremely disturbing to members of the family if their religious tradition opposes what they view as desecration of the body.

There is evidence that rituals can reduce anxiety. Often associated with religious practices, rituals provide a measure of comfort to the person who practices the rituals. In a study of 30 Catholic college students, Anastasi and Newberg (2008) found that reciting the Rosary significantly lowered anxiety as measured by the State-Trait Anxiety Inventory. In an Alcoholics Anonymous meeting the ritual of pronouncing, "My name is _____ and I am an alcoholic," serves to let people know they are not alone.

Often, culture is viewed as the set of lifeways, rituals, and values associated with a group of people who share ethnicity and geographic territory, for example, Navajo residents of a reservation, Bantu of Africa, and Bedouin tribes of the Middle East. We also conceptualize culture, however, as transcending geographic boundaries when people share the aspects that define culture. For example, the profession of nursing might be viewed as a culture. Nurses around the world often seem more alike than different in terms of their shared commitment to their patients, common goals to heal and prevent illness and injury, similar rituals such as uniforms, caps, and pinning ceremonies, and finally specialized education. Although some countries have higher standards of education, governance, and practice, it seems reasonable to state that nursing practice in widely diverse settings has the common origin of meeting the health needs of the community. Professional organizations such as Sigma Theta Tau and International Honor Society have a mission to bring nurses from diverse countries and cultures together.

Other groups that might be viewed as subcultures within a dominant culture include patients with similar illnesses, such as HIV/AIDS, the chronically mentally ill, disabled children, pregnant adolescents, and heart attack victims. Groups of people living in close proximity can also be considered subcultures when they are a tightly knit group with shared values and rules, such as street gangs, retirees living in a gated golf community, expatriate Americans living in Oaxaca, and migrant workers on California ranches.

Participant Observation: A Skillful Technique in the Process of Becoming Culturally Competent

A key skill of public health nurses is the ability to observe and make sense of their surroundings. In a clinical sense, **participant observation** is a technique in which the nurse makes careful observations of specific processes, actions, or communications while providing care as a participant in the activity. Usually, participant observation techniques are used as research methods in ethnographies conducted over time—often a year or more. The technique, however, can be useful to public health nurses who need to pay close attention to subtle changes in their client, family, and the population and group interactions.

Participant observation is also a key method in conducting participatory action research, which is one of the best ways to design new population-based health programs. Action research involves community stakeholders in all phases of planning programs targeting that community (Brown et al., 2008; Cashman et al., 2008). For example, a public health team wants to start a program to improve psychosocial outcomes for women in a cardiac rehabilitation program. They might interview consumers in a selected program such as the "Heart Awareness for Women Program" (Davidson et al., 2008) and conduct participant observation periods to see how women move through the program.

The literature has many examples of participant observation in research, but reviewing the technique can be helpful to students who are learning observation skills to understand culture in any setting. The techniques are particularly easy to do in public settings. The following are some examples from the research literature that demonstrate how culture can be learned by an outsider. In an ethnographic study involving both participant observation and interviews, Stevens (2006) studied 15 adolescent female parents about what "being healthy" meant to them. A key finding was that although the girls were aware of public health messages about health, their fundamental needs of safe living conditions, finding food, and paying bills took precedence over practicing health promotion. For example, the girls' attention was focused on their own needs, and the key concepts that emerged from the data related to how the young mothers were going to meet their own basic needs and the basic needs of their infants.

An example of how participant observation is a powerful supplement to interviewing in Stevens' study was food shopping. Although it seemed clear from interviews

that adolescent mothers understood that good nutrition involved eating fruits and vegetables, the pressures of long hours at work and exhaustion at taking care of an infant made fast food a much easier choice. Participant observation demonstrates exactly how and under what conditions the mothers shopped for food rather than what they stated they should buy.

Similarly, Kaplan, Calman, Golub, Ruddock, and Billings (2006) conducted participatory action research in the Bronx to identify best practices of promoting public health by faith-based institutions. Addressing racial and ethnic disparities, a coalition of 40 community-based programs, including 14 churches, was mobilized to change community members' attitudes about health practices and to influence health policy on behalf of racial and ethnic minorities. Although limitations to the study were identified, the team concluded that the faith-based leaders could have an enormous positive influence on the health of their communities.

In an ethnographic study of 30 rural African American women who used cocaine, Brown and Smith (2006) found that the women tended to be either child-focused or self-focused with a wide range of responses to explain their drug use. For example, through interviews and participant observation conducted over 4 years, the researchers found that living in a rural area or small town created a sense of boredom among some of the women, who did drugs for something to do. It is one thing for someone living in a small town to say they have nothing to do but quite another for the researcher to live there and experience first-hand what it feels like to be socially isolated.

In this study other women used their children as an excuse, saying they felt overwhelmed with the demands of mothering. Again, participant observation makes clear to the researcher what it is like to live under the conditions required of the population being studied. Imagine a working single mother who arises at 5:00 a.m., goes to work at 6:00 a.m. as a waitress in a café until 3:00 p.m., picks up her children from school, helps them do homework, and then has to fix dinner and get them to bed by 8:00 p.m. while doing laundry and getting clothes ready for the next day. At what point in this busy day does she have time to shop for healthy food, take care of her own needs, and indulge in relaxing activities such as exercise or reading?

Similarly, in public health nursing having a client say she is bored or overwhelmed by the demands of a growing family is much more meaningful if the nurse has visited the community and sees there are no social outlets for young mothers. An example of how the public health nurse might use this information is to start a series of group meetings about health topics (with child care provided) that could also serve as a support group for women. In the case of the population of adolescent mothers, the nurse might begin a support group that involves other professionals who could teach job training skills such as computer classes, crafts classes, or gardening. The point is that any successful intervention program can be made culturally specific by focusing on the needs and interests of the population served. Complete the field exercises in **Box 7-1** as part of your learning.

Culturally Competent Care

The body of literature on cultural competence has grown since this term was determined to be the desired outcome of simple awareness of cultural differences. At its most basic level, cultural

---

BOX **7-1**   **Field Exercise 1**

Choose one or more of the following and keep field notes about your observations and interpretations. Field notes are simply a kind of journal (use a small notebook) in which you would document the date and setting of the observation period and then describe your observations.

1. Have lunch at an ethnic restaurant in your community and observe the interactions of staff with each other and with patrons.
2. Identify a subcultural group within your community and visit their territory. Some examples might be an Amish farm, a Native American reservation, a juvenile court detention center, or a homeless shelter. Document your observations.
3. Visit a health clinic and observe the rituals of signing in, waiting room behavior, and payment processes. Document your observations.

competence is a set of attitudes and behaviors by the public health nurse to take into account that the client or population has cultural beliefs, values, health practices, and ways of behaving in social interactions that may differ widely from expectations of the health providers. The public health nurse uses knowledge of the culture, which may be limited, and key informants, the client being the most important, to accomplish the goals of care without violating the rights of the client or population so as to maintain their cultural traditions.

One interpretation of cultural competence is to practice the traditions of the client population, but the danger here is that these attempts to blend into the culture are unnatural and providers might appear to be making fun of the population. Mimicry can be insulting, and so the provider inadvertently creates problems instead of preventing them. Showing respect for the other's culture does not mean trying to be someone you are not.

The American Academy of Nursing (2008) emphasizes the importance of including cultural material in nursing education. Several theorists (Campinha-Bacote, 2002; Kim-Godwin, Clarke, & Barton, 2001; Purnell, 2000, 2002; Purnell & Paulanka, 2003) have published extensively on the topic. Wells (2000) wrote that cultural competence is not sufficient and argued for cultural proficiency to replace it as the desired goal.

Regardless of how the concept is viewed, best practice in providing culturally competent care should involve the most fundamental characteristic of respect (de Chesnay, Peil, & Pamp, 2008). Respect for differences on the part of both provider and client population leads to open communication about customs and values, and openness in the relationship leads to

problem solving about how best to meet the health needs of the population. A good rule of thumb is to be as respectful, polite, and considerate as one can under the rules of one's own culture. In this way most clients of diverse populations understand the nurse's intentions as honorable and respond accordingly.

CULTURAL COMPETENCE AND CONFLICTS

It is all well and good to say we should practice cultural competence, but what if the rights of the client population conflict seriously with the values or morals of the provider? The practice of female circumcision is an example. Abhorrent to Western practitioners, female circumcision affects millions of girls and is widely practiced in some cultures. Members of these cultures often immigrate to the United States. The United Nations has called for an end to the practice of female circumcision, also called female genital mutilation. The World Health Organization has studied the public health consequences of the procedure, and Little (2003) discussed the effects of hemorrhage, abscesses, sepsis, long-term problems with voiding, painful intercourse, and childbirth difficulties.

From a public health standpoint, it is a legitimate argument that eliminating the practice of genital mutilation is good policy. Support for the procedure, however, is ingrained in the culture and attitudes of millions of poor families who do not have access to educational programs on the public health issues and who perpetuate the practice by using a variety of practitioners who use unsterile instruments without anesthesia (Momoh, 2004; Morison, Dirir, Elmi, Warsame, & Dirir, 2004).

Even for male circumcision, which does not have the stigma associated with female circumcision, the unsterile use of implements exacerbates the spread of one of the world's most virulent pandemics, HIV/AIDS, in areas where traditional healers and religious leaders practice cutting rituals. These rituals are not only for circumcision, but also for symbolism (family bonding) and marking (curing illness), and often many boys are cut by the same tools in a short time period (Ndiwane, 2008). The cutting leads to sepsis and scarring if left untreated.

The world is becoming less a set of individual countries that are autonomous and more a global village in which there is extensive immigration and sharing of resources. Consequently, it is increasingly likely that healthcare providers and their patients find their cultural values in conflict. Respect for differences needs to be negotiated on a personal basis when providers come into conflict with clients over health issues, and education about each other's culture can certainly help prevent misunderstandings. Open discussion of these issues while maintaining the rights of the other to hold differing views is both respectful and culturally appropriate.

One way to look at whose cultural values take precedence is to view the relationship between provider and client as a contract in which the client comes to the provider as an expert to provide a specific service. The two then agree to disagree on anything not relevant to the contract. For example, a public health nurse in an inner-city immigrant neighborhood of Somali refugees wants to design a program to address diabetes management. Everyone agrees that diabetes is a major health issue for the population, but this is also a population in which female circumcision is practiced. For the nurse to try to get the women to stop this practice is inappropriate because female circum-

cision is a health issue that is not part of the contract. However, being open to discussing with leaders of the population the health risks without judging or trying to eliminate the cultural practice might be well received.

LEARNING PROCESS ON BECOMING
CULTURALLY COMPETENT

Learning to provide culturally competent care is a complex process and starts with the respect for cultural differences that is fundamental to interaction with people of a different culture than one's own. One of the best ways to learn about different cultures is immersion in which a professor takes a group of students to a foreign country or medically underserved area of the United States to practice. There are many examples of programs in which this is an integral part of nursing education (Bennett & Holtz, 2008; de Chesnay, 2005; Nauright, 2005).

Although it is certainly desirable to be proficient in the language of the group with whom one is working, lack of language skill should not be used as an excuse not to interact with people, even in immersion programs in foreign countries. Adequate translators are often available in communities with large ethnic populations, and sometimes younger members of a family can translate for older members, although this practice is not often the best choice. Taking the time to learn a few words or phrases helps greatly in establishing trust and rapport.

Other approaches to consider in the process of learning and designing culturally competent programs for English-speaking ethnic minority groups within a city might include the following:

1. Project directors read as much as possible about the target population and have informal conversations

with key informants. *Key informants* are members of the group or population of interest who are trusted members of the representative culture and who are willing to educate the staff in how best to approach community leaders and stakeholders in a respectful way.

2. Key project staff members meet with community leaders to identify the stakeholders. *Stakeholders* include all those who have a vested interest in the project such as the consumers who will be the recipient of the interventions and the gatekeepers—individuals who must give permissions for access to consumers, such as ministers for their congregations.

3. Staff members meet with stakeholders to identify issues related to the topic. An excellent way to talk about issues is in focus groups. *Focus groups* are conducted with small homogeneous groups of people within the target population. The focus group leader asks specific questions to elicit the group's perceptions to design appropriate aspects of the program.

4. Staff members meet with key informants or stakeholders on an ongoing basis to share developments and to plan, implement, and evaluate the unfolding process of the program "together."

5. Staff members put in place evaluation measures that capture the perceptions of the stakeholders.

Complete the exercises in **Box 7-2** as part of your learning.

Culture and Public Health Nursing

Cultural considerations for public health nurses far exceed the implementation of

---

BOX 7-2   Field Exercise 2

1. Assume you are a client in a community far from your home. Write a short essay on what it means to you to have a provider who is culturally competent.

2. Interview one member of an ethnic or racial minority group different from your own and ask about the person's attitude toward the practice of female circumcision. Note that it is not necessary to identify someone from a culture that practices female circumcision. Compare and contrast how your own attitude differs or is similar.

3. Imagine you are developing a diabetes education program for a group of poor African American, Asian, or Latina women in your community. How would you go about designing the program? Next, speak to a member of the cultural group you chose and ask them how they would develop the same program. What are the similarities and differences?

---

cultural competence strategies needed to care for individuals and families. In addition to individual and family care, public health nurses focus on population health and the community as the client (Racher & Annis, 2007). The skill set necessary to integrate culture in providing health care is extended to identifying diverse cultures found in different communities. Examples of community cultures include the culture of farm workers, domestic violence, substance abuse, poverty, prisons, and rural communities.

Public health nurses are concerned with the culture and healthcare needs of underserved populations, for example, migrant farm workers and their families. Migrant farm workers make a valuable contribution to the everyday lives of the American people, and they and their "uprooted" children have numerous health problems not seen in the general population (Wilson, Pittman, & Wold, 2000). Research conducted among migrant workers and children of migrant farm workers provides insight into their perceptions of culture and health. The adults noted in the aforementioned research identify priority issues centered on the need for health information, English lessons, available community resources, and legal information, whereas the children viewed health as well-being and had a good knowledge of what to do to be healthy. The children did voice concerns about the difference in access to health care in the United States and the threat of deportation (Perilla, Wilson, Wold, & Spencer, 1998; Wilson, Wold, Spencer, & Pittman, 2000). Knowledge of the culture of migrant farm workers enables public health nurses to develop and implement community projects based on the culture of this population.

Domestic violence is no stranger to public health nurses and is present in most societies and age groups. Unfortunately, the signs of violence often go unrecognized while multiple acts of physical and psychological abuse are continually perpetrated. Educational level is associated with increased acts of violence, and findings suggest the possibility of educating girls as a potential for preventing domestic abuse (Ergin, Bayram, Alper, Selimoglu, & Bilgel, 2005).

Reactions to domestic violence between Latina and non-Latina women were studied, and the results showed cultural implications for the Latina women. Treatment responses that include a bicultural or bilingual counselor who focused on the family and children were demonstrated to be desirable for Latina women (Edelson, Hokoda, & Ramos-Lira, 2007). Public health nurses must consider the individual differences in women of any culture when planning programs for domestic violence.

Other types of public health programs targeting substance abuse (Hopson & Steiker, 2008; Kulis et al., 2005; Lange, 2007; Walle, 2004), poverty (Pearson, 2003; Wood, 2003), prison programs (Cervantes, Ruan, & Duenas, 2004; Devieux et al., 2005), and rural communities (Hartley, 2004; Jensen & Royeen, 2002; Savage et al., 2006) are found in the literature. The common theme in all these programs is emphasis on cultural considerations.

Substance abuse programs have been targeted at Native Americans (Walle, 2004) and women learning to care for themselves (Lange, 2007). Two evidence-based substance abuse prevention programs targeted students in alternative schools (Hopson & Steiker, 2008) and middle school students with a Mexican heritage (Kulis et al., 2005). Both programs emphasized the importance of culturally grounded curriculums. It is unlikely that curriculums will be implemented or sustained if interventions are not culturally congruent with those receiving the intervention. For example, Hopson and Steiker (2008) allowed students in alternative schools to read workbook exercises and reword them to capture their lifestyles and culture to facilitate student participation.

The culture of poverty has also been reported in the literature (Pearson, 2003;

Wood, 2003). Poverty is complex and encompasses many factors, such as not having basic needs like adequate food, clothing, and housing. These situations may lead children to developmental delays, dropping out of school, and giving birth during the teen years. Some examples of cultural rules of poverty are living in the present and not planning for the future, sharing money with others rather than trying to get ahead to guarantee that others will share in their need, and not expecting change because of a strong belief in fate and destiny (Pearson, 2003). Wood (2003) encourages community-based advocacy to enhance the health of children who are most vulnerable in poor families.

One intervention program for adolescent juvenile offenders provides insight into the ability to decrease recidivism and increase substance abuse resistance (Cervantes et al., 2004). Much of the success of the Program Shortstop was attributed to cultural sensitivity aimed at Hispanic youth who came from low-income immigrant families. There were four prevention/intervention sessions using videos, homework, legal education, a simulation incarceration, activities to improve family communication and conflict resolution, drug information, self-esteem building drills, parent workshops on family communication, legal rights and responsibilities, and youth mentoring. Eighty-nine percent of the youth who completed the program were not rearrested within 1 year. Also, the participants gained legal knowledge and effective ways to deal with substance abuse and delinquency at school. In a follow-up study most parents reported that their child's high-risk behavior had decreased.

Other researchers studied the differences among African American and Cuban American adolescent juvenile offenders, predominately male, related to preventing drug and sexually risky behaviors while focusing on culture. These researchers examined levels of drug and sexually risky behaviors to determine if there were any differences among the two groups. Language in the focus groups and in-depth interviews was culturally sensitive, using the local terminology of the participants. The results in part indicated that both groups of youth engaged in risky behaviors that could lead to HIV infection and had about the same level of sexual activity and number of partners. The Cubans in this sample had higher levels of unprotected sex and higher levels of sex while using drugs than the African American youth. Some of the differences in this sample may be related to acculturation, communication with parents, and media-targeted efforts. Adolescents who are more acculturated tend to engage earlier in risky sexual behaviors, and Hispanic youth may not talk about risky behaviors at home. Specific media protective health messages may have been targeted more toward the African American youths than Cuban American youths (Devieux et al., 2005).

It is well established that rural communities may have limited resources and inadequate numbers of healthcare providers. A challenge for healthcare providers is to provide health services for vulnerable populations in rural areas (Jensen & Royeen, 2002). The *Health United States 2001 Urban and Rural Health Chartbook* (Eberhardt et al., 2001) identified risky behaviors among rural populations that may be attributed to a rural culture health determinant. There is evidence of increased risk behaviors among rural residents such as obesity, smoking, poverty, and decreased exercise and nutritional diets. In addition, environmental and cultural factors and economic issues can contribute to health behaviors and health (Hartley, 2004). Other researchers have described interdisciplinary rural health projects as "best practice" in rural health projects (Jensen & Royeen, 2002). Public health nurses can be leaders in implementing population-based models for improving the quality of health care in rural communities with particular emphasis on the unique cultural aspects of each community. Furthermore, public health nurses are uniquely positioned to participate in community-based participatory research in that they subscribe to the four principles of building trust, collaboration, excellence in science, and ethics associated with community-based participatory research (Savage et al., 2006).

CASE STUDIES

Three case studies are presented below as examples of programs in which culturally competent interventions are predominant:

1. Migrant family project
2. Rural Georgia domestic violence project
3. Project IDEAL—diabetes

A description of the project and discussion about cultural material precedes suggested field activities that students might find useful to give a sense of the public health implications when using culturally competent interventions.

Migrant Farm Workers and Their Families Case Study

The Farm Worker Family Health Program (FWFHP) has been in existence for over 15 years in a rural area of southern Georgia.

The program is a health-focused academic community partnership where faculty and students provide health screening and referrals and community organizations provide access to migrant farm workers at their work sites, trailer parks where they live, and to their children attending a county summer school program. In addition, the local Farmworker Health Clinic provides client health records, assessment forms for documentation, and some medications and serves as the referral source for clients requiring follow-up treatment from the FWFHP.

The 2-week cultural immersion program provides a unique opportunity for interdisciplinary students (undergraduate nursing, nurse practitioner, dental hygienists, physical therapy and psychology) to gain needed cultural sensitivity while providing health-related screenings to this uninsured at-risk population. Since the inception of the program, about 10,000 episodes of care have been provided to migrant farm workers and their families. Adult screening includes vital signs, hemoglobin and glucose tests, dental screening, and physical therapy if desired. The most frequent diagnoses among adults are low back pain, dental caries, and diabetes, which is on the rise in this vulnerable population.

The child health screenings include a physical examination, height and weight measurements (body mass index), hearing and vision screening, glucose screening if indicated by increased body mass index, and hemoglobin screening. In addition, nursing students present health classes to migrant children in pre-kindergarten to ninth grade related to basic hygiene, dental care, nutrition, and smoking risks. The teaching strategies include discussion, lecture, videos, handout materials, games, and poster presentations. The most frequent diagnoses among the children were dental caries, anemia, vision problems, and upper respiratory tract infections.

Other students also participate. Dental hygiene students perform dental checks and fluoride treatments on all children and tooth sealants to retard decay. If needed, children are referred to a local dentist. The psychology students perform developmental assessments and provide counseling and referral if indicated. Physical therapy students assess gross motor development.

CULTURAL CONSIDERATIONS

The FWFHP noted specific cultural considerations for this particular population:

- Before attending the FWFHP, all faculty and students are required to participate in a series of modules related to the history and culture of migrant farm workers and their families.
- Communication barriers were addressed by having an interpreter available at all screenings to assist with clients who did not speak English.
- Services to be rendered in the evenings and at work sites were incorporated into the program.
- The need for educational materials in Spanish was identified and materials were made available.
- Counseling services for migrant farm workers was made available.

IMPACT ON THE HEALTH OF THE PUBLIC

The impact of this culturally congruent public health initiative included the following:

- The major impact of the FWFHP is the health care that is provided to this uninsured, vulnerable population. Even though the program runs

only 2 weeks in the summer, other health programs are provided throughout the year by the local Farmworker Health Clinic. The health services are positively received by the migrant farm workers and their children.

- Community participation and resources are available for this uninsured population and for the faculty and students. Different churches in the area provide chairs and tables for the screenings and lunch for the students, faculty, and other volunteers.
- The immersion experience facilitates student understanding of the Hispanic and rural cultures. Specifically, this experience with migrant farm workers and their families can be used in students' future practice when encountering patients with a Hispanic or migrant farm worker background.
- A major positive outcome for the children is the establishment of a medical health record that is available year after year for those children who return and attend the summer program. Parents are provided with health records related to screenings and immunization schedules and are encouraged to immunize their children at appropriate times.
- Another positive outcome for the population is the referral system that is in place that enables the healthcare providers to arrange future health care in the community. One example was a man who presented with a deep laceration that had become infected and led to septicemia. The man was taken to the emergency department

---

BOX **7-3**   Field Exercise 3

1. Interview a person whose first language is not English (or any other language you speak) about experiences with healthcare professionals who do not speak his or her language. What feelings do these experiences evoke?
2. Develop a brief training module for migrant workers or their children on a topic similar to one of the following: dental hygiene, foot care for the elderly, HIV/AIDS prevention, prenatal nutrition, infant bathing, child immunizations, anxiety prevention, substance abuse, or domestic violence. In what way(s) would you ensure that the individual or population's particular cultural values and beliefs are addressed?
3. Conduct a participant observation session at a clinic that serves the migrant population. Observe rituals, values, and folk practices. For example, who speaks for the family to the healthcare professional? How are children disciplined? Are they told to sit still or allowed to run around? Are any foods brought in, and if so, what are they? What language do they use?

---

at a local hospital at once and treatment began immediately, thus preventing a potential amputation or death. Ultimately, the wound began healing.

Complete the exercises in **Box 7-3** as part of your learning.

Rural Domestic Violence Project Case Study

A unique program in north Georgia serves both urban and rural populations by providing assistance to victims of domestic violence for over two decades. It has grown into a center with diverse services ranging from crisis intervention, legal advocacy, transportation, child care, household establishment assistance, life skills workshops, children's programs, referral, transitional housing (hopefully leading to permanent housing), to community education.

The mission of the center is focused on the safety of women and children who are victims of domestic violence by providing the above free services. Emergency shelter and crisis intervention are paramount when domestic violence occurs, but the program provides so much more to the victims. In addition to the 24-hour hotline in English, there is now a 24-hour hotline in Spanish.

The groups receiving services include whites, African Americans, Hispanics, refugees, immigrants, and human trafficking victims. In the last 2 years the Multi-Cultural Program has provided support services to 50 women from Mexico, 7 from Guatemala, 4 from Venezuela, 3 from Honduras, 3 from Salvador, 2 from Peru, 2 from Brazil, 2 from Russia, 2 from Nicaragua, 1 from Honduras, 1 from Greece, 1 from Panama, 1 from the Netherlands, and 1 from Columbia. In addition, transitional housing was provided to 17 women from Mexico, 3 from Jamaica, 3 from Puerto Rico, 2 from Panama, 1 from Libya, 1 from Ghana (refugee), 2 from Haiti (human trafficking victim), 1 from Cameroon (refugee), 1 from Ethiopia (human trafficking victim), and 1 from Liberia (refugee).

The staff at the center remain sensitive to individual cultural backgrounds and try to meet needs within that framework. One example was a woman from Liberia who had walked all her life before coming to the United States and had never driven in a car, nor had anyone from her village. Nevertheless, she wanted to learn how to drive, and the center provided driving lessons, which was a life-changing event. Other life-changing events include the ability to have employment and afford and maintain an apartment, leading to a sense of achievement and self-satisfaction.

CULTURAL CONSIDERATIONS
The Rural Domestic Violence Project notes specific cultural considerations for this particular population:

- The culture of poverty is incorporated into the services provided to help the victims break their cycle of poverty. Women in the rural Domestic Violence Project who use the transitional housing and progress to long-term housing, find employment, and pay their rent and other bills expressed their satisfaction that they could maintain a home for their families and no longer had to live homeless and in adverse poverty.
- Cultural competence workshops are provided for the staff.
- Hiring of bilingual staff enhances effective communication, eliminating the need for interpreters.

- A support group was developed and implemented for the Latina population.
- Immigration and residency status information are provided.
- Sensitivity to special dietary needs, clothes, and other cultural norms is developed.
- Brochures in Spanish are provided.
- Age-appropriate services are provided for children and adolescents.

IMPACT ON THE HEALTH OF THE PUBLIC
The impact of this culturally congruent public health initiative included the following:

- Transitional housing for 3 years is available at the program's relatively new 72-unit apartment complex. The gated community consists of two-, three-, and four-bedroom units and provides low-cost housing and on-site support services. After 3 years the low-cost housing is available permanently, thus providing much-needed support for this specific population.
- Free crisis and counseling services are available for women and children who are victims of domestic abuse. The ability for women and children to have a safe shelter from an otherwise traumatic situation allows the women a respite from their immediate distress. They are in a safe place with capable counselors who can help them make necessary choices to restart their lives in an abuse-free environment.
- Legal advocacy services assist with obtaining protective orders to ensure safety for the women and their children. The advocacy services enable restraining orders to be

put in place and allow the women and children to be safe at the center. Many women do not initiate these orders but are glad when someone empowers them to take necessary legal action.

- Emergency services provide for the immediate safety of the family and help the victims to develop ways to be safe and initiate these safety measures themselves.
- Immigration services are rendered to combat human trafficking and the Internet mail-order bride business.
- The special needs of children who have been living in homes with domestic violence are addressed in the program such as support groups, early literacy programs, immunizations, play therapy, special outings, organized activities, and individual or group counseling sessions. Emotional distress and other psychological issues are effectively worked out among most of the children. The support groups help the children to realize they are not the cause of domestic violence in their homes and they are not alone but rather other children experience some of the same things they do.

Complete the exercises in **Box 7-4** as part of your learning.

Project Ideal

Project Ideal is a program of the WellStar School of Nursing at Kennesaw State University that began in 2003 and is focused on providing diabetes prevention and self-management education for Latinos. This is a significant program because Latinos are the largest minority in Georgia, numbering almost 576,000. Latinos

---

BOX **7-4** **Field Exercise 4**

1. Volunteer at a shelter. Journal about your observations and reflect on these observations.
2. Identify and review three films about domestic violence and observe the interactions between abusers and victims. What are your observations?
3. Interview an administrator of a shelter or a therapist who specializes in violence to address the questions you have about domestic violence.

---

have a high risk for developing diabetes, and as many as 1 in 10 Latinos may have diabetes. There are ways to prevent or postpone diabetes by maintaining a healthy lifestyle, such as eating healthy foods and exercising.

The classes are conducted in small groups and focus on maintaining a healthy lifestyle, needed medications, meal planning, blood sugar monitoring, and exercise. Coupled with the classes are the support group meetings. The support group meetings consist of special education sessions with guest speakers for adults, separate educational sessions for children, blood pressure, weight and height screening, and follow-up, and currently participants are encouraged to take part in English as a second language classes.

Project Ideal also provides a forum for educators and healthcare providers to study the concepts of diabetes self-management education and the American Diabetes Association criteria for recognition. Included in the program are materials for diverse Latino groups, pre-diabetes education materials, consultation with a Latino healthcare educator, and program development consultation and oversight.

CULTURAL CONSIDERATIONS

Project Ideal facilitates specific cultural considerations for this particular population:

- Understanding and respecting the cultural aspects of eye contact is essential when working with Latinos, such as being aware not to get too close initially until you have eye contact and avoiding direct eye contact unless they initiate it first. This is not as critical in the younger population as it is in the older generations. With length of time and acculturation, the necessity for avoiding eye contact diminishes with some individuals.
- Understand and respect the demonstrative use of hugs in welcoming.
- Identify participants' perceptions and value of health to best foster maintenance of diabetes.
- Know that there are differences within Latino groups, and some prefer not to be in groups with Latinos from different countries, whereas others enjoy the cultural exchange that occurs.
- Consider eating habits and the cultural names of different foods in different Latino populations. The words "naranja" and "chino" can both mean orange. The use of the metric system and traditional systems can be found among Puerto Ricans, such as measuring height in inches and weight in kilograms, and

the Mayans measure height in centimeters and weight in kilograms. This cultural information is essential when teaching nutrition classes such as weighing food for diets.
- Understand how people like to get information and use the "word of mouth method" in Latino populations.
- Know that some members in the Latino groups, in this project, trust individuals who survived a condition over a physician's word or teachings. Families and friends who have diabetes are trusted more than a healthcare provider and information is sought from them.
- Many Latinos prefer health providers who speak Spanish.

IMPACT ON THE HEALTH OF THE PUBLIC

The impact of this culturally congruent public health initiative included the following:

- The major impact of this program is the reduction of HbA_{1c} levels among participants with diabetes. This is significant because studies have shown that for every 1% reduction in HbA_{1c} levels, an approximate 35% reduction in the risk for the microvascular complications of diabetes occurs.
- This program provides a service to an underserved population.
- Nursing students are provided with the opportunity to develop culture competence skills when participating in the program.
- Although weight reduction has not been a statistically significant benefit of the program, there is evidence that the participants are maintaining their weight and not gaining weight while in the program.

- Diabetes prevention and education to children and teens participating in the program is provided.
- Quality of life is improved for Latinos who live with diabetes.

Complete the exercises in **Box 7-5** as part of your learning.

Discussion of Cultural Issues in the Community Projects

The three projects presented are diverse and meet different health needs of selected populations, yet there are common cultural issues evident in the projects. Cultural competence is needed

---

BOX 7-5 Field Exercise 5

1. Identify a similar program in your own community and ask to observe several intake interviews. How do the individual clients respond to the healthcare provider? How does the program reach out to the specific population being served?

2. Eat several meals at a local restaurant frequented by members of the Latino population and examine the types of foods on the menu. Prepare a nutritional analysis of these foods.

3. Identify a cultural group of interest and a particular health issue experienced by this group. Attend a support group meeting that addresses this particular issue and prepare a summary of the themes of the discussion.

---

among those providing care to these populations. Cultural themes in common with all three projects are respect, immersion, and communication. Respect for the recipients of care encompasses allowing them to express themselves and finding ways to incorporate their desires into the plan of care. One example of respect is being sensitive to special dietary needs, clothes, and other cultural norms. Considering the farm workers' schedules by providing services in the evening and acknowledging their need for materials in Spanish illustrates respect. Respect is also shown by being conscious of the cultural aspects of eye contact and the demonstrative use of hugs in welcoming in the Hispanic culture.

Immersion in a culture helps healthcare providers understand the cultural traditions that can assist in the planning and delivering of culturally appropriate health care. Gaining an understanding of diverse cultures enhances one's own ability to practice in an appropriate culturally sensitive manner. Much of the success of Project Ideal can be attributed to the in-depth understanding of the Latino culture and paying attention to participants' perceptions and values about health to best foster management of their diabetes.

Providing culturally specific workshops and preparation for staff, faculty, and students is another way to become familiar with a culture. Speakers might be invited to a panel presentation at which culturally appropriate food is served and music played.

Communication is essential in planning health care and services for diverse populations and can be a challenge because of many barriers that impede communication. Communication barriers are addressed in the case studies by the use of interpreters, hiring bilingual staff, and acknowledging the differences within Latino groups. In addition, understanding how people like to get information, such as the word-of-mouth method, in Latino populations and using key informants they trust are helpful in facilitating desired communication. Cultural considerations found in the case studies are essential for the health of the public.

CONCLUSION

The purpose of this chapter was to provide a cultural framework for public health nursing to best promote culturally competent health care to diverse populations. Several case studies were presented that demonstrate aspects of cultural considerations in implementing population-based projects. Public health nurses are encouraged to make use of participant observation and participatory action research methods to design programs that are culturally relevant to the stakeholders. Taking the time to learn the cultural lifeways, values, and traditions of the populations served is critical to providing health care, not only to patients and their families but also to populations.

ACKNOWLEDGMENTS

We gratefully acknowledge the contributions of the project staff who shared information about their programs.

References

American Academy of Nursing. (2008). *Cultural competency in baccalaureate education*. Washington, DC: AACN.

Anastasi, M., & Newberg, A. (2008). A preliminary study of the acute effects of religious ritual on anxiety. *Journal of Alternative and Complementary Medicine, 14*(2), 163–165.

Bennett, D., & Holtz, C. (2008). Building cultural competence: A nursing practicum in Oaxaca, Mexico. In C. Holtz (Ed.), *Global health care* (pp. 601–614). Sudbury, MA: Jones and Bartlett.

Brown, D., Hernandez, A., Saint-Jean, G., Evans, S., Tafari, I., Brewster, L., et al. (2008). A participatory action research pilot study of urban health disparities using rapid assessment response and evaluation. *Health Policy and Ethics, 98*(1), 28–38.

Brown, E. J., & Smith, F. B. (2006). Rural African American women who use cocaine: Needs and future aspirations related to their mothering role. *Community Mental Health Journal, 42*(1), 65–76.

Campinha-Bacote, J. (2002). The process of cultural competence in the delivery of health care services: A model of care. *Journal of Transcultural Nursing, 13*(3), 180–184.

Cashman, S., Adeky, S., Allen, A., Corburn, J., Israel, B., Montano, J., et al. (2008). The power and the promise: Working with communities to analyze data, interpret findings and get to outcomes. *American Journal of Public Health, 98*(8), 1407–1417.

Cassar, L. (2006). Cultural expectations of Muslims and Orthodox Jews in regard to pregnancy and the post-partum period: A study in comparison and contrast. *International Journal of Childbirth Education, 21*(2), 7–30.

Cervantes, R. C., Raun, K., & Duenas, N. (2004). Program Shortstop: A culturally focused juvenile intervention for Hispanic youth. *Journal of Drug Education, 34*(4), 385–405.

Davidson, P., Digiacomo, M., Zecchin, R., Clarke, M., Paul, G., Lamb, K., et al. (2008). A cardiac rehabilitation program to improve psychosocial outcomes of women with heart disease. *Journal of Women's Health, 17*(1), 123–134.

de Chesnay, M. (2005). Teaching nurses about vulnerable populations. In M. de Chesnay (Ed.), *Caring for the vulnerable* (pp. 349–356). Sudbury, MA: Jones and Bartlett.

de Chesnay, M., Peil., R., & Pamp, C. (2008). Cultural competence, resilience and advocacy. In M. de Chesnay and B. Anderson (Eds.), *Caring for the vulnerable* (pp. 25–35). Sudbury, MA: Jones and Bartlett.

Devieux, J. G., Malow, R. M., Ergon-Perez, E., Samuels, D. Rojas, P., Khushal, S. R., et al. (2005). A comparison of African American and Cuban American adolescent juvenile offenders: Risky sexual and drug use behaviors. *Journal of Social Work Practice in the Addictions, 5*(1/2), 69–83.

Eberhardt, M. S., Ingram, D. D., Makuc, D. M. (2001). *Health United States 2001 urban and rural health chartbook*. Hyattsville, MD: National Center for Health Statistics.

Edelson, M. G., Hokoda, A., & Ramos-Lira, L. (2007). Differences in effects of domestic violence between Latina and Non-Latina Women. *Journal of Family Violence, 22*, 1–10.

Ergin, N., Bayram, N., Alper, Z., Selimoglu, K., & Bilgel, N. (2005). Domestic violence: A tragedy behind the doors. *Women & Health, 42*(2), 35–51.

Hartley, D. (2004). Rural health disparities, population health, and rural culture. *American Journal of Public Health, 94*(10), 1675–1678.

Hopson, L. M., & Steiker, K. H. (2008). Methodology for evaluating an adaptation of evidence-based drug abuse prevention in alternative schools. *Children & Schools, 30*(2), 116–127.

Jensen, G. M., & Royeen, C. B. (2002). Improved rural access to care: Dimensions of best practice. *Journal of Interprofessional Care, 16*(2), 117–128.

Kaplan, S., Calman, N., Golub, M., Ruddock, C., & Billings, J. (2006). The role of faith-based institutions in addressing health disparities: A case study of an initiative in the Southwest Bronx. *Journal of Health Care for the Poor and Underserved, 17*(2), 9–20.

Kim-Godwin, Y. S., Clarke, P., & Barton, L. (2001). A model for delivery of culturally competent care. *Journal of Advanced Nursing, 35*(6), 918–926.

Koffman, J., Morgan, M., Edmonds, P., Speck, P., & Higginson, I. J. (2008). Cultural meanings of pain: A qualitative study of Black Caribbean and White British patients with advanced cancer. *Palliative Medicine, 22*, 350–359.

Kulis, S., Marsiglia, F. F., Elek, E., Dustman, P., Wagstaff, D. A., & Hecht, M. L. (2005). Mexican/Mexican American adolescents and keeping it REAL: An evidence-based substance use prevention program. *Children & Schools, 27*(3), 133–145.

Kwong, E. W., & Lam, I. O. (2008). Chinese older people in Hong Kong: Health beliefs about influenza vaccination. *Nursing Older People, 20*(7), 29–33.

Lange, B. (2007). The prescriptive power of caring for self: Women in recovery from substance use disorders. *International Journal for Human Caring, 11*(2), 74–80.

Little, C. M. (2003). Female genital circumcision: Medical and cultural considerations. *Journal of Cultural Diversity, 10*(1), 59–65.

Momoh, C. (2004). Attitudes to female genital mutilation. *British Journal of Midwifery, 12*(10), 631–635.

Morison, L., Dirir, A., Elmi, S., Warsame, J., & Dirir, S. (2004). How experiences and attitudes relating to female circumcision vary according to age on arrival in Britain: A study among young Somalis in London. *Ethnicity and Health, 9*(1), 75–100.

Nauright, L. (2005). Preparing nursing professionals for advocacy: Service-learning. In M. de Chesnay (Ed.), *Caring for the vulnerable* (pp. 357–362). Sudbury, MA: Jones and Bartlett.

Naved, R. T., & Persson, L. (2008). Factors associated with physical spousal abuse of women during pregnancy in Bangladesh. *International Family Planning Perspectives, 34*(2), 71–78.

Ndiwane, A. (2008). Laying down the knife may decrease risk of HIV transmission: Cultural practices in Cameroon with implications for public health and policy. *Journal of Cultural Diversity, 15*(2), 2004–2008.

Pattison, N. (2008). Caring for patients after death. *Nursing Standard, 22*(51), 48–56.

Pearson, L. (2003). Understanding the culture of poverty. *Nurse Practitioner, 28*(4), 6.

Perilla, J., Wilson, A. H., Wold, J. L., & Spencer, L. (1998). Listening to migrant voices: Focus groups on health issues. *Journal of Community Health Nursing, 15*(4), 251–264.

Purnell, L. (2000). A description of the Purnell model for cultural competence. *Journal of Transcultural Nursing, 11*(1), 40–46.

Purnell, L. (2002). The Purnell model for cultural competence. *Journal of Transcultural Nursing, 13*(3), 193–196.

Purnell, L., & Paulanka, B. (2003). *Transcultural health care: A culturally competent approach* (2nd ed.). Philadelphia: F. A. Davis.

Racher, F. E., & Annis, R. C. (2007). Respecting culture and honoring diversity in community practice. *Research and Theory for Nursing Practice: An International Journal, 21*(4), 255–270.

Savage, C. L., Xu, Y., Lee, R., Rose, B. L., Kappesser, M., & Anthony, J. S. (2006). A case study in the use of community-based participatory research in public health nursing. *Public Health Nursing, 23*(5), 472–478.

Stevens, C. A. (2006). Being healthy: Voices of adolescent women who are parenting. *Journal for Specialists in Pediatric Nursing, 11*(1), 28–41.

Tsai, J. H. (2006). Xenophobia, ethnic community, and immigrant youths' friendship network formation. *Adolescence, 41*(162), 285–299.

Turton, C. L. (1995). Spiritualized needs of hospitalized Ojibwe people. *Michigan Nurse, 68*(5), 11–12.

Wald, L. (1908). Best helps to the immigrant through the nurse. *American Journal of Nursing, 8*(6), 464–467.

Walle, A. H. (2004). Native Americans and alcoholism therapy: The example of Handsome Lake as a tool of recovery. *Journal of Ethnicity in Substance Abuse, 3*(2), 55–79.

Wells, M. (2000). Beyond cultural competence: A model for individual and institutional cultural development. *Journal of Community Health Nursing, 17*(4), 189–200.

Wilson, A. H., Pittman, K., & Wold, J. (2000). Listening to the quiet voices of Hispanic migrant children about health. *Journal of Pediatric Nursing, 15*(3), 137–147.

Wilson, A., Wold, J., Spencer, L., & Pittman, K. (2000). Primary health care for Hispanic children of migrant farm workers. *Journal of Pediatric Health Care, 14*(5), 209–215.

Wood, D. (2003). Effect of child and family poverty on child health in the United States. *Pediatrics, 112*(3), 707–711.

CHAPTER 8

HITTING THE PAVEMENT:
INTERVENTION OF CASE FINDING
Outreach, Screening, Surveillance,
and Disease and Health Event Investigation

Margaret Macali
Karen Galanowsky
Monte Wagner
Marie Truglio-Londrigan

While visiting in a home recently to look up a case of a one-year-old child that was blind (and will be so permanently, but could have been given its sight if the proper medical care had been given it when born) I also found a seven-year-old boy whose leg was drawn up in a V-shape with the knee quite rigid. I found the child had fallen, broken the leg at the knee, and, never having had a physician, the bones knit in the position described. I referred the case to a specialist on children who performed an operation and, after lying in a hospital six months, the boy left using both his legs. . . . The great work of the visiting nurse, socially, lies in this field, not only relieving petty ailments and dealing with the common diseases, but searching out the cases that other wise go unattended (Steel, 1910, p. 341).

LEARNING OBJECTIVES

At the completion of this chapter, the reader will be able to

- Describe the red wedge of the Minnesota Department of Health Population-Based Public Health Nursing Practice Intervention Wheel Strategies, which includes case finding, outreach, screening, surveillance, and disease and health investigation.

- Verbalize culturally appropriate and congruent ways to initiate these intervention strategies.
- Explore the various ways that public health nurses apply and perform the strategies of case finding, outreach, screening, surveillance, and disease and health investigation.

KEY TERMS

- Case finding
- Disease and health event investigation

- Outreach
- Screening
- Surveillance

The strength of the Minnesota Department of Health Population-Based Public Health Nursing Practice Intervention Wheel Strategies (Keller, Strohschein, & Briske, 2008; Minnesota Department of Health, 2001) is in the identification of specific intervention strategies and the level of practice (systems, community, and individual/family) that are applied by public health nurses who are charged with protecting the public's health. "Protecting the public" are words that have historically inspired a few so that the many may live healthy lives. The purpose of this chapter is to present to the reader one section of the intervention wheel (red section) which includes case finding, outreach, screening, surveillance, and disease and health event investigation. **Case finding**, as an intervention strategy, takes place at the individual/family level of practice.

This chapter is divided into several sections. The first is the description of these key intervention strategies. The second is a demonstration of how these intervention strategies are applied within the context of several public health issues. The third is the presentation of a case study so that readers may understand the process of these interventions. The final section is a look at the case study and the application of the intervention strategies to the various levels of practice, including individual/family, community, and system.

MINNESOTA DEPARTMENT OF HEALTH POPULATION-BASED PUBLIC HEALTH NURSING PRACTICE INTERVENTION WHEEL STRATEGIES

Case Finding

Case finding is exactly what the words imply: to find new cases for early identification of a client with a particular disease or to find cases where particular contact person(s) may be at risk for developing a particular disease. Liebman, Lamberti, and Altice (2002) noted that case finding is important from several points of view. First, by identifying individuals with a particular disease, early treatment may

be provided in a timely way, thus resulting in reduced morbidity. Second, the identification of individual(s) prevents further transmission of the disease. Finally, in addition to the early identification of individual(s) with disease through case finding, the process of case finding is also significant in the identification of high-risk individual(s) and "serves as an important opportunity for health education and teaching to promote primary prevention of disease, even among those found not to be infected" (p. 345).

Case finding is essential to identify individuals at risk for disease. Case finding is also important for early diagnosis of those "with" infectious and noninfectious disease(s), including foodborne and waterborne illnesses. In recent years the process of case finding has also been instrumental in the identification of individuals experiencing still other noninfectious disease(s), including chronic illness, mental health issues such as anxiety and depression, and social, spiritual, emotional, or environmental issues including abuse, violence, and addictions. Skjerve et al. (2007), for example, studied the use of a cognitive case-finding instrument known as the seven-minute screen in a population of older adults for the identification of dementia. Jack, Jamuson, Wathen, and MacMillan (2008) explored public health nurse perceptions of **screening** for intimate partner violence and noted that "screening using a standard set of question is difficult to implement . . . the standard practice is to assess for mothers' exposure to IPV during in-depth assessment of the family; the nature of in-depth assessment having a case-finding rather than screening approach" (p. 150) is beneficial. Puddifoot et al. (2007) looked at anxiety as a treatable condition that frequently goes untreated because it is not diagnosed. The key question here is how to find the unidentified case. These researchers studied whether two simple written questions would aid in the identification of anxiety in a particular person, thus facilitating case finding and ultimate treatment. Similarly, Damush et al. (2008) noted how post-stroke depression is often undiagnosed and ultimately untreated, resulting in an increase in morbidity and mortality. The purpose of this study was to determine if detecting patients with post-stroke depression in administrative databases using a case-finding algorithm among veteran stroke survivors would be possible. The essence of case finding in these particular situations is that this process identifies individuals in need and connects those individuals to resources such as treatments, support groups, agencies, counseling, and other support services. This echoes the words of Keller and colleagues (2008), who stated "case finding locates individuals and families with identified risk and connects them with resources" (p. 199). There are various strategies that the public health nurse may use that facilitate and sustain this case-finding process. One only needs to ask how to find these cases. The answer is outreach, screening, surveillance, and disease and health event investigation.

Outreach

The public health nurse may use various strategies to engage in case finding. One of these strategies is **outreach**. The word "outreach" creates a vision for us in which the public health nurse or other public health practitioner actually reaches out into the community and connects with and helps those in need. Keller et al. (2008) noted that "outreach locates populations of interest or populations at risk and provides information about the nature of the concern, what can be done about it and how services can be obtained" (p. 199). Rajabiun et al. (2007) described a qualitative study in which they investigated the process of engagement in HIV medical care. Analysis of the data demonstrated that the participants frequently cycled in and out of care based on a number of influences. The researchers identified that those individuals who had cycled out of care must be found so that care could be reestablished. Outreach, however, was identified as an intervention that played a significant role in connecting participants back to the needed care, thus enhancing care of the individual and in the process protecting the public.

The process of outreach is not a simple one. The public health nurse must take into account the specific population of interest, the demographics of that population, the particular problem that needs to be addressed, where they live, the resources available to them, that particular population's values and beliefs, how they live in the world, and whether or not they want to be found. Although the entire process is rather complicated, the actual enactment requires four important steps.

The first is how the outreach will be carried out so that the public health nurse can gain access to the population and find those in need, hence case finding. Is it via mobile van, motorcycle, walking in the community, telephone calls, knocking on doors, or any other method of connecting with the population of interest? In a school-based community health course, Truglio-Londrigan et al. (2000) worked with community health nursing students in a senior housing project. To gain access to the population of older adults living in the senior housing project to identify their individual needs, the students knocked on the 99 doors of the building. The students in this course believed that the doors in the apartment buildings were there for protection by keeping people out, but they were actually a barrier to care and services. Their answer to this was to knock on every single door and meet every single person living in the apartment complex. Nandi et al. (2008) assessed access to and use of health services in Mexican-born undocumented individuals in New York City. To gain access to this population, recruitment took place in communities with large populations of Mexican immigrants. Areas were selected in two phases. In the first the U.S. Census data were used to identify neighborhoods with the highest numbers of the targeted population. The second step in the process was a walk-through of the key identified neighborhoods to conduct interviews. Finally, Liebman et al. (2002) noted that a mobile van was an innovative approach to case finding. The authors identified that the use of the van was a way for professionals to move out into communities and gain access to hard-to-reach populations who may not come into traditional health clinics.

The photo on this page provides an example on how one particular public health nurse reached out and gained access to populations of interest. As you examine this photo, look at the nurse and imagine that it is you in the photo. What are you thinking? Who are you visiting? Where do they live? What do you suppose you will find when you reach the end of your destination? What type of services do you suppose you will provide?

A second important consideration is the person who will be doing the out-

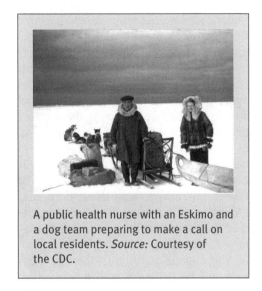

A public health nurse with an Eskimo and a dog team preparing to make a call on local residents. *Source:* Courtesy of the CDC.

reach. Will the person be a lay worker who lives in the community and a member of the population? Mock et al. (2007) wanted to promote cervical cancer screening among Vietnamese American women. To determine the effectiveness of this approach, a study was designed to look at lay workers who did the outreach plus media-based education (combined intervention) and media-based education only. Vietnamese woman acted in the role of lay outreach coordinators and lay health workers. Ultimately, the combined intervention motivated more Vietnamese American women to obtain their Pap tests than did media education alone, thus identifying that the person doing the outreach may have a significant impact on whether or not individuals in need will be found and ultimately connected with the needed care and/or resources. Findley et al. (2008) presented a coalition-led childhood immunization program that included an outreach component in which trained peer educators were used. Other elements of this initiative included bilingual and community appropriate materials as well as reminders to parents. Results demonstrated that students enrolled in this program were more likely to receive timely immunizations than children not enrolled in the program, again demonstrating the importance of finding cases and connecting those cases to needed care and resources. Toole et al. (2007) wanted to conduct a survey of homeless individuals to determine their needs. The difficult nature of this type of research is how to find these homeless individuals. The researchers enlisted former homeless, trained, research assistants to aid in the process.

A third consideration is how the message will be delivered to the population once the connection is established. Is it via the newspaper, flyers, booklets, television ads, songs, radio announcements, Internet advertisement, or some other technological advancement not yet discovered? The importance of knowing the target population is critical. The public health nurse may have a plan for an outreach process that is well developed and the population is identified and accessible. But, if the message is developed in a way that is not congruent with the population, the message will miss its mark. For example, several years ago community health nursing students identified a need in conjunction with a county department of health and the office on aging in a local county. That need was to deliver nutritional education to the population of older adults living in a particular community. The community students went to the nutrition center and spoke with the older adults, and indeed these older adults concurred that programs on nutrition would be very beneficial for those who use the nutrition center. The community students spent a great deal of time in the development of the program.

On the day in which the program was delivered, this author was conducting an observation and noted that students arrived in costumes of the "Fruit of the Loom Guys" traditionally seen on the television undergarment commercials. The costumes were great and the older adults loved them. When the students progressed up to the stage to deliver the message, it was very clear that while their presentation was intriguing to the older adults the minute they began to deliver their message they lost the attention of their population. The community students had developed a rap song about the food groups. In the audience the older adults began to look confused, many asking, "What are they saying?" The message was lost because the connection was lost. The message that the students developed was not congruent with the population they were targeting. This is similar to concepts pertaining to health teaching and educational programming, covered in greater detail in Chapter 10.

Finally, the fourth component for consideration is where the final point of contact or service in the outreach process is being rendered. The example given above concerning the presentation of a nutritional program for older adults in a community nutrition site is an example of the final point of contact for the program delivery. Toole et al. (2007) discussed the dilemma of the homeless and raised the question of where they may go when they first become homeless. The lack of access to services creates a situation where the homeless person will increasingly be more likely to experience poor health. The investigators of this research had to think about how they could access this population to hear the voices of this vulnerable population. The researchers knew if they were going to be successful in gaining access to this population and to find individuals, they must go to where they were. These areas included "(i) unsheltered enclaves (including abandoned buildings, cars and outdoor) and congregate eating facilities without sleeping quarters; (ii) emergency shelters; and (iii) transitional housing or single room occupancy (SRO) dwellings . . ." (p. 448). It is not unheard of for public health nurses to ride city buses day and night into neighborhoods where they know their clients travel, in an attempt to find them and give the care they may need. **Table 8-1** provides examples of point of contact for targeted populations.

SCREENING

Another strategy that public health nurses may decide to use in their process of case finding is screening. Keller et al. (2008) stated that "screening identifies individuals with unrecognized health risk factors or asymptomatic disease conditions in populations" (p. 199). Leavell and

Clark (1965) addressed the concept of screening as an intervention strategy that is beneficial in its ability to engage in case finding for individual(s). The overall purpose of this activity is to engage in early identification of a disease, thus facilitating prompt treatment. This early identification is considered in the secondary level of prevention during the early pathogenesis period of time when the person(s) is asymptomatic. The benefits of screening and early identification of disease are numerous:

- Early detection and diagnosis leading to early treatment
- Early detection breaking the chain of transmission and development of new cases
- Early detection leading to a decrease in morbidity and mortality
- Early detection leading to lower costs pertaining to treatments
- Early detection protecting the community and/or the targeted population

Table 8-1 Examples of Outreach and Gaining Access to Targeted Populations

Targeted Individuals, Families, and Populations	Mechanism of Outreach and Access
Mothers and caretakers of preschool-age children	Health promotion safety educational programs in park settings as children engage in play
Heads of households responsible for purchasing food and cooking	Health promotion educational programs on nutrition outside food stores and accompanying the person as they shop up and down the food aisle
Day workers waiting to begin their day	Health promotion programs on immunizations and the provision of such at pick-up sites
Adolescents engaging in extreme sports	Health promotion programs on use of safety pads at a skate park

This improvement in health and well-being is documented in the literature. Hartge and Berg (2007) noted that "women can improve their prospects for long-term health by being screened for several cancers with tests proved to decrease morbidity and mortality from colorectal, breast, and cervical cancer" (p. 66). Liebman and coworkers (2002) identified that case finding via screening not only is significant because it breaks the chain of further transmission to new diagnosed cases, but it may identify individuals who present with high-risk behavior. This knowledge therefore provides opportunities for education focusing on primary prevention and health promotion. This identification of individuals at risk for a disease through screening presents with the same benefits listed above and also includes the following:

- Early detection of high-risk behaviors and modifiable risk factors leading to prevention of disease
- Early detection leading to empowerment of the person or the population being targeted
- Early detection leading to improvement in lifestyle and quality of life

The application of screening to identify individuals at risk for developing disease takes us closer to health promotion and disease prevention. Wimbush and Peters (2000) described the implementation of a cardiovascular-specific genogram that may be used to identify persons at risk for cerebrovascular disease within families. These authors further described the complex array of risk factors associated with cerebrovascular disease and noted the differences between modifiable risk factors, such as lack of exercise, high fat and high sodium diets, high blood cholesterol,

obesity, smoking, high blood pressure, and stress, as compared with nonmodifiable risk factors, such as age, gender, and genetic predisposition. The application of the genogram, a tool used to illustrate family health and relationship patterns over generations, facilitates the public health nurse's understanding of risks present in a family and which of those risks are modifiable. The use of the genogram, in this way, demonstrated promise as a tool to obtain data to inform the public health nurse as to individuals at risk for cerebrovascular disease. Fedder, Desai, and Maciunskaite (2006) similarly presented a strategy that was based on an infectious disease management model that would improve early detection. The authors proposed that practitioners consider "a chronic disease event—e.g., a heart attack, breast cancer diagnosis, or diabetes mellitus diagnosis—as the index case and then screen the siblings and progeny (their brothers, sisters, and children), who are predictably at higher risk . . ." (p. 331). Again, the overall goal is to increase awareness and target risky behavior in others, facilitating prevention and health promotion.

Screening takes place in individual and mass screening models. Screening for the individual takes place as a public health nurse working with one person performs a screening test such as a blood pressure. Conversely, a mass screening may be a situation where a particular group is targeted for a particular screening program pertaining to one disease or even multiple diseases. The reason the particular group may be targeted has to do with data derived either from an assessment or surveillance data. These data are a source of information for the public health nurse and inform them in their decision making. The data may indicate that the particular group in question is at greater risk for the development of a particular disease such as diabetes. In this case the public health nurse may engage in an initiative to develop and implement a mass screening to identify new cases of this disease.

The benefits of screening are well documented; however, there are limitations as well. One such limitation is what happens to the individual once he or she is informed that the screening test just performed is positive. For example, in the mass screening above, what happens to an individual who is told that his or her blood sugar level is elevated? What type of follow-up is provided? What good is this type of mass screening if the public health nurse finds a case but there is no mechanism to ensure that the individual has access to care for diagnosis, treatment, and follow-up? The University of Medicine and Dentistry of New Jersey Mobile Health Care Project addressed this issue. They established a collaborative, joint partnership initiative with the Children's Health Fund where a nurse-faculty managed mobile healthcare unit provided care to the underserved population of Newark, New Jersey. One of the goals of this initiative was to provide health promotion services in the form of screenings. Individuals with positive findings were referred to the University of Medicine and Dentistry of New Jersey hospitals and affiliates for treatment and referral (McNeal, 2008), thus making sure people had access to the care they needed.

Although the benefits of screening are well known, the public health nurse and other public health practitioners must engage in continual dialogue in terms of

deciding if a disease is in fact screenable. Escriba-Aguir, Ruiz-Perez, and Saurel-Cubizolles (2007) discussed this issue and identified that if a screening program is to be undertaken, several assumptions must be met: "(a) existence of a test with good sensibility and specificity, (b) high incidence of the problem, (c) existence of appropriate intervention and support measures. . . , and (d) the diagnostic tool should be acceptable for the population to whom it is aimed and for professionals who apply it" (p. 133).

The issue of sensibility and specificity is an important one. The UK National Screening Committee (2008) offers advice and recommendations about screening based on evidence: "In any screening program, there is an irreducible minimum of false positive results (wrongly reported as having the condition) and false negative results (wrongly reported as not having the condition)" (n.p.). This concern is further defined by others when they speak to the concepts of sensitivity and specificity to address this issue. "Sensitivity quantifies how accurately the test identifies those *with* the condition or trait. . . . Specificity indicates how accurately the test identifies those *without* the condition or trait. . . ." (McKeown & Hilfinger Messias, 2008, p. 261).

It is evident that there are also ethical and economic considerations to be considered in these cases. For example, the public health nurse and other public health practitioners need to consider the following questions with regard to these possibilities. How ethical is it to conduct screening tests that may inform people they have a disease when they do not? Will these individuals engage in unnecessary testing? Who will pay for the cost of this unnecessary testing? Are there any adverse effects of this unnecessary testing? What is the emotional trauma that the individual will experience and is this important to consider? How ethical is it to conduct screening tests that may inform people that they do not have a disease when in fact they do? What will happen to these individuals? How much later will they be diagnosed and will the diagnosis be too late for any effective treatment modality? What is the emotional trauma that this individual will experience?

The UK National Screening Committee also addresses the final three assumptions put forth by Escriba-Aguir et al. (2007) in the development of the criteria that must be met before initiation of screening. These criteria are presented in **Table 8-2**.

Public health nurses and other public health practitioners may also refer to the work of the U.S. Preventive Services Task Force (USPSTF) for practice decisions with regard to the above. The USPSTF, sponsored by the Agency for Healthcare Research and Quality, is a panel of experts in prevention and primary care. The USPSTF conducts rigorous systematic assessments of evidence for the effectiveness of preventive services such as screening, counseling, and preventive medications. The mission of the USPSTF is to "evaluate the benefits of individual services based on age, gender, and risk factor for disease; make recommendations about which preventive services should be incorporated routinely into primary medical care and for which populations and identify a research agenda for clinical preventive care" (USPSTF, 2007, n.p). Based on these evaluations the USPSTF assigns one of five letter grades to each of its recommendations (A, B, C, D, or I). **Box 8-1** provides an explanation of this grading system and its application for practice.

As of October 2008 there were new screening guidelines for colorectal cancer. The USPSTF recommends screening for colorectal cancer using fecal occult blood testing, sigmoidoscopy, or colonoscopy in adults beginning at age 50 years and continuing until age 75 years. This guideline was given a grade A recommendation. As seen in Box 8-1, the grade A means that the USPSTF strongly recommends that clinicians routinely provide the service to eligible patients, thus providing guidance to healthcare providers in the clinical practice setting. The guidelines for this particular situation are listed as grade A recommendation for the age group 50 to 75 years but not for those ages 76 to 85 years. The USPSTF recommends against routine screening for colorectal cancer in adults ages 76 to 85 years. There may be considerations that support colorectal cancer screening in an individual patient. In this situation the grade of C recommendation means the USPSTF makes no recommendation for or against routine provision of the service. Again, these recommendations provide guidance to the healthcare provider in the clinical practice setting.

Screening is an important strategy for case finding; however, as identified above there are challenges that must be addressed. Wald (2007) addressed these challenges in an editorial, noting that the type of quantitative information needed on screening performance of the test is usually not even known. "The culture needs to change, so that screening is subject to professional scientific assessment before it is promoted to the public" (Wald, 2007, p. 1).

Table 8-2 Essential Criteria to Be Met When Deciding to Screen or Not to Screen

Disease	Test	Treatment	Cost	Programming
The condition should be an important health problem.	The test must be simple, safe, precise, and valid.	There must be evidence that there is an effective treatment for the condition and that early treatment will lead to better outcomes.	There is evidence as to the cost-effectiveness of the screening in relation to interventions and outcomes.	There is evidence from randomized controlled trials that the screening program is effective in the reduction of mortality and morbidity.
The epidemiology of the disease must be understood.	The test must be acceptable to both the population and the healthcare providers administering the test.			The benefits of the screening program outweigh the physical and psychological harm, if any.
	There should be criteria and/or a protocol on what the next steps are for further care if an individual tests positive.			There should be protocols for the implementation and evaluation of the screening program, including set standards for staffing, facilities, and program management.

Source: Adapted from UK National Screening Committee (2003).

BOX **8-1** USPSTF Grade Definitions

The USPSTF grades its recommendations according to one of five classifications (A, B, C, D, I), reflecting the strength of evidence and magnitude of net benefit (benefits minus harms).

A: The USPSTF strongly recommends that clinicians provide [the service] to eligible patients. *The USPSTF found good evidence that [the service] improves important health outcomes and concludes that benefits substantially outweigh harms.*

B: The USPSTF recommends that clinicians provide [this service] to eligible patients. *The USPSTF found at least fair evidence that [the service] improves important health outcomes and concludes that benefits outweigh harms.*

C: The USPSTF makes no recommendation for or against routine provision of [the service]. *The USPSTF found at least fair evidence that [the service] can improve health outcomes but concludes that the balance of benefits and harms is too close to justify a general recommendation.*

D: The USPSTF recommends against routinely providing [the service] to asymptomatic patients. *The USPSTF found at least fair evidence that [the service] is ineffective or that harms outweigh benefits.*

I: The USPSTF concludes that the evidence is insufficient to recommend for or against routinely providing [the service]. *Evidence that the [service] is effective is lacking, of poor quality, or conflicting and the balance of benefits and harms cannot be determined.*

Source: Adapted from U.S. Department of Health and Human Services, Agency for Healthcare Research and Quality, U.S. Preventative Task Force. (2007). Grade definitions: Strength of recommendations. Retrieved December 8, 2008, from http://www.ahrq.gov/clinic/3rduspstf/ratings.htm

---

SURVEILLANCE

The oldest **surveillance** systems date back centuries. John Snow's work with cholera in London in 1854 is an example of public health surveillance and disease and health investigation, discussed later in this chapter. These past surveillance processes focused on communicable diseases, leading to interventions such as quarantine. Today public health surveillance includes the monitoring of communicable diseases and chronic illness, birth defects, behaviors, and injury. Interventions have expanded to include disease control and prevention.

Klaucke et al. (1988) stated, "Epidemiologic surveillance is the ongoing and systematic collection, analysis, and interpretation of health data in the process of describing and monitoring a health event" (p. 1). The application of public health surveillance data is noted by the U.S. Department of Health and Human Services and Centers for Disease Control and Prevention (U.S. DHHS/CDC, 2006) as data that can be "useful in setting priorities, planning, and conducting disease control programs, and in assessing the effectiveness of control efforts" (p. 337). This public health surveillance provides data that informs the public health nurse about patterns of disease occurrence and the potential for disease in a population, thus facilitating initiatives in disease prevention. The term "public health surveillance" is presently used in reference to the monitoring of health events in populations as opposed to medical surveillance, which describes the monitoring of individuals (U.S. DHHS/CDC, 1992, 2006).

A review of the definition of public health surveillance informs the public health nurse of the exact nature of the process. This process may be viewed in **Box 8-2**.

The first step in the systematic public health surveillance process is that of *data collection*. This collection takes place as data are reported by those individuals in practice. Each state has a system of reporting that guides those in practice as to the disease and/or conditions that must be reported, who is responsible for reporting, what information is reported, to whom and how quickly the information must be reported (U.S. DHHS/CDC, 1992, 2006). Diseases that are reported are known as notifiable diseases. These diseases are revised periodically because diseases are added to the list and others are deleted. **Box 8-3** is an example of notifiable diseases.

Those responsible for reporting notifiable diseases generally include physicians, dentists, nurses, medical examiners, administrators of hospitals, clinics, nursing homes, schools, and nurseries, to name a few. The type of disease and the threat to the public determine how quickly the person doing the reporting has to submit the case report. For example, a disease that poses great threat may have to be reported immediately, whereas others may have a longer period of time. The case report is usually sent to the local department of health, which then forwards the case report to the state department of health. In some cases information may then be sent to the CDC and the World Health Organization. In a situation where the healthcare provider sends the case report to the department of health, passive surveillance is taking form. In a situation where a member of the department of health goes out into the community to obtain information, active surveillance is taking form.

The second step in the surveillance process is the analysis of data. As data are collected, they are continually being monitored and analyzed. Sources of data that may be analyzed include those listed in **Box 8-4**.

According to the U.S. DHHS/CDC (1992, 2006), the data are first monitored and analyzed for descriptive information such as time, place, and person. In addition, the public health nurse and other public health practitioners, such as the epidemiologist, must monitor and analyze the data and determine if what they are viewing is expected or different. They must also be able to determine what that difference is. One way of doing this is to look at the recent reported data and to compare those data to previous years, looking for trends and patterns.

BOX **8-2** **Systematic Public Health Surveillance Process**

Collection of data

Analysis of data

Interpretation of data

Dissemination of data

Public health action

Source: U.S. DHHS/CDC (2006).

BOX 8-3 Nationally Notifiable Infectious Diseases: United States 2008

Acquired immune deficiency syndrome (AIDS)

Anthrax

Arboviral neuroinvasive and non-neuroinvasive diseases

- California serogroup virus disease
- Eastern equine encephalitis virus disease
- Powassan virus disease
- St. Louis encephalitis virus disease
- West Nile virus disease
- Western equine encephalitis virus disease

Botulism

- Botulism, foodborne
- Botulism, infant
- Botulism, other (wound and unspecified)

Brucellosis

Chancroid

Chlamydia trachomatis, genital infections

Cholera

Coccidioidomycosis

Cryptosporidiosis

Cyclosporiasis

Diphtheria

Ehrlichiosis/anaplasmosis

- *Ehrlichia chaffeensis*
- *Ehrlichia ewingii*

- *Anaplasma phagocytophilum*
- Undetermined

Giardiasis

Gonorrhea

Haemophilus influenzae, invasive disease

Hansen disease (leprosy)

Hantavirus pulmonary syndrome

Hemolytic uremic syndrome, postdiarrheal

Hepatitis, viral, acute

- Hepatitis A, acute
- Hepatitis B, acute
- Hepatitis B virus, perinatal infection
- Hepatitis, C, acute

Hepatitis, viral, chronic

- Chronic hepatitis B
- Hepatitis C virus infection (past or present)

HIV infection

- HIV infection, adult($\geq$13 years)
- HIV infection, pediatric (<13 years)

Influenza-associated pediatric mortality

Legionellosis

Listeriosis

Lyme disease

Malaria

Measles

Meningococcal disease

Mumps

BOX **8-3**   **Nationally Notifiable Infectious Diseases: United States 2008 (continued)**

Novel influenza A virus infections

Pertussis

Plague

Poliomyelitis, paralytic

Poliovirus infection, nonparalytic

Psittacosis

Q Fever

Rabies

- Rabies, animal
- Rabies, human

Rocky Mountain spotted fever

Rubella

Rubella, congenital syndrome

Salmonellosis

Severe acute respiratory syndrome–associated coronavirus (SARS-CoV) disease

Shiga toxin-producing *Escherichia coli* (STEC)

Shigellosis

Smallpox

Streptococcal disease, invasive, group A

Streptococcal toxic shock syndrome

Streptococcus pneumoniae, drug resistant, invasive disease

Streptococcus pneumoniae, invasive disease non–drug resistant, in children < 5 years of age

Syphilis

- Syphilis, primary
- Syphilis, secondary
- Syphilis, latent
- Syphilis, early latent
- Syphilis, late latent
- Syphilis, latent, unknown duration
- Neurosyphilis
- Syphilis, late, non-neurological
- Syphilitic stillbirth

Syphilis, congenital

Tetanus

Toxic shock syndrome (other than streptococcal)

Trichinellosis (trichinosis)

Tuberculosis

Tularemia

Typhoid fever

Vancomycin-intermediate *Staphylococcus aureus* (VISA)

Vancomycin-resistant *Staphylococcus aureus* (VRSA)

Varicella (morbidity)

Varicella (deaths only)

Vibriosis

Yellow fever

Source: Adapted from Centers for Disease Control and Prevention. (2008). Notifiable disease surveillance system. Retrieved December 7, 2008, from http://www.cdc.gov/ncphi/disss/nndss/PHS/infdis2008.htm

---

BOX 8-4 Examples of Sources of Data and Reports

Mortality reports

Morbidity reports

Vital statistics

Notifiable disease reports

Laboratory data

Specific topics (cancer registry, adverse drug reactions,

injury surveillance systems, occupational illness)

Birth defects monitoring programs

Surveys (National Health Interview Survey, National Health
and Nutrition Examination Survey)

Source: Adapted from U.S. DHHS/CDC (1992, 2006).

The *interpretation of data* is the next step in the surveillance process. As the public health nurse and/or the epidemiologist notes a difference in the expected pattern in a particular population, this is a signal to those involved that additional investigation is necessary and that the information must be disseminated to those in practice for action.

The *dissemination* of this surveillance data, the fourth step, takes place as information is sent to those in the practice setting to "inform and motivate" (U.S. DHHS/CDC, 2006, p. 367). During an outbreak, epidemic, natural disaster, or potential terror event, interpretation and dissemination of data are both ongoing and circular, thus affecting public health actions.

The final step in the systematic public health surveillance process is that of *action*. The entire process would be useless if no action was taken. The action signifies the response to the data, and this response is in the form of an intervention for change. These interventions may be in the form of a coalition whose members work together in a partnership to target a particular population and pool their resources for action and change. The action for change may also be in the form of targeting of monies for programming, research, and policy development.

The material presented above signifies that the public health surveillance process is really a circular process. **Figure 8-1** is a pictorial of this process.

EFFECTIVENESS/TECHNOLOGY

The World Health Organization (2003, p. vii) identified key factors that are essential if a systematic public health surveillance system is to be effective:

1. Useful
2. Efficient
3. Flexible

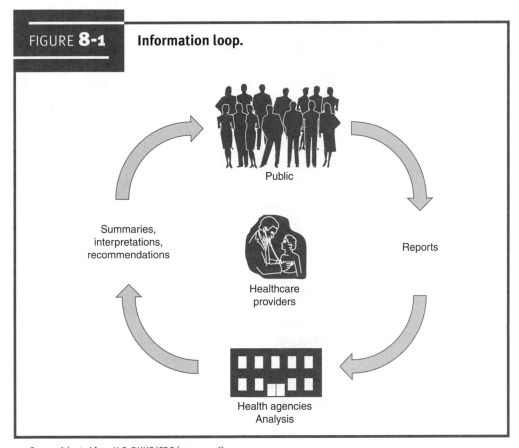

FIGURE **8-1** **Information loop.**

Public

Summaries,
interpretations,
recommendations

Healthcare
providers

Reports

Health agencies
Analysis

Source: Adapted from U.S. DHHS/CDC (1992, 2006).

4. Representative
5. Simple

The use of technology is critical to this. Technology as a tool that facilitates, tracks, and disseminates data and other sources of health information is addressed by the World Health Organization (2008, p. 86) in the following statement: "A well functioning health information system is one that generates reliable and timely strategic health information on which to base decisions at different levels of the health system." Chapter 6 is dedicated to technology and public health.

Disease and Health Event Investigation

The final intervention is that of disease and health investigation. Keller et al. (2008) noted that disease and health investigation "systematically gathers and analyzes data regarding threats to the health of populations, ascertains the source of the threat, identifies cases and others at risk, and determines control measures" (p. 199). The entire process may be viewed in **Box 8-5**.

For public health nurses and other public health practitioners, the start of

---

BOX **8-5**   **Process of Disease and Health Event Investigation**

Identifying the source of the threat

Identifying cases

Identifying the contacts

Identifying others at risk

Determining control measures

Communication with individuals, families, and populations

Source: Adapted from Minnesota Department of Health (2001).

---

any investigation begins with an event, such as disease, that presents in an individual(s). The public health nurse and/or other public health practitioner begin the task of investigation by asking questions. These questions serve as a reminder to the epidemiological concepts of the agent, host, and the environment discussed earlier in this text. For example, the investigator may ask these questions: Who is affected? Are there any other people affected? Have these people anything in common or are they connected in any way? Where do the people live? Did they venture into any other areas that they do not commonly go to? Where do they live, work, go to school, play etc.? Is there a particular time that is presenting as a pattern, for example during the summer when it is very humid with much rain?

Other data are essential to gather in this systematic process. For example, the public health nurse and other public health practitioners need to go out into the field and conduct direct observation and speak to people in the communities. This is critical to the process because

subjective information from individuals in the community may bring forth information that is important to the success of the investigation. Collecting specimens is also of importance to determine what the offending agent is. It is very important to realize that this process is not a one-time deal. In other words, as the public health nurse engages in this investigation, he or she may have to go out into the field not once or twice but multiple times to ensure that the data gathered are reliable and valid. They must share the information with others and confer findings. Critical thinking is key to the success of the investigation.

At the completion of the investigation, the public health nurse will come to know what the problem is and what intervention will correct the issue. Because the public health nurse is dealing with a population, any education and communication that take place must be done from a population perspective. This perspective is discussed in Chapter 10. Of course, as with any process, once the interventions are initiated, there must be careful monitoring and surveillance to see what the outcome is and if the intervention is a success or not. One of the most famous examples of this **disease and health event investigation** took place in the middle of the 19th century. The investigator was an anesthesiologist by the name of John Snow. **Box 8-6** describes the disease and health investigation of cholera.

PUBLIC HEALTH ISSUES IN PRACTICE

Public health nursing combines nursing practice and public health sciences, focuses on populations even when dealing with individuals, and is always connected with government at a local, county, state, and/or federal level. Public health nursing may start at the population level, working down to the individual index case, which Venes (2005) defined as "the individual whose condition leads to an investigation" (p. 1090); or it may start with the index case, working up to the population at risk. Either way, the population is always the main focus and the governmental and/or legal relationship is always a part of what guides the practice. Keller, Stohschein, Lia-Hoagberg, and Schaffer (2004) described public health nursing services to "individuals or families as population based because those individuals are part of a targeted constituency" and services to them "clearly contribute to improving the overall health status of that population" (p. 457). Much of public health practice, including public health nursing practice, is based on legislation such as sanitary and communicable disease laws. It is because federal, state, and local laws require enforcement that public health nursing can be described as a combination of nursing practice and public health sciences, including the enforcement of federal, state, or local health laws. The U.S. DHHS and the CDC guide public health practice, including public health nursing at the federal level, whereas the State Commissioner of Health and each state's legislated Standards of Performance for Local Boards of Health guide the practice at a local level. As a result many public health nurses may find they first consult with their state health department rather than the CDC for direction in case finding, surveillance, outreach, and disease investigation. Because of this, certain examples provided within this chapter relate to the specific state health department within which the writers function.

Tuberculosis (TB) control, investigation of foodborne illnesses, and rabies prevention, exposure, and follow-up are examples of practice areas guided by the aforementioned federal regulatory agencies and each state's legislative practice standards. TB, foodborne illness, and rabies are all listed as notifiable at the federal level (see Box 8-3), but enforcement of this mandate occurs at the local and state levels. Public health nurses participate in this mandate by ensuring that those individuals already ill receive the appropriate treatment, that contacts to index cases are adequately managed, and by investigating and intervening in outbreaks (CDC, 2006). A presentation of these diseases along with an exploration on the application of the Minnesota Department of Health intervention wheel follows.

Public Health Issue: TB

The New Jersey Department of Health and Senior Services (NJDHSS, 2004)

BOX **8-6** Disease and Health Investigation of Cholera by John Snow

In 1854 John Snow conducted an investigation of a cholera outbreak in London's Golden Square. Initially, John Snow determined who was afflicted with the signs and symptoms of the cholera, then he identified where they lived. Next, Snow took this information and placed it on a map of Golden Square. By doing this he had a clear picture of all the cases of cholera in front of him. The picture with all the spots created a visual image that permitted him to "see" more clearly the patterns and clusters of cases. The map is shown on page 207.

Snow believed that the source of the cholera was water, and because of this he also marked on the map the locations of water pumps used by the population of Golden Square to get their daily water supply. He immediately noted that more cases were around pump A than around pumps B and C.

Snow knew he must talk with the people of Golden Square, so he went out into the community and asked questions. What he found was that the people of Golden Square knew that something was wrong with pump B and as a result they stayed away from it and would not use the water. He also found out that pump C was not accessible to the people of Golden Square; thus they did not use it. At that point he had an idea. He thought that pump A, known as the Broad Street Pump, might be the source for the cholera. But, he also noticed that directly east of pump A there were no cholera cases.

This did not make any sense to him, so once again he investigated by asking key questions and making observations. He discovered that the people directly to the east of pump A obtained their water from a very deep well situated in a local brewery. He also found that people who worked in the brewery had a daily allotment of malt liquor. Thus these people were protected because their source of water was derived from two safe supplies. To further his investigation Snow then returned to those who were afflicted with cholera or who had lost loved ones and determined that the one item that all these individuals had was that they obtained their water from pump A. This investigation led to changes in that people who knew that pump A was the contaminated source ceased using this pump and therefore halted the cholera outbreak.

(continues)

Source: From U.S. DHHS/CDC (1992, 2006).

defines *Mycobacterium tuberculosis* complex as the etiologic agent that causes the communicable disease of TB. This TB complex includes *M. tuberculosis* and *Mycobacterium africanum*, both primarily from humans, and *Mycobacterium bovis*, which originates from cattle (NJDHSS, 2004). In concert with the CDC, the

BOX **8-6** **Disease and Health Investigation of Cholera by John Snow (continued)**

NJDHSS (2004) describes the occurrence of TB as a result of or contact with airborne droplet nuclei from infectious persons when they cough, sing, or sneeze. "Tuberculosis is a mycobacterial disease, which starts as a pulmonary infection. Early lung lesions commonly heal and leave no residual changes except occasional pulmonary or tracheobronchial lymph node calcifications" (p. 1). In es-

sence, the person has become infected by the bacilli, but this is a latent foci; the individual is neither sick nor communicable and the diagnosis is latent TB infection. Acute pulmonary TB is a result of reactivation of the latent TB infection or a reinfection. A sputum positive for acid-fast bacilli with abnormal chest x-ray leads to a presumptive diagnosis, and the pulmonary TB diagnosis is confirmed by isolating *M. tuberculosis* on culture. Pulmonary and laryngeal TB are the most contagious, and close prolonged exposure to the index case can lead to infection of the contacts (NJDHSS, 2004).

The NJDHSS (2004) provides surveillance case definitions of TB as confirmed and probable. *Confirmed* requires a positive Mantoux tuberculin skin test (TST) and presenting symptoms compatible with active TB that improve while receiving antitubercular medication or with abnormal chest radiographic consistent with active TB while receiving antituberculosis medications and/or one of the specific and acceptable positive laboratory criteria such as isolation of *M. tuberculosis* from a clinical specimen. *Probable* is any suspected case meeting some of the confirmed criteria but still under further evaluation (NJDHSS, 2004, pp. 2–3).

Health providers are expected to report within 24 hours to the state department of health any confirmed or probable TB case(s). This type of reporting is considered *passive surveillance* because the state receives the report without any specific action on its part. This reporting then initiates a series of activities such as *case finding, outreach, active surveillance,* and *disease investigation*, all located under the banner of TB control.

TB control starts with an individual index case; outreaches to family and other close contacts; expands to workplace, school, or other potential exposure sites; and ultimately relates to the population at large. It is the larger population that public health nursing wants to keep safe. In helping specific individuals achieve health, the public health nurse protects the population.

During the case finding and contact disease investigation stages, population groups are considered at risk based on their exposure to the index case. Each person's closeness to the index case, length of exposure time, and the specific exposure environment are all factored into determination of risk. During the ensuing disease and health event investigation, at-risk populations are interviewed and skin tested (*screened*) to determine their health status. Data information is circular as viewed in Figure 8-1; during this process surveillance is active.

For pulmonary and laryngeal TB cases, treatment is required by law and includes medical management and the potential for directly observed therapy. Directly observed therapy is based on standards of care developed from practice-based research. NJDHSS (2007) defined directly observed therapy as the "direct observation by a health care worker of a patient's ingestion of anti-TB medications at a frequency prescribed by the treating physician" (p. 24). In addition, it "provides the opportunity to identify previously unknown contacts to infectious TB cases, [may help to] identify undisclosed substance abuse [and] allows [for] the health care worker to build a therapeutic relationship with the client" (NJDHSS, 2007, p. 24).

Treatment is based on the diagnosis and on the state of resistance exhibited by the bacilli on culture. In addition, the answers to the following questions are important. Is this an active case or a latent TB infection? Is it infectious or noninfectious? Pulmonary or nonpulmonary? Is the person coinfected with HIV? Is the individual pregnant or a child 6 years of age or younger? Goals of treatment are to cure the case and prevent transmission to other individuals. It is important to note that noncompliance by the individual can result in court-ordered confinement until a noninfectious state is achieved.

Public Health Issue: Foodborne Illnesses

Although TB is an example of airborne transmission of disease, foodborne illness is usually transmitted person to person via the fecal–oral route, although vector transmission can occur. Vector transmission takes place, for example, if a fly lands on food after being contaminated by the causative agent. If that food then becomes contaminated, it could become a vehicle for foodborne illnesses such as *Escherichia coli, Salmonella, Shigella*, or hepatitis A if ingested into the human system.

Foodborne illnesses may be reported as a singular event (one individual) or a family/community event (individuals who attended a family picnic, specific restaurant, or day care). Foodborne illness *surveillance* is passive until a report(s) comes in. Depending on the specific event, surveillance quickly becomes active. The resulting *disease and health event investigation* begins with the reported event (index case); extends to potential contacts; *outreaches* to the food supplier, restaurant, day care agency, school, and/or treating hospital; is *screened* and diagnosed by stool and food samples; and ends with remedial methods to prevent further illness. When commercial food handlers are involved, registered environmental health specialists or sanitarians are also involved. The sanitarian is a state-licensed individual responsible for environmental health inspections and ensuring that compliance is upheld with public health laws. These environmental health specialists work with the food supplier, restaurant, and/or food handler by providing food management education, conducting inspections, and collecting food samples. Legal interventions that may occur include fines, suspension of license, and/or food-handlers course requirements.

The public health nurse works with all public health practitioners throughout the entire process outlined above, including the strategies noted in the intervention wheel. To illustrate this involvement, the specifics of shigellosis are examined.

Transmitted by the fecal–oral route and usually person to person, shigellosis is caused by the *Shigella* bacteria (NJDHSS, 2009a). Its most common symptoms are diarrhea that can be bloody, nausea, vomiting, stomach cramps, and fever that usually develop between 1 and 7 days after swallowing the bacteria. Its spread usually occurs among household contacts, children in preschools or day care, persons living in residential facilities, homosexual men, and with contact of a contaminated object or food through ingestion or via direct contact with an infected person. (NJDHSS, 2009a). Diagnosis occurs after finding the *Shigella* bacteria in the stool. A person may continue to transmit the *Shigella* bacteria as long as long as these bacteria are present (NJDHSS, 2009a).

As noted in Box 8-3, shigellosis is a reportable illness. Many states, including New Jersey, use the same shigellosis surveillance case definition as the CDC, which is classified as confirmed or probable. *Confirmed* requires "isolation of Shigella from any site of the human body, regardless of symptoms" and *probable* requires a "clinically compatible case that is epidemiologically linked to a confirmed case" (NJDHSS, 2009b, n.p.).

When the local health department receives a *Shigella* report, the case finding, outreach, surveillance, and disease investigation processes are initiated. Although the responsibility in this case primarily lies with the health officer, it is often the public health nurse who outreaches to the index case to obtain the history and gather important information pertaining to the signs and symptom. The date when symptoms first appeared is critical because it informs the public health nurse as to the incubation period. For shigellosis the incubation period may vary from 1 to 3 days but can also range from 12 to 96 hours and up to 1 week (NJDHSS, 2009b). This disease investigation would then need to include specific index case information up to 4 days before symptom onset. Other important information the public health nurse needs to secure includes a food history (what foods were eaten, when they were eaten, where they were eaten), travel history, types and location of outside activity, work history, and inclusion of household contacts. The public health nurse also needs to ask additional questions: Did others eat the same food? Have they also become ill? Did they need to see a doctor? What are the foods common to all who became ill? Are the numbers of reported cases increasing and are they part of a community group, such as day care or school? Is the index case or subsequent cases a person who directly prepares or handles food? The answers to these questions then direct the continued processes of disease investigation, case finding, outreach, and surveillance.

As shown in Figure 8-1, the informational loop is circular. Surveillance continues to be active until all aspects of the disease or outbreak are closed. Specific treatment should focus on fluid and electrolyte replacement to prevent dehydration and antibiotics use; however, care must always be rendered because of the possibility of drug resistance (Heymann, 2004). All persons infected with *Shigella* need to use enteric precautions and perform frequent hand-washing. When a foodborne illnesses, such as shigellosis, involves a food handler, a day care center, or a school, special management is necessary and the environmental health specialist or sanitarian needs to be involved.

Primary prevention is always a first priority in public health practice when it comes to foodborne illness. For example, when an environmental health specialist conducts a restaurant inspection, he or she also provides food handling education. Both practices are meant to prevent any contamination with the management of food. Public health nurses frequently find themselves in situations where the provision of health education is essential for prevention. The following example illustrates this point. Public health nurses conduct immunization school audits, and at the same time they may find themselves in the position of providing education in infection control and prevention of communicable diseases. In this one particular circumstance, a public health nurse was provided a table located in the dining area of the preschool to review the infants'/children's immunization records. While conducting this audit, the public health nurse observed one of the child care workers changing a baby's diaper on a changing table located in the same room near the food preparation area. In addition, before and after diaper change hand-washing was not observed. What educational and prevention opportunities presented themselves with this observation? Besides what the public health nurse should do, what type(s) of referrals could be made to further enhance the infection control interventions for this nursery/preschool?

Public Health Issue: Rabies

Whereas TB and *Shigella* are communicable diseases for which no preventive vaccination exists, rabies can be prevented by vaccination, but not by the vaccination of humans. It is the routine vaccination of domestic animals that can help prevent rabies. "Pre-exposure vaccination [for humans] should [only] be offered to persons in high-risk groups, such as veterinarians and their staff, animal handlers, rabies researchers, and certain laboratory workers" (CDC, 2008a, p. 21).

Rabies can be described as "a rhabdovirus of the Genus Lyssavirus" (NJDHSS, 2008, p. 2) that is typically present in the saliva of clinically ill mammals and is transmitted through a bite. Although all warm-blooded hosts can be susceptible to the virus, in the United States distinct variants have been found in coyotes, foxes, raccoons, skunks, and several species of bats (CDC, 2007).

The CDC (2008a) report on human rabies prevention indicated that improved dog vaccination programs coupled with enhanced stray animal control has resulted in a considerable decrease of rabies cases in domestic animals since World War II:

In 1946, a total of 8,384 indigenous rabies cases were reported among dogs and 33 cases in humans. In 2006, a total of 79 cases of rabies were reported in domestic dogs, none of which was attributed to enzootic dog-to-dog transmission, and three cases were reported in humans, [none of which] was acquired from indigenous domestic animals. (p. 2)

Even with this decline rabies still causes concern among public health professionals, because *confirmed* human exposure to the rabies virus is generally always fatal unless appropriate postexposure prophylaxis is provided.

The management of potential human exposure requires an accurately assessed risk for infection (CDC, 2008a). Human incubation for rabies may range from days to years but is usually weeks to months. Because of this the CDC (2008a) considers "administration of rabies postexposure prophylaxis [as] a medical urgency, not a medical emergency, but [stresses] that decisions must not be delayed" (p. 3). The application of the intervention wheel strategies is presented here to demonstrate the processes that the public health nurse is involved with in cases of human exposure to rabies.

Rabies postexposure follow-up starts with receiving the report of a bite, scratch, or exposure to saliva from a potentially infected animal and extends to *outreach* and *case finding* with the individual(s) exposed. Determination of risk often falls to the public health nurse, especially if the victim did not present to a medical care provider. Other times the assessment may be shared when an emergency room primary care provider reports to the local health department. Containment and quarantine of the domestic animal falls to animal control with enforcement shared by the licensed environmental specialist or sanitarian. The animal is quarantined and observed for "ten days after a bite" (CDC, 2008a, p. 18) to ensure it is not rabid. This quarantine occurs whether the animal was vaccinated or not. Any untoward signs and symptoms compatible with rabies result in the animal being euthanized and the head removed and sent to the state laboratory for testing. Should the exposure be a result of a wild animal, the capture and securing the head for testing comes under the jurisdiction of animal control and veterinarian services.

The public health nurse's responsibility includes obtaining health/event information, providing postexposure-related information to the individual(s) involved, and securing, tracking, and documenting the required postexposure treatment for the exposed client. As with foodborne illness, *surveillance* is passive until the report is received, at which time it becomes active. Recommendations for postexposure prophylaxis include the following:

> Prompt and thorough wound cleansing, followed by passive rabies immunization with human rabies immune globulin and vaccination with a cell culture rabies vaccine. . . . A regimen of five 1-ml. doses of HDCV or PCECV administered intramuscularly to previously unvaccinated persons. The first dose of the 5-dose course should be administered as soon as possible after exposure (day 0). Additional doses should then be administered on days 3, 7, 14, and 28 after the first vaccination. (CDC, 2008a, p. 2)

As mentioned above, the disease and health event *investigation* is shared with health officers, environmental sanitarians, animal control officers, and veterinary professionals who control the animal-related sequence of events. It may also be shared with the state departments of health and the CDC. An example of this occurrence happened in July 2007 during the South Atlantic Summer Showdown softball tournament held in Spartanburg County, NC. The CDC (2008b) provided a report regarding this interstate public

health response to a rabid kitten. A summation of that report is as follows.

From July 13 through 15, 2007, approximately 60 teams with 12 players each from multiple states participated in the South Atlantic Summer Showdown softball tournament. On July 14 one of the North Carolina coaches, upon finding "an apparently healthy and alert kitten" (CDC, 2008b, p. 1337) in a garbage bin, placed the kitten in a box, brought it to six or more different games at two different facilities, and at the end of the day took the kitten to her home. On July 15 the coach's housemate took the kitten to an emergency animal hospital because it had become increasingly lethargic, was behaving abnormally, and had bitten her. When the housemate presented the kitten to the attending veterinarian, however, she did not report the bite. Instead, she signed a routine release form that indicated "the kitten had not bitten anyone during the preceding 10 days" (CDC, 2008b, p. 1337). Because the kitten was severely ill, this release allowed for the kitten to be euthanized with cremation scheduled for July 18.

On July 18 a softball player's mother contacted the emergency animal hospital upon learning the kitten had become sick. Because this mother had also been bitten by the kitten when it was at the tournament, she asked whether the kitten had been tested for rabies. Learning that it had not, she picked up the cat's body and brought it to the local health department, which sent the head to North Carolina's State Laboratory for rabies testing. A positive rabies diagnosis was made. That fact became the starting point for what was eventually a four-state rabies investigation. "Of the approximately 60 teams participating in the tournament, 38 had players and associated family and friends who reported exposure to the rabid kitten" (CDC, 2008b, p. 1338). Of that number, 27 individuals were assessed as having exposures that warranted postexposure prophylaxis because they "had reported actual exposure to the kitten's saliva, either through a bite, a lick on the oral or nasal mucosa, or a claw scratch" (CDC, 2008b, pp. 1338–1339). Cooperation of investigators within the four affected states and CDC "enabled the expeditious identification and prophylactic treatment of exposed persons while preventing unnecessary administration of PEP" (CDC, 2008b, p. 1339).

CASE STUDY APPLICATION: WHEN TIME IS OF IMPORTANCE

Thus far this chapter has presented for the reader three different public health issues. The case described here is a detailed account of one of the issues presented, TB, and the application of the intervention wheel strategies of case finding, surveillance, disease and health event investigation, outreach, and screening.

The Case

On June 14 a 39-year-old woman was admitted to the hospital with complaints of cough, fever, decreased appetite, night sweats, and a weight loss of 23 pounds over the last month. The admission chest x-ray revealed bilateral upper lobe infiltrates. The physician ordered immediate respiratory isolation and a bronchoscope with bronchial wash. The latter took place on June 17 and was 3+ positive for acid-fast bacillus. A probable diagnosis of pulmonary *M. tuberculosis* was made; treatment was started on June 19 with

first-line anti-TB medications. A report to the local health department occurred on June 21, 7 days after the hospital admission, thus initiating an active surveillance. One month later the final culture was identified as *M. tuberculosis* with pan-sensitivity to the TB medications that had been prescribed.

TB Interview and Plan

On June 22 the public health nurse began the disease and health event investigation when she reached out into the community as she arrived at the hospital to interview the newly reported TB index case. During this communication she learned the patient had been a part-time volunteer for a local day care center, working approximately 2 to 5 hours per week. Reporting that her sister was the center's director, the patient stated her work was mostly secretarial with little exposure to the children. The public health nurse also learned the index case had been coughing for approximately 2 months—1 month longer than noted on admission. Therefore, she may have been infectious longer than previously thought. Due to this important information, further investigation was needed and in a timely manner.

The state TB nurse manager was called in. Both public health professionals realized that the first steps in the subsequent contact investigation was to identify the infectious period, develop a list of contacts, and then visit the day care center, again signaling the importance of outreach. In talking to the public health nurse and reviewing the medical record, the state TB nurse manager determined the infectious period to be February 17 to June 14. This conclusion set the beginning of the infectious period at 3 months before the cough onset and ended it when the patient was hospitalized in respiratory isolation. The following day both the public health nurse and TB nurse manager met with the day care director to discuss potential exposure to children and staff, conduct an on-site assessment of environmental factors, identify high-priority contacts during the infectious period, and provide TB education to the key individuals involved.

On-Site Assessment and Identification of Contacts

Because index case confidentiality is always a consideration in work site or congregate setting investigations, the state TB nurse manager obtained a signed written statement from the director of the day care center indicating her obligation to respect the issues of confidentiality as related to the index case and this investigation. The index case also signed a written consent for the health department to conduct the investigation at her work site.

The on-site assessment, which is so important to this disease and health event investigation, again demonstrated the importance of outreach. This assessment revealed a small day care center with low ceilings and only one window located in the kitchen. The play area room measured 17 by 23 feet; ceiling height was 6 feet 5 inches. There were 35 children, 4 years of age or younger, all born in the United States; there were five staff members. The director reported that the index case had spent most of her time in the play area room.

Given the size of the rooms, poor ventilation, the age of the children, and the infectiousness of the index case, all chil-

dren and staff were considered high-priority contacts. During the meeting the director also indicated she had a 6-month-old infant who did not attend the day care but spent approximately 5 to 6 hours with the index case on weekends. This infant, also considered a high-priority contact, was available for the public health nurse to plant a TST that same day. When the screening test was read 48 hours later, the reaction was 15 mm, a reaction considered positive. A follow-up chest x-ray revealed infiltrates. The infant was admitted to the hospital with a tentative diagnosis of probable pulmonary TB, and anti-TB medications were started.

Contact Investigation Continues

The disease and health event investigation process continued as the public health professionals collected the names and located information of all identified contacts, in all exposure settings, including household, social, and workplace. Outreach and notification of all contacts was required because they needed TSTs and screening. Educational sessions were also provided to parents of all day care children. In addition to the 39 children and staff contacts at the day care center, the index case also named nine other high-priority contacts, seven household and two social. Active surveillance and outreach continued as the public health nurse visited the patient's household to verify the contacts, provide education, and conduct TST screening. This visit determined that all household contacts had been identified, and none was immune compromised. The nurse then conducted a home visit to the identified social contacts' residences. There it was discovered that one social contact had a 6-month-old infant not named on the initial index case interview. During this home visit and contact interview, the nurse realized this baby had approximately 70 hours of exposure per week to the index case, during the determined infectious period. Furthermore, the infant had been presenting with signs and symptoms of what the mom thought were a "cold"; she was thinking of calling the baby's doctor. The TB clinic was called, and the infant was referred to the emergency room and then subsequently admitted to the hospital. Probable pulmonary TB was the diagnosis, and treatment was started.

Summary

In the day care center 14 of 35 children were TST positive; 50%, or 7 of these children, were diagnosed with confirmed pulmonary TB disease. All TB cases were treated and later placed on directly observed therapy upon hospital discharge. The remaining seven children were placed on treatment for latent TB infection.

Of the household and social contact population, 70% were found to be TST positive; the two infants were diagnosed with confirmed pulmonary TB disease and treated in the same manner as the day care children. The remaining TST-positive adults were placed on treatment for latent TB infection.

As you reflect on this case study, do you see the intervention strategies discussed in this chapter being carried out by the two public health nurses? What exactly did they do and how did they do it?

MINNESOTA DEPARTMENT OF HEALTH POPULATION-BASED PUBLIC HEALTH NURSING PRACTICE INTERVENTION WHEEL: LEVELS OF PRACTICE

As public health nurses work with their target populations, they must always keep in mind the cultural context of those they serve. With TB, *Shigella*, and rabies they are concerned about the individual, family, and population's relationship to the index case and how best to reach out to all in the most effective way so that case finding, screening, surveillance, and disease intervention may take place. It is important to note that for these interventions to be effective, the nurse must be a part of the community, not in an office behind a desk. The public health nurse must combine nursing practice and public health sciences, including the enforcement of federal, state, or local laws. The public health nurse must be able to apply and perform the 17 intervention strategies of the intervention wheel and also apply those skills and initiate change at the individual/family, community, and system levels of public health practice. How may the public health nurse apply these 17 strategies at the three various levels of practice? Public health nurses need to examine and explore what ways are best received by the individual/family, population, and community.

Consideration of the case study above illustrates how the public health nurse worked on the individual and family level. On the individual/family level, the public health nurse developed a trusting relationship with each person. Considering the fear that is often associated with a diagnosis of TB, the public health nurse's ability to reach out and connect with the index case especially in the questioning phase was critical. The case study also illustrates the importance of working with each individual, given the sensitivity and the need for confidentiality. This again highlights the importance of trust development in the public health nurse's relationship with each individual contacted during the investigation. Once this relationship is established, the public health nurse may engage in health teaching and counseling, two additional strategies discussed in other chapters, that assist with the disease and health investigation.

On the community level, the public health nurse worked with multiple community organizations. For example, the emergency department, hospital, day care center, state department of health, and the local department of health were all actively involved in the disease and health investigation. This particular case study does not delve into the way the educational sessions were provided; however, this may be a potential example of how a community may step in to assist in this process. For example, if the population involved did not speak English and the public health nurses were not fluent in the population's primary language, this would have been an opportunity to reach out into the community and receive outside assistance from another agency or organization.

On the systems level, policy and law sustain the process in the case study. For example, TB is one of the many diseases presented on the Nationally Notifiable Infectious Diseases list. This system-level strategy assures that newly diagnosed cases are sent to the departments of health, local and state, for follow-up and case finding via disease event investigation. This assures the identification of others at risk or active cases yet to be diagnosed, thus protecting the public.

CONCLUSION

This chapter presents the red sections of the Minnesota Department of Health Population-Based Public Health Nursing Practice Intervention Wheel. The section discussed is that of case finding, outreach, screening, surveillance, and disease and health event investigation. The chapter was divided in a way that permitted the reader to first learn about these four particular public health nursing interventions. The second section presented various public health issues: TB, foodborne illnesses, and rabies. A third section presented a case study that demonstrated how the public health nurse applied these interventions throughout the levels of public health practice. Public health nursing is not a linear practice. It is a challenging practice that requires the public health nurse to think, apply, and do on multiple levels and spheres. It is forever changing and challenging.

References

Centers for Disease Control and Prevention [CDC]. (2006). Summary of notifiable diseases— United States, 2006. *Morbidity and Mortality Weekly Report, 55*, 1–9. Retrieved December 29, 2008, from http://www.cdc.gov/mmwr/preview/mmwrhtml/mm5553al.htm

Centers for Disease Control and Prevention [CDC]. (2007). Natural history of rabies. Retrieved December 29, 2008, from http://www.cdc.gov/rabies/history.html

Centers for Disease Control and Prevention [CDC]. (2008a). Human rabies prevention—United States. *Morbidity and Mortality Weekly Report, 57*(RR03), 1–26, 28. Retrieved December 29, 2008, from http://www.cdc.gov/mmwr/preview/mmwrhtml/rr5703al.htm

Centers for Disease Control and Prevention [CDC]. (2008b). Public health response to a rabid kitten—four states. *Morbidity and Mortality Weekly Report, 56*, 51. Retrieved February 6, 2009, from http://www.cdc.gov/mmwr/preview/mmwrhtml/mm5651a1.htm

Damush, T. M., Huanguang, J., Ried, L. D., Quin, H., Cameon, R., Plue, L., et al. (2008). Case-finding algorithm for post-stroke depression in veterans health administration. *International Journal of Geriatric Psychiatry, 23*, 517–522.

Escriba-Aguir, V., Ruiz-Perez, I., & Saurel-Cubizolles, M. J. (2007). Screening for domestic violence during pregnancy. *Journal of Psychosomatic Obstetrics & Gynecology, 28*(3), 133–134.

Fedder, D., Desai, H., & Maciunskaite, M. (2006). Putting a public health face on clinical practice: Potential for using an infectious disease management model for chronic disease prevention. *Disease Management Health Outcome, 14*(6), 329–333.

Findley, S. E., Irigoyen, M., Sanchez, M., Stockwell, M. S., Mejia, M., Guzman, L., et al. (2008). Effectiveness of a community coalition for improving child vaccination rates in New York City. *American Journal of Public Health, 98*(11), 1959–1962.

Hartge, P., & Berg, C. (2007). Improving uptake of cancer screening in women. *Journal of Women's Health, 16*(1), 66–67.

Heymann, D. L. (2004). *Control of communicable diseases manual* (18th ed.). Washington, DC: American Public Health Association.

Jack, S. M., Jamuson, E., Wathen, C. N., & MacMillan, H. L. (2008). The feasibility of screening for intimate partner violence during postpartum home visits. *Canadian Journal of Nursing Research, 40*(2), 150–170.

Keller, L., Strohschein, S., & Briske, L. (2008). Population-based public health nursing practice: The intervention wheel. In M. Stanhope & J. Lancaster (Eds.), *Public health nursing: Population-centered health care in the community* (pp. 186–214). St. Louis, MO: Mosby Elsevier.

Keller, L. O., Stohschein, S., Lia-Hoagberg, B., & Schaffer, M. A. (2004). Population-based public health interventions: Practice-based and evidence-supported. Part 1. *Public Health Nursing, 21*(5), 453–468.

Klaucke, D. N., Buehler, J. W., Thacker, S. B., Parrish, R. G., Trowbridge, F. L., Berkelman, R. L., & the Surveillance Coordination Group. (1988). Guidelines for evaluation surveillance systems. *Morbidity and Mortality Weekly Report, Supplements, 37*(S-5), 1–18.

Leavell, H., & Clark, E. (1965). *Preventive medicine for the doctor in his community: An epidemiologic approach.* New York: McGraw-Hill.

Liebman, J., Lamberti, M. P., & Altice, F. (2002). Effectiveness of a mobile medical van in providing screening in services for STDs and HIV. *Public Health Nursing, 19*(5), 345–353.

McKeown, R., & Hilfinger Messias, D. K. (2008). Epidemiology. In M. Stanhope & J. Lancaster

(Eds.), *Public health nursing: Population-centered health care in the community* (7th ed., pp. 241–277). St. Louis, MO: Mosby Elsevier.

McNeal, G. (2008). UMDNJ School of Nursing mobile healthcare project: A component of The New Jersey Children's Health Project. *The ABNF Journal,* Fall, 121–128.

Minnesota Department of Health, Division of Community Health Services, Public Health Nursing Section. (2001). *Public health interventions: Application for public health nursing practice.* St. Paul: Minnesota Department of Health.

Mock, J., McPhee, S., Nguyen, T., Wong, C., Doan, H., Lai, Ky, et al. (2007). Effective lay health worker outreach and media-based education for promoting cervical cancer screening among Vietnamese American women. *American Journal of Public Health, 97*(9), 1693–1700.

Nandi, A., Galea, S., Lopez, G., Nandi, V., Strongarone, S., & Ompad, D. C. (2008).Access to and use of health services among undocumented Mexican immigrants in a US urban area. *American Journal of Public Health, 98*(11), 2011–2020.

New Jersey Department of Health and Senior Services [NJDHSS]. (2004). Tuberculosis (*Mycobacterium tuberculosis*). Retrieved December 22, 2008, from http://www.state.nj.us/health/cd/manual/tb.pdf

New Jersey Department of Health and Senior Services [NJDHSS]. (2007). Standards of care for tuberculosis disease and latent TB infection. Retrieved February 8, 2009, from http://www.state.nj.us/health/cd/documents/complete_standards_of_care.pdf

New Jersey Department of Health and Senior Services [NJDHSS]. (2008). Rabies (human and animal). Retrieved December 22, 2008, from http://www.state.nj.us/health/cd/manual/rabies.pdf

New Jersey Department of Health and Senior Services [NJDHSS]. (2009a). What you should know about shigellosis. Retrieved February 6, 2009, from http://www.state.nj.us/health/cd/f_shigell.htm

New Jersey Department of health and Senior Services [NJDHSS]. (2009b). Shigellosis case definition. Retrieved February 6, 2009, from http://www.state.nj.us/health/cd/cd_shigell.htm

Puddifoot, S., Arroll, B., Goodyear-Smith, F. A., Kerse, N. M., Fishman, T. G., & Gunn, J. M. (2007). A new case-finding tool for anxiety: A pragmatic diagnostic validity study in primary care. *International Journal of Psychiatry in Medicine, 37*(4), 371–381.

Rajabiun, S., Mallinson, R. K., McCoy, K., Coleman, S., Drainoni, M., Rebholz, C., et al. (2007). The public health approach to eliminating disparities in health. *American Journal of Public Health, 98*(3), 400–403.

Skjerve, A., Nordhus, I. H., Engedal, K., Pallesen, S., Braekhus, A., & Nygoord, H. A. (2007). The seven minute screen (7MS). *International Journal of Geriatric Psychiatry, 8,* 764–769.

Steel, A. (1910). Neighborhood nursing. *American Journal of Nursing, 10*(5), 340–342.

Toole, T., Conde-Martel, A., Gibbon, J., Hanusa, B., Freyder, P., & Fine, M. (2007). Where do people go when they first become homeless? A survey of homeless adults in the USA. *Health and Social Care in the Community, 15*(5), 446–453.

Truglio-Londrigan, M., Arnold, J., Santiao, M., De Sevo, M., Higgins Donius, M. A., Valencia Go, G., et al. (2000). "Knocking on 99 doors": The experience of The College of New Rochelle (New York). In P. S. Matteson (Ed.), *Community-based nursing education: The experience of eight schools of nursing* (pp. 57–75). New York: Springer.

UK National Screening Committee. (2003). National screening criteria for appraising the viability, effectiveness and appropriateness of a screening program, Retrieved December 5, 2008, from http://www.nsc.nhs.uk/uk_ncs/uk_ncs_ind.htm

UK National Screening Committee. (2008). What is screening? Retrieved December 6, 2008, from http://www.nsc.nhs.uk/whatscreening/whatscreen_ind.htm

U.S. Department of Health and Human Services [DHHS], Public Health Service, Centers for Disease Control and Prevention [CDC]. (1992). *Principles of epidemiology: An introduction to applied epidemiology and biostatistics* (2nd ed.). Washington, DC: American Public Health Association.

U.S. Department of Health and Human Services [DHHS]/Centers for Disease Control and Prevention [CDC]. (2006). *Principles of epidemiology: An introduction to applied epidemiology and biostatistics* (3rd ed.). Washington, DC: American Public Health Association.

U.S. Preventive Services Task Force [USPSTF]. (2007). About USPSTF. Retrieved February 7, 2009, from http://www.ahrq.gov/clinic/uspstfab.htm

Venes, D. (2005). *Taber's cyclopedic medical dictionary* (20th ed.). Philadelphia: F. A. Davis.

Wald, N. J. (2007). Screening: A step too far. A matter of concern. *Journal of Medical Screening, 14*(4), 163–164.

Wimbush, F., & Peters, R. (2000). Identification of cardiovascular risk: Use of a cardiovascular-specific genogram. *Public Health Nursing, 17*(3), 148–154.

World Health Organization. (2003). *WHO-recommended standards for surveillance of selected vaccine-preventable diseases.* Geneva: World Health Organization.

World Health Organization. (2008). *Priority interventions HIV/AIDS prevention, treatment and care in the health sector.* Geneva: World Health Organization.

RUNNING THE SHOW: REFERRAL AND FOLLOW-UP, CASE MANAGEMENT, AND DELEGATED FUNCTIONS

JANNA L. DIECKMANN

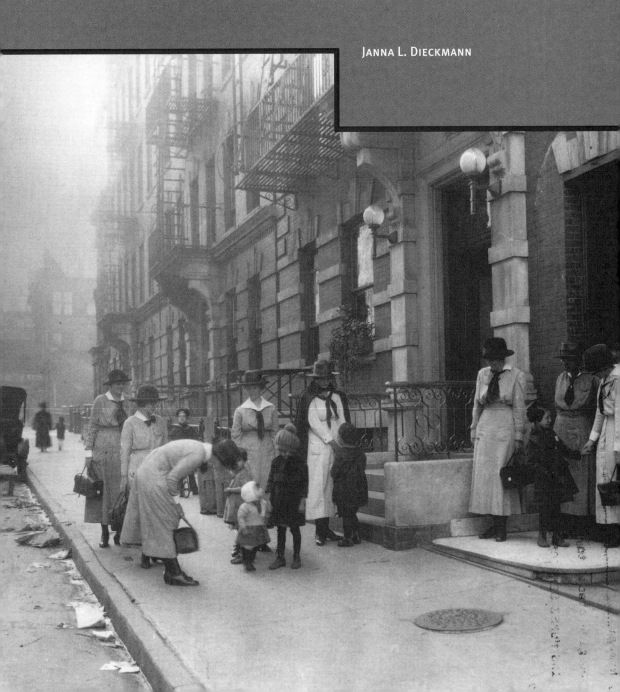

To meet the rightful demand of the children for play, we conducted in our back yards one of the first playgrounds in the city. It was an experimental station in a way, as well as an enlightenment of the general public, and was instrumental in helping to develop public feeling in the matter. After a time the interests of the residents of the settlement were directed to the "Out-Door Recreation League," share being taken in its executive work . . . (Wald, 1902, p. 569).

LEARNING OBJECTIVES

At the completion of this chapter, the reader will be able to

- Identify referral and follow-up, case management, and delegation as public health intervention strategies.
- Identify how intervention strategies may be implemented at the individual/family, community, and system levels.

- List the steps of the referral and follow-up process.
- Describe the case management process.
- Apply the public health intervention strategies of referral and follow-up, case management, and delegation to the case study presented in the chapter.

KEY TERMS

- Case management
- Delegation

- Referral and follow-up

The public health nurse designs and implements interventions within a complex network of health, social welfare, housing, and other services. Maximizing nursing services requires nurses' comprehensive knowledge and effective interface with a complex and well-functioning systems of multiple services that are available, accessible, and culturally competent. Public health nurses have understood that the determinants of health and the multiple causation of disease mean that individual change must have multiple foci. Public health nursing services work best by collaborating with other community-based caring and helping systems. Our clients—patients, families, populations of interest, systems, and communities—require more than public health nurses can directly provide. We have become experts in identifying client need and connecting clients to community services providers and services systems.

This chapter addresses three important public health interventions in the green wedge of the Minnesota Department of Health Population-Based Public Health Nursing Practice Intervention Wheel: referral and follow-up, case management, and delegated functions. These interventions have similarities, may overlap, and may be addressed toward similar objectives. All three interventions draw the public health nurse to working beyond the nurse–client dyad, as the nurse seeks to add the contributions of other community services and health providers to improve the system for client support and change. At the community practice level, this means public health nurse participation in initiating services or expanding availability and access to meet an identified need. At the systems practice level, the public health nurse modifies organizations and policies that shape systems of care. At the individual/family practice level, this includes interventions to change knowledge, attitudes, beliefs, practices, and behaviors (Rippke, Briske, Keller, Strohschein, & Simonetti, 2001).

The first of the three public health interventions addressed in this chapter, *referral and follow-up*, "assists individuals, families, groups, organizations, and/or communities to identify and access necessary resources in order to prevent or resolve problems or concerns" (Keller, Strohschein, & Briske, 2008, p. 199). *Case management* "optimizes self-care capabilities of individuals and families and the capacity of systems and communities to coordinate and provide

services" (Keller et al., 2008, p. 199). *Delegated functions*, the third intervention, "are direct care tasks a registered professional nurse carries out under the authority of a health care practitioner as allowed by law. Delegated functions also include any direct care tasks a registered professional nurse entrusts to other appropriate personnel to perform" (Keller et al., 2008, p. 199).

MINNESOTA DEPARTMENT OF HEALTH POPULATION-BASED PUBLIC HEALTH NURSING PRACTICE INTERVENTION WHEEL STRATEGIES AND LEVELS OF PRACTICE

Referral and Follow-Up

Referral and follow-up interventions are hallmarks of public health nursing. The referral process is defined as "a systematic problem-solving approach involving a series of actions that help clients use resources for the purpose of resolving needs" (Clemen-Stone, McGuire, & Eigsti, 2002, p. 316). As a practice expectation and as an ongoing intervention, the public health nurse seeks to link individuals/families, populations, communities, and systems to resources. New public health nurses quickly gain knowledge of the interfaces between target populations and assistive resources. Experienced public health nurses have extensive information, experiences, and facility in establishing linkages between and among community members, groups, and organizations. Individuals/families, populations, communities, and systems often seek the knowledge and advice of public health nurses when they want to know where to go for help or when they want to improve systems and services that provide resources (Rippke et al., 2001, p. 81).

Referral and follow-up interventions are related to other public health nurse interventions and generally occur in the context of ongoing nursing service. For example, health teaching for weight reduction provided by the public health nurse to a group of adults at a community center may encourage group members' interest in increasing their physical activity and muscle strength. Based on group members' expressed need, the public health nurse would seek and explore appropriate resources and provide group members with a tailored recommendation of relevant resources. At a later point the public health nurse would evaluate or follow up on the referral to determine the extent and character of the contacts between group members and the resources to which they were referred. In this example referral and follow-up interventions further the goals of the health teaching intervention but remain a separate intervention characterized by unique guidelines, practices, and values. The referral process is most effective when it is linked to other public health nurse interventions.

Referral and follow-up interventions may be applied with counseling or consultation interventions to link the individual/family, population, community, or system to a resource to prevent or resolve a problem or concern. The more information the public health nurse has about the expressed concern and the targeted intervention, the better and more sustainable the referral and follow-up is likely to be. Referral and follow-up is also used after screening and case finding (related to surveillance, disease investigation, and/or outreach) to address a need identified by this particular public health nurse intervention. The ethics of both screening and case finding direct the public health nurse to make formal plans to respond to newly identified needs. For example, when the individual or family has a positive screening result or a "case" is identified, linkage to a relevant resource is required. Advocacy interventions also generally demand linkage(s) to services and resources to address aspirations and needs at any practice level.

The two other intervention approaches addressed in this chapter, case management and delegated functions, are also interrelated with the referral and follow-up intervention. Case management is a goal-oriented process that uses available resources to achieve case management objectives. Referral and follow-up interventions occur jointly with the case management plan. Delegated function interventions shift care responsibility to an eligible resource or provider of care. The interface with this resource requires the public health nurse to apply referral and follow-up strategies. Additional elements of case management and delegated functions interventions are described in later sections of this chapter.

PUBLIC HEALTH NURSES AS "SENDERS" AND "RECEIVERS" OF REFERRALS

Public health nurses make referrals and receive referrals. Public health nurses may send or initiate a referral on behalf of a client or may receive a referral for a new or already known client. The process of receiving referrals at a public health nursing organization is generally formal to accommodate the frequency of requests and to provide a means to track data and referral outcomes. Referrals are received as part of an intake process at the public health nurse organization, both formal referrals from organizations and professionals and informal referrals from the client or the client's network. In some agencies public health nurses are permanently assigned to receive referrals, and in some agencies the intake function rotates among nurses. For cost or effectiveness reasons, intake may be alternatively delegated to skilled non-nurse staff members under the direction of a public health nurse. Once a referral is received, it is weighed and a plan to respond is established. The referral may be accepted for services from the public health nurse organization. On the other hand, referrals may be determined to require resources or services not available from the public health nurse organization. In this situation the referral may be declined and the referring agency or person promptly notified by intake public health nurses.

The intake public health nurse may also make recommendations for more appropriate, alternate agencies to receive the referral. Most communities have organized systems of information and referral, generally directed by social workers educated in this specialty area. Contacts with information and referral systems, sometimes called "First Call for Help," are available by telephone and increasingly online for specific geographic communities. Most states now have a "211" switchboard to connect callers to community resources. These systems request specific information about the client and the need to closely match the request with an appropriate resource. Information and referral differs from the public health nurse intervention of referral and follow-up in that information and referral provides only information on available resources. Even though

information and referral agencies may provide comprehensive information, information and referral does not make a referral or conduct follow-up. Based on information provided by the information and referral agency, the public health nurse or the group/family must select a possible resource and contact the suggested service agency to initiate a request for assistance.

It is important to note that the intake function of public health nurse agencies provides nurses and organizations with information about community needs and about gaps in resource availability, affordability, and appropriateness. Even when a public health nurse organization is unable to respond to an intake request, each request helps build a description of current community needs. When a mismatch between community need and existing resources is found, public health nurses and public health nurse organizations will seek to meet emerging or newly defined needs by developing new resources or by modifying or improving existing resources. Analysis of the needs may also suggest that resources exist but a barrier prevents relevant resources from providing assistance. For example, a community organization providing HIV/AIDS prevention and care services has historically targeted a defined geographic area. Now a neighboring area requires resources because it has experienced increased HIV incidence and AIDS prevalence. One solution would be to expand the existing HIV/AIDS service area into the neighboring community.

GAINING KNOWLEDGE ABOUT AVAILABLE FORMAL RESOURCES

Public health nurses must gain a working knowledge of available community resources to make effective referrals and must develop working relationships with resource organizations to fulfill follow-up obligations. How does a public health nurse build knowledge of community agencies and resources? Descriptive and contact information about community agencies and resources should be included in the public health agency orientation and public health staff development programs. Information can be shared in print or electronic formats, especially when there are changes in eligibility or availability of services. Many public health nurses maintain contact lists or active files of potential community resources. Public health nurse agencies may also develop relationships with specific resources, which may include formal strategies for interagency contact, referral, and follow-up (Allender & Spradley, 2005). Consultation with public health nurse supervisors or agency social workers can assist public health nurses to identify relevant resources.

In addition to formal structures for gaining information about community agencies, organizations, and resources, public health nurses learn about agencies through their informal networks. Informal networking with other public health nurses is often the most fruitful source of resource information. Clients, families, and other health professionals can provide information about resources, which is especially helpful when it is from the resource user's viewpoint. Observing the presence and activities of other agencies and organizations in a community also suggests who is operating in an area and the types of services offered. For example, home-delivered meals are a strategic service for homebound elders and the chronically ill. Before referring a client, a public health nurse would pose questions about the service to colleagues and

clients. Perhaps a home-delivered meal program provides excellent meals at the promised time at an inexpensive cost. On the other hand, perhaps the service's waiting list is 10 months, meals are too salty for many recipients, and delivery drivers get lost and miss deliveries. Knowing what to expect from a potential resource, as well as whether the client can accept the pros and cons of resource operations, enables the public health nurse to weigh the value of making an actual referral.

IDENTIFYING REFERRAL NEEDS: WHEN AND WHO?

A referral must have merit. "Merit" takes into consideration whether a referral is the *right* referral at the *right* time for the *right* client. Determining the merit of a referral is heavily influenced by community values and expectations and (1) whether or not referrals are an effective strategy, (2) the timing of a referral, (3) whether the referral is to prevent a problem or address an existing problem, and (4) the nature of the "match" between the referral resource and the client.

Among public health nurses in some agencies, developing and making referrals is an infrequent activity. Client needs may have been overlooked, resources are scanty, or the nurses are overwhelmed. On the other hand, most public health nurses would agree that use of community resources extends the effectiveness and quality of public health nurse interventions and is well worth the time and attention required to prepare and complete a referral.

The actual timing of making referrals may vary among public health nurses and across public health nurse organizations. Some public health nurses wrap referrals into case closure activities, whereas others ensure that referrals are made early enough in the nurse–client relationship that new community resources have begun client services before public health nurse service termination. In the latter case the public health nurse is well situated to conduct follow-up activities as the nurse maintains contact with the client before case closure. The public health nurse can both observe the impact of the community resource's contacts with the client and directly ask the client about the use and success of the referral agency's services.

Public health nursing approaches also vary in whether community resources are applied early to prevent client crises or in a more targeted fashion to address client crises once present. Many public health nurses prefer to target preventive activities to avoid client crises, although some would rather reserve community resources to address emergent crises. Both perspectives are based in ethical judgments about when and how services are best involved, and both raise questions about cost-effectiveness. In prevention, lower cost can be spread over a wider population, whose members may or may not be at risk. Public health nurses often base interventions on the ethic that suffering should be prevented whenever possible. When addressing crises that have already occurred, individual costs are likely higher, but these costs are directed only at individuals having actual health problems.

Some client groups are seen as more deserving than others of receiving resources. Some clients can be viewed in a more favorable light than other clients, because their concerns or needs are interpreted in a more sympathetic manner. For example, a person with alcoholism, living on the street, might be viewed less sympathetically than a stable

couple with a young child. Or those making every effort to improve their health would be viewed more positively than those with the same health concern but who make no effort to help themselves. Society is more willing to provide aid and assistance when clients are sympathetic, are deemed "moral," and are seen as trying to help themselves. When the public views a client group as being more "deserving," they are willing to provide greater resources for resolving their needs and are more open to paying for more expensive resources (Dieckmann, 1999; Katz, 1996). For example, as AIDS has become more mainstream, since the mid-1980s, communities are more willing to commit resources to people living with HIV/AIDS. When clients are viewed as sympathetic and deserving, it is more acceptable to fund services and more resources become available. These principles have implications for individual/family use of referral resources but also for the overall availability of resources at the community and systems practice levels.

Steps to Conducting Referral and Follow-Up

Implementing the steps of the referral and follow-up intervention assumes active client participation and client control. Assistance in planning is offered *to* the client, and the public health nurse collaborates *with* the client. Because the referral process is client centered, the public health nurse avoids making decisions *for* the client but seeks to establish a working partnership that uses a problem-solving approach to achieve shared goals.

Individual/family clients, populations, communities, and systems vary across a continuum as to their ability to contribute to the referral process. Some clients are dependent on the public health nurse for gathering information, weighing options, and requesting the referral. In these situations public health nurses use referral planning and implementation to build relevant skills and independence in clients. Other clients are more independent in considering and implementing referrals, placing the public health nurse in almost a consultative role. In this situation the public health nurse validates and extends these clients' independent problem-solving behaviors. The public health nurse provides clients with the opportunity to learn and adopt new behaviors to achieve their next steps to full independence.

The steps to conduct referral and follow-up are sequential; these steps are based on the outline provided by Clemen-Stone and colleagues (2002) and McGuire, Gerber, and Clemen-Stone (1996). If a need or resource cannot be identified or if the client declines referral, it may be useful to revisit earlier steps. These steps are appropriate for individuals/families, populations, communities, and systems. Additional comments about the implications of the referral and follow-up intervention for communities and systems are found at the end of this section (see Referrals and Follow-Up at Systems and Community Practice Levels, below).

Step 1: Establish a Nursing Relationship With the Client. Nursing interventions begin with establishing a respectful working relationship with the client as a basis for individualizing or targeting care. The referral and follow-up intervention is often used with existing clients for whom the public health nurse has provided other public health interventions. Here the professional relationship has already been established. On the other hand, a public health nurse may initiate a profes-

sional relationship with a new client solely to develop and implement referral and follow-up. Whether based in an ongoing collaborative intervention or in a brief encounter, the public health nurse must similarly establish trust and gain the client's agreement to engage in the referral process. Public health nurses may quickly assess and develop working hypotheses about the client that may later be confirmed, but the nurse should not establish fixed assumptions in the initial step.

Step 2: Identify Client Need and Set Objectives for Referral. Based on a caring professional relationship with the client, the public health nurse gathers information about the client and the client's context. Listening to the client's perspective of his or her current situation and larger context is crucial (Wolfe, 1962). What is the client's need and what are the parameters of the need? Clients may benefit from a thorough discussion of the need. Allowing the client to review and describe a need provides essential information for the nurse, but the process of verbally articulating needs also enhances client comprehension of the need, investment in the referral process, and self-efficacy in securing a solution. Because one intention of the referral process is to increase client independence, incorporating strategies that facilitate client em-powerment are beneficial to strengthening current decisions for self-care and later self-determination.

When the public health nurse has secured an apparent understanding of the client's needs, the nurse reflects a synthesis of the need back to the client to confirm that what has been heard is what the client meant to convey. Probing for further client information or perspective may be helpful. After brief consideration the public health nurse presents his or her summary of the client's expressed need and proposes options for addressing this need. Critically important at this point is the nurse's determination whether the client's need is in practice one need or several. If several, then the public health nurse proposes at least two ways of posing the need and gains client agreement with one interpretive approach. Given a favored approach, the nurse and client work collaboratively to establish objectives for the referral.

This give-and-take process may be quite brief, or it may be lengthy. If the referral and follow-up intervention is conducted with an individual/family, organization, community, or system, more than one well-organized meeting may be required to share information, make decisions, and gain a working consensus about objectives. As the process of making a referral proceeds, the nurse and client may choose to return to this step for further clarification of need(s) and redetermination of objectives.

Step 3: Search for Resources and Explore Resource Availability. A systematic search for resources to meet the need and the identified referral objectives is conducted by the nurse, sometimes with participation of the client. Public health nurses familiar with meeting needs similar to the client's may quickly establish a group of options, either from personal experience or from consulting personal or agency resource files. Addressing more complex client needs may require consultation with professional colleagues or with information and referral specialists. Although the principles of making a good referral can guide the public health nurse, a nurse's experi-

ence and confidence in making referrals contributes to a prompt and personalized outcome. A nurse's ability to apply the *art* of nursing is especially relevant in the selection of potential referral resources. The client and the resource must *fit* together in both tangible and intangible ways for the referral to effectively accomplish the identified goals.

Step 4: Client Decides Whether to Agree to Referral. Information about potential referral resources is presented and discussed with the client. The client may select a resource(s), may wish to consider the resource(s), or may decline to agree to any referral. It can be helpful to provide clients with written information to allow later review of potential resources or later communication with the resource by the client. Application of the referral and follow-up intervention is based on ethical principles of client self-determination that places decision making in the hands of the client (McGuire, Gerber, & Clemen-Stone, 1996). When a client is uncertain or declines referral, the public health nurse may explore the client's feelings and reasons, identify factors that might facilitate or deter resource use, negotiate use of identified resources, propose a wider variety of referral resources, and/or reassess the client's needs and objectives for service. If a client declines referral at whatever point, no referral is made. The nurse must balance encouragement with an open ear that the client does not wish a referral.

Step 5: Public Health Nurse Matches Client With Resource and Makes the Referral to the Resource. The client and the nurse select a resource or resources that best match client needs and preferences. Does the client believe

the resource will work for them? The public health nurse's knowledge of the client and client's needs is important in making the referral to the identified resource and in explaining the client to the agency. If the client is a population, community, or a system, a referral might be a grant application or application to secure program funding. When clients are more experienced or skilled, they may make the referral themselves; this increased skill in self-managing care is a factor in client empowerment. Other clients may lack experience, be self-doubting, or be overwhelmed and emotionally fragile. As the nurse makes the referral, he or she asks questions and gains more information to assist the client to maximize interactions with the resource. The public health nurse also provides the client with tailored information about the resource and with anticipatory guidance on using the agency's resources.

Some agencies require detailed application information; the nurse gathers information and confirms with the client what information should be shared. Some communities use written interagency referral forms that have been developed to address system and resource needs for sharing information. Although patient privacy laws now prevent their use, in the past the agency that received a written referral would respond in writing to the referral source to describe initial contacts and plans for the referred individual or family (Cady, 1952; Kraus, 1944).

Step 6: Follow-Up to Facilitate Client Utilization of Resource. Nursing interventions at this step, alternatively called "following along," can ease the client's experience with the resource. Soon after the client follows through and contacts the resource, the public health nurse contacts the client to determine the client's progress and engagement with the resource. Is the client using the resource as planned? Is the resource agency engaged with the client? The public health nurse can reemphasize the purpose of the referral, interpret the resource to the client and the client to the resource, and promote linkages between client and resource. If signs of a weak linkage are found, the nurse may advocate for the client with the resource. The public health nurse can also directly address any barriers to seeking or using the resource (Will, 1977).

Step 7: Evaluation of Referral Process and Outcome, Client Outcome, and Resource Assistance. Did the client receive services and what was provided by the resource? In what ways did the client's status change as a result of working with the resource? Obtaining adequate information and data for evaluation can be challenging but is an essential element in the ongoing process of making referrals. Whether the client is an individual/family, population, community, or system, evaluation of referral and client outcomes has system-level implications. Lack of resources or poor service from resources in the community suggests gaps that public health nurses should address. Because the referral and follow-up intervention is a continuous process, public health nurses learn from each referral and provide feedback to improve the system itself and nurses' utilization of system resources.

Barriers to Successful Referral and Follow-Up

Successful follow-through on any referral frequently depends on the resources of clients and is based on several factors. Wolfe's classic analysis (1962) identified the central role of client motivation in initiating resource utilization: To what extent does the client see the referral and resource use as important? Does the referral appear to be practical and relevant to the client's situation? Individualizing the referral for the client or the family and tailoring the referral to the client's expressed preferences enhance referral utilization.

The concepts of *perceived benefits* and *perceived barriers* in the health belief model can assist in facilitating client follow-through for resource use. Clients accept a recommended referral only when they expect a benefit that is greater than the perceived barriers. Public health nurse interventions are designed to enhance perceived benefits by clarifying the expected positive impact of accepting the referral and by explaining specific actions to engage with the referral resource. At the same time public health nurse interventions are directed toward reducing perceived "tangible and psychological costs" of accepting the referral by identifying perceived barriers and reducing their impact through clarifying misinformation and applying reassurance, incentives, and concrete assistance to use the resource (Champion & Skinner, 2008, pp. 47–49). Referral follow-through by patients at risk for cancer was improved when diagnostic/treatment appointments were scheduled within 2 weeks, when patients received clear instructions, and when patients received careful attention from the clinic staff (Manfredi, Lacey, & Warnecke, 1990).

Public health nurse interventions at the system and community practice levels seek to reduce institutional and systemic barriers, such as reducing barriers to clinic utilization through improved accessibility by adding evening and weekend service hours or through enhanced language accessibility by providing more trained interpreters (Office of Minority Health, 2001).

A wide variety of factors may delay or obstruct clients' participation in the referral process or in using the referred resource, despite initial agreement with the significance of the problem, plans for solution, and selection of and referral to the resource. From an individual or family viewpoint, differences in religious/cultural beliefs or practices can increase uncertainty and reduce trust of a new resource. Or clients may become uncertain about why they were referred to a resource or doubt that it is a priority and so postpone or forget to engage with services. Structural barriers, such as geographic barriers, may make certain resources unusable, or resources may simply be unavailable. Appointment times may be inconvenient or require a long wait. Financial barriers may place good resources outside clients' reach or may delay the resource's acceptance of the client so long that clients lose motivation to make change.

These barriers may also suggest ineffective or flawed systems due to lack of financial or professional resources or due to lack of community consensus to address individual/family or community problems or concerns. Public health nurses may need to advocate at the community or system levels. For example, this advocacy may include screening services or enhancing existing services to improve utilization, such as translation or handicap accessibility.

STRATEGIES FOR FOLLOW-UP

Several effective strategies are helpful to use in following up on client referrals. If resources are limited, public health nurses may establish priorities for whom to contact, based on complexity of need or family situation, or on frequency or intensity of client contacts during the referral process. On the other hand, it may be helpful to invest in following up on all referrals. For example, until 1937 public health nurses in New York City delivered infants' birth certificates to the family home, because this provided an opportunity to refer newborns for prompt health supervision (Bokhaut & Mahoney, 1960).

Follow-up postcards or letters can be sent to clients, but responding to mailed forms can require significant effort. On the other hand, past programs have found responses above 85%, which has also reduced need for home visits (Bokhaut & Mahoney, 1960). Electronic mail may provide easier communication exchanges, but this technique is more available to those in higher socioeconomic groups. Telephone calls provide a framework for effective intervention, with a focus on reviewing the referral and its outcomes, supportive listening, additional teaching, or identifying/making additional referrals (Cave, 1989). This additional contact can reconfirm the appropriateness of the referral and resource for the client and allows for additional assessment of the client and context. Rather than promoting dependence, follow-up telephone calls promote independent decision making and critical thinking by encouraging client reflection and providing a means to reinforce client choices and actions (Donaldson, 1977). Follow-up home visits can be extremely useful but are also expensive in staff time and travel costs; reserving this approach for higher risk groups requiring intensive services and multiple referrals may best balance costs (Brooten, 1995; Wingert, Teberg, Bergman, & Hodgman, 1980).

One teen pregnancy program found that home visiting led to significant increases in the proportion of prenatal adolescents who identified and kept prenatal appointments, enrolled in the Women, Infants, and Children program, and applied for Medicaid (Flynn, Budd, & Modelski, 2008). Additionally, the technological advancements of today's healthcare environment provide additional evidence of how this technology may be put to use with regard to follow-up (Lillibridge & Hanna, 2008).

Ethics of Referral and Follow-Up
Public health nurses must also navigate several ethical conflicts or challenges embedded in the referral and follow-up intervention at any practice level. The first conflict lies in the potential gap between what the client wishes/wants and the public health nurse's professional determination of need. Should the client's view or the nurse's view prevail? Some conflicts may arise from a lack of communication or misunderstanding. In this situation the public health nurse may have to revisit the process of determining need and selecting objectives to meet the need. Perhaps the client's need has become more complex or multifaceted than originally determined. Or perhaps as a result of the referral process the client has become more sophisticated in self-identifying the need and has now become more assertive in directing criteria for a reasonable solution. Clients may also be surprised at the lack of actual resources to meet their need or feel a right to "their share" out of a belief that others with similar needs have received more assistance.

A second type of ethical conflict in referral and follow-up is determining whether society can or should provide the resources or services that clients want. Many resources have eligibility criteria that can seem arcane to clients and families or even to communities. Is a client's selected option a *need* or a *want?* Differentiating between needs and wants is often a matter of perspective of our "needs" contrasted against their "wants." But public health nurses may have ethical obligations to both client and the wider societal system: On what basis do public health nurses make judgments about resource access and distribution? Balancing individual rights to resources against ensuring the wider public good is difficult. The public health nurse must recognize when to protect limited resources and when to strongly advocate for meeting client needs.

Mandated or legally-required referrals are a third type of ethical conflict for the public health nurse. In contrast to a voluntary referral that clients themselves decide whether to accept or reject, public health nurses must make legal reports or referrals to protect individuals or society from certain diseases and health conditions or from violence, abuse, or neglect. Parents may neglect immunizations or physically abuse their child. An individual may receive a positive screen for a reportable disease. Or a frail older adult may have money stolen by a relative. When referral is mandated, it may be better to directly discuss the mandated referral with the individual/family. If a threat to the nurse is a concern, the discussion may take the form of notification through telephone or written formats. The nurse–client relationship can survive a mandated referral, thus allowing the public health nurse to be in an excellent position to contribute to and support a solution.

The last ethical conflict occurs when clients firmly decline a referral. But based on the ethic of self-determination, the solution is extremely clear. The client always and at any time maintains a right to decline referral. Coercive referrals, or referrals based on subterfuge, have no place in an ethical nursing practice. On the practical side, if clients oppose a referral, they are very unlikely to engage with or use a resource effectively. Unwelcome referrals are more likely to waste the referral agency's staff time and financial resources. Certainly, public health nurses may provide these clients with written information about a referral or may call back to check on clients' subsequent status, but client refusals of referral are clear and must be respected.

Referrals and Follow-Up at Systems and Community Practice Levels

The principles of referral and follow-up for the individual/family level of practice have been discussed previously in this text. However, referral and follow-up also have implications for public health nursing interventions at the systems and community levels. Community- and systems-focused practices contribute to the context of referral and follow-up for individuals, families, and populations. Public health nurse engagement at the community and systems practice levels is often based on direct knowledge gained from individuals/ families, of the strengths and weakness of referral, and of follow-up practices in a particular geographic area. Experienced public health nurses often identify weak areas that have potential to be strengthened through community and systems changes.

Public health nurses must move outside familiar programs and agencies to build linkages with both health and nonhealth resources that seek to monitor and address neighborhood and community needs at the systems level. Thinking broadly and creatively can increase potential for problem solution, through modification of organizations, policies, laws, and/or power relationships. Public health nurse participation in these groups can lead to involvement in community assessment and intervention to reduce or remedy barriers to client/family access to resources. Perhaps new resources and services will be established in the community, or perhaps nursing organizations will seek support and broaden their existing services. The search for effective and appropriate resources to meet local, contemporary needs is ongoing; attention to evaluation of existing programs and systems is a useful first step.

Acknowledging a need for additional resources and/or greater coordination and linkages among existing agencies may result from careful assessment but also from events that capture community concern. Our daily news often includes tragic reports; one community responded to the murder of a 7-year-old girl by her 12-year-old sister by first gathering and reflecting on the events and how this might have been prevented. Several agencies had known and worked with this family, but breakdowns in referral and follow-up resulted in inadequate assistance. As a short-term system response, the community nursing service coordinated monthly interagency conferences to discuss cases, problems, and linkages. As a long-term system change, community agencies agreed to work toward improving county mental health services.

The public health nurse also has a role in shaping community norms, attitudes, awareness, practices, and behaviors for referral and follow-up. Are referral systems working well enough that individu-

als, families, and populations who require assistance are able to locate and use appropriate resources. Public and private health insurance does not address this expense, but do communities acknowledge these needs? Voluntary charitable groups, such as United Way, provide funding for information and referral services, but many community residents are unfamiliar with this resource and its use. Economic retrenchment in healthcare facilities and agencies discourages building and maintaining referral and follow-up systems, even when there is evidence that costs of care can be reduced. Individuals, families, and populations who require referral are often those who least know how to navigate contemporary community resources. Public health nurses have a role in raising their clients' needs and in reflecting the deficits of the current referral and follow-up system to the widest community audience. Individuals do need help—and want help—to change, although community attitudes may frame this positive, optimistic quality as overburdening services. Community attitudes and community willingness to make financial commitments is key to improving linkages between those needing resources and existing resources.

Case Management

Case management "optimizes self-care capabilities of individuals and families and the capacity of systems and communities to coordinate and provide services" (Keller et al., 2008, p. 199). According to the American Nurses Credentialing Center (2008–2009):

Nurse case managers actively participate with their clients to identify and facilitate options and services, providing and coordinating comprehensive care to meet patient/client health needs, with the goal of decreasing fragmentation and duplication of care, and enhancing quality, cost-effective clinical outcomes. Nursing case management is a dynamic and systematic collaborative approach to provide and coordinate health care services to a defined population. Nurse case managers continually evaluate each individual's health plan and specific challenges and then seek to overcome obstacles that affect outcomes. A nurse case manager uses a framework that includes interaction, assessment, planning, implementation, and evaluation. . . . To facilitate patient outcomes, the nurse case manager may fulfill the roles of advocate, collaborator, facilitator, risk manager, educator, mentor, liaison, negotiator, consultant, coordinator, evaluator, and/or researcher. (para. 1)

Case management takes place in a variety of settings. Some of these settings may include acute care, school-based programs, public health such as departments of health and/or visiting nurse practices, long-term care, and independent practices. Additionally, the individuals, families, and populations served generally present with complexity of needs and thus may be at high risk and are vulnerable in their ability to access needed services. As such, a model of case management where there is a care manager who advocates for the client and family serves the system as well as clients, families, and populations (Bower, 1992).

Case management is often conducted in conjunction with other public health

nursing interventions, including both the referral and follow-up intervention and the delegated functions intervention. Depending on client/family need, a public health nurse using the case management intervention may apply the delegated functions intervention to shift care provision to achieve improved quality or reduced costs or perhaps to secure more culturally relevant care providers fluent in the family's preferred language and knowledgeable of their cultural practices.

The case management intervention shares some aspects with the referral and follow-up intervention; some have suggested that referral is a component of case management, and others see case management as a more intensive application of referral. This chapter interprets case management and referral/follow-up as separate practices that share some elements. For example, the timeline of nurse–client interactions is quite different between the two. In referral the public health nurse may have limited contacts with the individual/family; after implementing the referral plan, the public health nurse conducts follow-up to facilitate referral resource utilization and to conduct evaluation. But case management suggests frequent interactions over a long period. Ongoing nurse–family interactions permit the case manager to shadow the individual/family as they use resources to work toward their goal; this approach can be conceptualized as "following along" with the family to facilitate individual/family change.

Case management relates to several other public health nursing interventions. Outreach or case finding interventions may precede case management to identify individuals/families in need of services; case finding may also follow case management. Case management implementation may include the public health interventions advocacy, collaboration, consultation, counseling, and health teaching. And at the provider level of intervention, case management may lead to advocacy or collaboration and is closely associated with provider education (Rippke et al., 2001).

FRAMING CASE MANAGEMENT

The characteristics of case management can be seen through two contrasting "frames." One approach to framing case management relies on its objective financial outcomes, which are driven by goals of cost containment, efficient use of resources, and reduced fragmentation of care. Case management may be focused "primarily on maintaining quality while controlling costs of health care through coordination and management of care" (Kersbergen, 1996, p. 169), through programs in which services are managed rather than cases. Because it is difficult to resist societal pressures to restrain spending, cost containment can easily become the driving force in case management. But care rationing may be structurally and ethically inconsistent with nursing professional precepts and with the goals of quality care and thus possibly compromise the professional values of its nurse case managers (Beilman, Sowell, Knox, & Phillips, 1998). Knollmueller cautions about the risk of "turning case management into a scheme for rationing services if we limit the scope of service to a management of the benefit or a funding package and disregard the human faces behind the service" (1989, p. 42).

The second contrasting frame for case management relies on meeting the needs and enhancing quality of life for individuals, families, populations, and communities; increasing service quality across the continuum and developing new services when needs are revealed; and developing the capacity of systems and communities to coordinate and provide services (Rippke et al., 2001). This approach to case management reflects public health nursing values in that it is client centered and relationship based but may yet be a vision rather than a working model.

CASE MANAGEMENT AT THE INDIVIDUAL/ FAMILY PRACTICE LEVEL

Case management "describes a process more than it defines a structure or an outcome" (Knollmueller, 1989, p. 38) and is frequently directed toward particular populations, especially populations with multiple needs, such as the frail elderly, people living with HIV/AIDS, or children with congenital illness (Tahan, 1998). As such, the first step in case management at the individual/family practice level is to conduct outreach and case finding to all individuals/families considered at risk and to offer case management services. As this step unfolds, the public health nurse seeks to develop a trusting professional relationship as a basis for effective case management. With the involvement of clients and families who respond to outreach and meet priority criteria for the agency's case management services, the nurse assesses their functional level to identify their needs. How and what do individuals and families identify as an adequate quality of life, and what is the gap between these goals and their current status? Note that this step should include assessment of financial resources, especially to ensure adequate financial support.

Using strategies similar to the referral/ follow-up intervention, the public health nurse next works with individuals and families to identify helpful resources and to design a detailed plan to access these resources. An effective planning process outlines each step to link the client to services and resources. Because families with multiple needs often require complex resources to meet their needs, the plan should incorporate strategies to form a multidisciplinary team. Early linkages across helping professions facilitate coordination and collaboration to meet individual/ family needs. The individual/family remains part of this multidisciplinary team to assist with "troubleshooting" to resolve actual or potential barriers to service acquisition and use. Periodic formative evaluations of service organization, coordination, and case management are conducted with providers and the individual/ family target of care (Rippke et al., 2001).

CASE MANAGEMENT INTERVENTION AT THE SYSTEM AND COMMUNITY PRACTICE LEVELS

Application of the case management intervention at the system and community practice levels is similar to those for the referral/follow-up intervention. The primary goal is "to create needed resources where resources do not exist or are inadequate" (Rippke et al., 2001, p. 97). The public health nurse intervening at the system or community practice level first identifies population subgroups whose quality of life is at risk and then conducts a resource assessment (similar to a community assessment) to determine availability, accessibility, acceptability, and cultural competence of existing community resources. Having identified any gaps in community services or in the service system, the nurse collaborates with community organizations and systems to develop a plan to address existing gaps. In collaboration with community partners,

the public health nurse also ensures that new resources and services are adequate and equitable. Periodic community assessment seeks to determine this "community's capacity to meet the quality-of-life needs of identified populations-at-risk" (Rippke et al., 2001, p. 97).

Delegated Functions

Delegated functions are direct care tasks "a registered professional nurse carries out under the authority of a health care practitioner as allowed by law. Delegated functions also include any direct care tasks a registered professional nurse entrusts to other appropriate personnel to perform" (Keller et al., 2008, p. 199). In relation to the delegated functions intervention, the public health nurse may initiate **delegation** of functions to others as the *delegator* or receive delegated function from others as the *delegatee*. Because the focus of delegated functions is on direct care tasks, this public health nursing intervention occurs primarily at the individual/family level of practice. Consultation, collaboration, coordination, and communication have important impacts on care and services, but these are not delegated functions. No other public health nursing intervention discussed in this book requires another health professional's authority; all other interventions are nursing functions conducted independently under the local state's nurse practice act (Rippke et al., 2001).

A public health nurse might delegate to unlicensed assistive personnel such as outreach workers conducting home visits in a maternal health program. In this case the public health nurse delegates, for example, prenatal education to the outreach worker. In situations in which a public health nurse trains lay health advisors, the nurse does not delegate nursing functions to them, and the lay health advisors share health information to their peers on an informal, "every mother knowledge" basis (Watkins et al., 1994). A school nurse may, in some states and for some skills, delegate to a school secretary, but the school nurse cannot delegate to parents assisting with vision screenings, because they are not operating in an official capacity.

The delegated functions intervention also differs from the referral and follow-up intervention. Neither a referral from a hospital to a public health agency nor a referral from a school nurse to a support group is delegation. A referral given to an individual or family to seek additional services from a community agency does not involve delegation of skilled care tasks. In the same sense coordination of care with a multidisciplinary team does not include transfer of nursing functions to others. Referrals from a physician or nurse practitioner for maternal–child home visiting or for home health care visits are not delegation, because home visiting is an independent nursing function. In this case the physician or nurse practitioner orders meet insurance reimbursement requirements rather than the legal requirements of delegation.

Public Health Nurse as Delegator

The National Council of State Boards of Nursing (NCSBN) and the American Nurses Association (ANA), as well as nursing specialty areas (Timm, 2003), have demonstrated heightened interest in delegation since the late 1980s (ANA & NCSBN, 2005; NCSBN, 1995, 2005). Because every healthcare worker's contributions are necessary to address "the public's increasing need of accessible, affordable, quality health care" (NCSBN, 1995, para. 1), appropriate delegation of responsibilities and tasks must be ensured. Because NCSBN and ANA have been most concerned with nurse delegation to others (rather than the nurse as delegatee), delegation is defined as "Transferring to a competent individual the authority to perform a selected nursing task in a selected situation. The nurse retains accountability for the delegation" (NCSBN, 1995, para. 5). In this context a nurse cannot delegate the practice functions of assessment, evaluation, and nursing judgment. This means that a specific task cannot be "routinely and uniformly delegated" (NCSBN, 2005, para. 9); the nurse must determine the individual needs of each patient for each event of delegation.

Five Rights of Delegation

When the public health nurse contemplates delegating a function to another licensed profession or to unlicensed assistive personnel (Zimmerman & Kirkpatrick, n.d.), the nurse must consider the five rights of delegation to determine whether delegation can be done. The first right is whether it is the "right task": Is this a task that may be delegated? Nursing assessment, for example, cannot be delegated under most states' nurse practice acts. In school nursing the appropriateness of delegating medication administration has received increased attention (National Association of School Nurses, 2006). A 2008 California Supreme Court decision concluded that unlicensed school employees may not administer insulin, based on a provision of the California Nurse Practice Act that specifically prevented nurse delegation of insulin administration (Block, 2009).

The second right is whether "the care setting, available resources, and other relevant factors [are] conducive to assuring client safety" (Rippke et al., 2001, p. 115). Especially when there is low potential for harm, low task complexity, minimal problem solving, and predictable task outcomes, a task is more likely to be appropriate to delegate. For example, many school systems do not provide a school nurse for each school, resulting in hours or days when a nurse is unavailable to children requiring health services. One New Jersey nonpublic school system developed and implemented a careful plan to allow delegation of epinephrine administration by unlicensed school personnel when the registered professional nurse was unavailable. Public health nurse consultants and the school system established detailed policies that balanced the risk of epinephrine injection against the benefit of its administration in carefully defined situations with carefully constructed checks and balances (Truglio-Londrigan et al., 2002).

In the third right the nurse considers the characteristics of the delegatee: Does the potential delegatee have "reasonable knowledge, training, and experience to assure consistent and safe performance of the task" (Rippke et al., 2001, p. 115). A nurse may delegate any nursing functions to another registered nurse, as long as the second nurse has appropriate knowledge, training, and experience for safe and consistent performance of the delegated task. An advantage of delegating to another registered professional nurse is that the nurse delegator can pass both responsibility and accountability to the second nurse, because both have the same

licensure. This third step also requires the delegator to consider whether the patient's condition is sufficiently stable and whether potential patient responses to the delegated task are sufficiently predictable that the delegatee's knowledge and judgment are sufficient.

The fourth right considers whether the task's objectives, directions, and expectations can be clearly communicated (Hansten & Washburn, 1992): What is the right communication? If the task is unfamiliar to the delegatee or requires multiple steps and complex decision making, the task is less likely to be delegated. Maternal outreach workers, who provide antepartal and postpartum health education and support to women at risk for delivering low-birth-weight infants, are selected based on their experiences in working with pregnant and postpartum women and are provided significant additional training. These programs have demonstrated effective and predictable contexts in which to delegate public health nursing functions to unlicensed assistive personnel.

Supervision and surveillance by the public health nurse delegator is the fifth right. The delegator must be available to monitor, provide feedback, and answer questions. In public health nursing when services are delivered in a variety of locations and delegator and delegatee may be in different places, a plan for ensuring opportunities for supervision and evaluation should be concrete. For example, in home healthcare services the public health nurse supervises a home health aide at regular intervals and is available for questions by telephone. New or emerging patient or home health aide needs can be addressed with supplemental home visits, if needed.

PUBLIC HEALTH NURSING AS DELEGATEE

The public health nurse must also consider the implications of these principles when the nurse accepts delegation from other healthcare professionals, including physicians and advanced practice nurses. For nurses working in population health and working under independent statutory authority, there may be confusion about whether the public health nurse actions are delegated by a physician under relevant laws. One state supreme court determined that public health nurses were independently liable when they provided long-term medication management of a patient with diagnosed tuberculosis but failed to identify and respond to clear symptoms of a severe medication reaction that required liver transplantation. In this case the court determined that the health department physician was immune from prosecution as a public official and that this physician owed a duty to the public and no particularized duty to the patient (*State ex rel. Howenstine v. Roper,* 155 S.W. 3d 747 [Mo. Sup. Ct. 2005]).

When the public health nurse accepts delegation from a healthcare professional and the delegation is allowed by law, the five rights of delegation should be considered to guide the nurse in determining whether or not to accept the delegation. First, is the task to be delegated within a professional nurse's legal scope of practice? Although a nurse may have the knowledge or skill to complete a task, whether or not it is legal may vary according to state nurse practice acts. Second, a public health nurse must consider whether the circumstances are right to implement a task. A hospital-based physician seeking to delegate the task may be unaware or may not appreciate the complexity of the proposed task if it is implemented in this individual's home. The task must also be consistent with the public health nurse's agency policies and procedures, with which the delegator may be unaware or unfamiliar (Rippke et al., 2001).

The third right focuses on the public health nurse's "knowledge, training, and experience to assure safe performance of the task" (Rippke et al., 2001, p. 116). The nurse should not accept responsibility for a task when the nurse lacks or doubts his or her ability to ensure safe and effective care. And the nurse must also consider whether the task is appropriate for this individual client and whether this client is stable enough at this time to attempt the proposed task given this public health nurse's knowledge, training, and experience. Fourth, the public health nurse must consider whether the orders, directions, and communications from the physician or nurse practitioner are clear and accurate. The fifth right is ensuring the right supervision is available: Who is responsible and accountable? The nurse must be clear that the task is within the nurse's legal scope of practice.

Whether public health nurses are the delegator or the delegatee, registered professional nurses retain professional accountability for their decisions. As the delegatee it is insufficient for a client task to be ordered; it must also be within the scope of nursing practice. As a delegator the registered professional nurse may delegate responsibility for task completion but retains accountability for the task—unless the nurse is delegating to another registered professional nurse (Rippke et al., 2001). Concerns for ensuring appropriate public health nursing interventions for delegated functions go well beyond exact performance of tasks. The scope of nursing practice, the relevant state nurse practice act, and legal decisions shaping nursing practice must all be considered.

MINNESOTA DEPARTMENT OF HEALTH POPULATION-BASED PUBLIC HEALTH NURSING PRACTICE INTERVENTION WHEEL: APPLICATION TO PRACTICE

Frequently, the frail elderly population is at increased risk for neglect and abuse. In this population it is essential to have providers who understand their distinctive needs and clinical presentation of disease. A percentage of the elderly will be found in the nursing home or adult home. Within the walls of these nursing homes is a subpopulation of poor minority older adults who present with a complexity of needs.

In caring for the geriatric population, nurse practitioners face numerous challenges, such as clinical presentation of disease, limited access to specialists, and limited access to care. For example, the clinical presentation of a specific disease process in an older adult may be very different from a younger adult, such as a urinary tract infection. In a younger adult a urinary tract infection most likely presents with urinary urgency, urinary frequency, and supra pubic tenderness, whereas in an older adult it can present as confusion, delirium, or fever. The American adult population is growing older, yet the specialists in this field have not kept pace with this growth.

The Case for Case Management

The following is a case study that exemplifies one of the intervention wheel's population-based strategies known as case management. After the case study there is a discussion as to the process of the case management and an exploration as to the application of case management in relation to the three levels of practice: individual/family, community, and system. In addition, **Box 9-1** provides questions for further contemplation by the reader after reading the case study.

Case Study

Shirley Franco, MSN, FNP
President, NP in Family Health, Gericine NPs Enhancing Geriatric Medicine

Gericine, a nurse practitioner primary healthcare group, was created to provide quality care to the underserved population. The nurse practitioners at Gericine care for and manage one of the most vulnerable populations, older adults residing in long-term care. This practice is located in the northeast outside of New York City. The Gericine model provides accessible health care while facilitating and planning treatment options that meet the resident's need. Nurse practitioners provide a comprehensive and individualized treatment plan and become the care manager for the population they serve.

Care managers are licensed healthcare providers who combine advanced practice nursing care with case management. The care manager becomes the primary care provider, advocate, and facilitator for the resident. He or she is responsible for providing residents with options and available resources while understanding the resident's status and life to death trajectory. Ultimately, the nurse practitioner care manager promotes quality, cost-effective outcomes. A nurse practitioner functioning in the care manager role commonly is faced with providing care for a resident like the situation described below.

An 87-year-old Hispanic man with a history of hypertension, chronic obstructive pulmonary disorder, chronic heart failure, gastric paresis, and recent gastrostomy tube placement for significant weight loss is newly admitted to a long-term care facility. This resident has been seen multiple times by a gastrointestinal specialist who suggested to the family that a gastrostomy tube may stabilize his weight. Despite the gastrostomy tube, the resident is losing weight and has had a 5-pound weight loss in 2 weeks. The resident's weight before the gastrostomy tube placement was 112 pounds, but now he is 107 pounds. The resident's wife is Spanish speaking and does not understand why her husband is still losing weight.

The nurse practitioner is challenged with providing cultural competent care to this resident with multiple comorbid conditions while trying to help the wife understand the disease process and where the patient is in the life-to-death trajectory. The nurse practitioner has carried out a comprehensive assessment including a family and a community assessment where the resident has lived the past 50 years of his life. The nurse practitioner notes that both the resident and his wife were active in their community church and that the resident has been an active member of the "Green Thumb" club. In fact, the resident has won many awards for the flowers and vegetables that he has successfully tended over the years.

The nurse practitioner decides that she will need a multidisciplinary approach to provide comprehensive care for the resident and his wife. The nurse practitioner seeks out the assistance of the social worker to support her need for advance care planning, and she requested that the gastrointestinal specialist be present and also the dietary and nursing staff. Together the multidisciplinary team is able to present to the resident and his wife the options and available resources located within the long-term care facility and the local community. They are able to create a plan to change the current feedings to a higher caloric concentration and a slower infusion rate for easier absorption and explain in detail the disease processes of gastroparesis and diabetes so the wife and resident understand the issues and concerns that are currently plaguing them and those that may occur in the future and have a comprehensive advance care plan that encompassed many of the aspects that the resident stated he wanted.

In this case the nurse practitioner focused on delivering a collaborative, communicative, and comprehensive plan of care to the resident and his wife. As the nurse practitioner care manager, the focus is on the quality of the care that is delivered while balancing the most cost-effective positive outcome for the resident.

BOX **9-1**   Field Exercise

- Who is the population of interest in this case?
- Why would this population be considered a "vulnerable" population?
- What were the major issues for this particular resident and his wife?
- How would you describe the processes of case management taking place in the case study?
- What roles did the nurse practitioner exemplify in this case study?
- Can you think of any other healthcare team members that could have been engaged?
- Would there be a situation in which referral and follow-up was necessary? If yes, explain.
- Would there be a situation when delegation would be beneficial? If yes, explain.
- As the nurse practitioner engaged in the process of case management, what other ways could she be engaged at the community and systems level to enhance the care of the resident and his wife?

In the case study described above, it is the nurse practitioners who are involved in the case management process as they care for their population of older adults and their families. This process begins with the assessment that is beyond the individual assessment but includes the family members with a look out into the community from where the resident was admitted. It is evident that the nurse practitioner works together with other members of the healthcare team but that this collaboration also includes family members. There is a give and take between all members with the focus being the resident and the resident's wife. The role of the nurse care manager is very evident as an educator, communicator, collaborator, and provider of care.

The nurse practitioner who is working as the care manager in this situation practices at the individual/family level as evidenced by the education taking place

with the resident and the resident's wife as well as the support and counseling. In addition, work at the community level may also be explored as this nurse practitioner care manager can reach out into the community and encourage members of their church and the Green Thumb club to come to visit the resident. In fact, the nurse practitioner may also encourage the community members to do more than just visit but to be engaged. For example, the members of the Green Thumb club may consider planting with the resident in small pots on the resident's unit or if possible work with administration to have a small section of the grounds dedicated to resident gardening. In this way the nurse practitioner is attempting to change attitudes of the community to look at the long-term care organization as a building that people can walk into and engage the residents rather than walk by the building door. The nurse practitioner may also carry out the intervention of case management on the system level in the following way. From her experience she may note that for some individuals in this vulnerable population the complexity of their problems may warrant more than the already established multidisciplinary team meetings as directed by Medicare and Medicaid. The nurse practitioner may request and lobby for a change in the long-term care system. The request may be in the form of a suggestion that for newly admitted long-term care residents with multiple needs that for the first 6 months these meetings may take place on a weekly basis to ensure a smooth transition.

CONCLUSION

This chapter addresses three public health interventions in the green wedge of the intervention wheel: referral and follow-up, case management, and delegated functions. Each intervention was discussed in detail along with exploration as to how these interventions may be implemented at the individual/family, community, and systems levels of practice. The argument for case management exemplified a nurse practitioner case management model where the nurse functioned as a care manager for an older adult living in a nursing home. This case presents a real-life experience for the reader where the intervention of case management was explored as well as how the nurse practitioner practiced at the individual/family, community, and system levels. The field exercise provided the context where the reader was able to reflect on the case and think beyond the field exercise box. In general, the green wedge offers the public health nurse additional strategies for the provision of care to populations.

References

Allender, J. A., & Spradley, B. W. (2005). *Community health nursing: Promoting and protecting the public's health* (6th ed.). Philadelphia: Lippincott Williams & Wilkins.

American Nurses Association [ANA] & the National Council of State Boards of Nursing [NCSBN]. (2005). Joint statement on delegation. Retrieved April 1, 2009, from https://www.ncsbn.org/Joint_statement.pdf

American Nurses Credentialing Center. (2008–2009). Nursing case management. Retrieved April 22, 2009, from http://www.nursecredentialing.org/NurseSpecialities/CaseManagement.aspx

Beilman, J. P., Sowell, R. L., Knox, M., & Phillips, K. D. (1998). Case management at what expense? A case study of the emotional costs of case management. *Nursing Case Management, 3*(2), 89–95.

Block, D. (2009). Reflections on school nursing and delegation [Editorial]. *Public Health Nursing, 26,* 112–113.

Bokhaut, T., & Mahoney, I. E. (1960). A referral plan that serves babies. *American Journal of Nursing, 60,* 824–827.

Bower, K. A. (1992). *Case management by nurses.* Washington, DC: American Nurses Publishing.

Brooten, D. (1995). Perinatal care across the continuum: Early discharge and nursing home follow-up. *Journal of Perinatal and Neonatal Nursing, 9*(1), 38–44.

Cady, L. L. (1952). Planning referral forms. *American Journal of Nursing, 52*, 175–176.

Cave, L. A. (1989). Follow-up phone calls after discharge. *American Journal of Nursing, 89*, 942–943.

Champion, V. L., & Skinner, C. S. (2008). The health belief model. In K. Glanz, B. K. Rimer, & K. Viswanath (Eds.), *Health behavior and health education: Theory, research, and practice* (4th ed., pp. 45–65). San Francisco: Jossey-Bass.

Clemen-Stone, S., McGuire, S. L., & Eigsti, D. G. (2002). *Comprehensive community health nursing: Family, aggregate, and community practice* (6th ed.). St. Louis, MO: Mosby.

Dieckmann, J. L. (1999). *Caring for the chronically ill: Philadelphia, 1945–1965*. New York: Garland Publishing.

Donaldson, N. E. (1977). Fourth trimester follow-up. *American Journal of Nursing, 77*, 1176–1178.

Flynn, L., Budd, M., & Modelski, J. (2008). Enhancing resource utilization among pregnant adolescents. *Public Health Nursing, 25*, 140–148.

Hansten, R., & Washburn, M. (1992). What do you say when you delegate work to others? *American Journal of Nursing, 92*, 48–49.

Katz, M. B. (1996). *In the shadow of the poorhouse: A social history of welfare in America* (rev. ed., 10th anniversary ed.). New York: Basic Books.

Keller, L. O., Strohschein, S., & Briske, L. (2008). Population-based public health nursing practice: The intervention wheel. In M. Stanhope & J. Lancaster (Eds.), *Public health Nursing: Population-centered health care in the community* (7th ed., pp. 186–214). St. Louis, MO: Mosby Elsevier.

Kersbergen, A. L. (1996). Case management: A rich history of coordinating care to control costs. *Nursing Outlook, 44*, 169–172.

Knollmueller, R. N. (1989). Case management: What's in a name? *Nursing Management, 20*(10), 38–40, 42.

Kraus, B. C. (1944). The patient referral system. *American Journal of Nursing, 44*, 387–391.

Lillibridge, J., & Hanna, B. (2008). Using telehealth to deliver nursing case management services to HIV/AIDS clients. *Online Journal of Issues in Nursing, 14*(1). Retrieved April 21, 2008, from http://www.nursingworld.org/MainMenu Categories/ANAMarketplace/ANAPeriodicals/ OJIN/TableofContents/Vol142009/No1Jan09/ ArticlePreviousTopic/TelehealthandHIV AIDSClient.aspx

Manfredi, C., Lacey, L., & Warnecke, R. (1990). Results of an intervention to improve compliance with referrals for evaluation of suspected malignancies at neighborhood public health centers. *American Journal of Public Health, 80*, 85–87.

McGuire, S., Gerber, D. E., & Clemen-Stone, S. (1996). Meeting the diverse needs of clients in the community: Effective use of the referral process. *Nursing Outlook, 44*(5), 218–222.

National Association of School Nurses. (2006). Position statement: Delegation. Retrieved April 8, 2009, from http://www.nasn.org/Default .aspx?tabid_349

National Council of State Boards of Nursing [NCSBN]. (1995). Delegation concepts and decision-making process: National Council position paper. Retrieved April 1, 2009, from https:// www.ncsbn.org/323.htm#

National Council of State Boards of Nursing [NCSBN]. (2005). Working with others: A position paper. Retrieved April 1, 2009, from https:// www.ncsbn.org/Working_with_Others.pdf

Office of Minority Health, U.S. Department of Health and Human Services. (2001). National standards for culturally and linguistically appropriate service in health care. Final report. Retrieved February 20, 2009, from www.omhrc.gov/assets/pdf/checked/ finalreport.pdf

Rippke, M., Briske, L., Keller, L. O., Strohschein, S., & Simonetti, J. (2001). Public health interventions: Applications for public health nursing practice. Public Health Nursing Section, Division of Community Health Services, Minnesota Department of Health. Retrieved December 15, 2008, from http://www.health.state.mn.us/divs/cfh/ophp/resources/docs/phinterventions_manual2001.pdf

Tahan, H. A. (1998). Case management: A heritage more than a century old. *Nursing Case Management, 3*(2), 55–62.

Timm, S. E. (2003). Effectively delegating nursing. *Home Healthcare Nurse, 21,* 260–265.

Truglio-Londrigan, M., Macali, M. K., Bernstein, M., Kaider, G., Peterson, S., & Tumnio, M. C. (2002). A plan for delegation of epinephrine administration in nonpublic schools to unlicensed assistive personnel. *Public Health Nursing, 19,* 412–422.

Wald, L. D. (1902). The nurses' settlement in New York. *American Journal of Nursing, 2*(8), 567–575.

Watkins, E. L., Harlan, C., Eng, E., Gansky, S.A., Gehan, D., & Larson, K. (1994). Assessing the effectiveness of lay health advisors with migrant workers. *Family Community Health, 16,* 72–87.

Will, M. B. (1977). Referral: A process, not a form. *Nursing 77, 7*(12), 44–55.

Wingert, W. A., Teberg, A., Bergman, R., & Hodgman, J. (1980). PNPs in follow-up care of high-risk infants. *American Journal of Nursing, 80,* 1485–1488.

Wolfe, I. (1962). Referral—A process and a skill. *Nursing Outlook, 10,* 253–256.

Zimmerman, P. G., & Kirkpatrick, C. (n.d.). Delegating to unlicensed assistive personnel. Retrieved April 10, 2009, from http://222.nurse.com/ce/CE124–60/CoursePage?

WORKING IT OUT: CONSULTATION, COUNSELING, AND HEALTH TEACHING

LIN DRURY

One of the most important points of a visiting nurse's work is the instructions she must give in the homes. The people must be taught some of the rules of hygiene and sanitation, and something of how to care for their sick. . . . Indeed, all of these people are not ignorant of what good nursing is, and I am sure every nurse has learned something from some one of them (Moore, 1900, pp. 19–20).

LEARNING OBJECTIVES

At the completion of the chapter, the reader will be able to

- Describe the Minnesota Department of Health Population-Based Public Health Nursing Practice Intervention Wheel Strategies of counseling, consultation, and health teaching.

- Differentiate between individual/ family, community, and system levels of public health practice.
- Analyze the application of the population-based public health nursing intervention strategies of counseling, consultation, and health teaching to the presiding case study.

KEY TERMS

- Consultation
- Counseling

- Health teaching
- Vulnerable populations

The Minnesota Department of Health Population-Based Public Health Nursing Practice Intervention Wheel Strategies (Keller, Strohschein, & Briske, 2008; Minnesota Department of Health, 2001) exemplifies how public health nurses work with individuals/ families and populations in communities to promote health, prevent disease, and limit the impact of illness. The population-based public health nursing practice intervention wheel is used to demonstrate public health nursing practice, to generate evidence on the best practices concerning public health nursing services, and ultimately to promote funding for research and health initiatives that public health nurses develop, initiate, and evaluate. The population-based nursing practice intervention wheel specifies 17 distinct intervention strategies that are initiated through three levels of practice: individual/family, community, and systems that are population based. In this text these 17 strategies are grouped into five themes. This chapter focuses on the blue wedge, termed "working it out." Specifically, these intervention strategies are counseling, consultation, and health teaching. The purpose of this chapter is to first define and describe these strategies, then to identify an issue in public health practice, and finally to demonstrate via a case study the "applying" and the "doing" of these interventions.

This intervention wheel also serves as a tool for conceptualizing public health nursing and facilitating a cognitive and practice shift from individual to population-based nursing. Providers and the general public are more than likely to envision the healthcare system as it is depicted on television—high technology interventions delivered to individuals in life-threatening situations. This vision, however, overlooks the health care that is delivered outside of acute care settings to individuals/families, populations, and the communities within which they live.

Throughout the 20th century diagnosis and treatment of acute illness has driven reimbursement and shaped unsystematic services focused on sickness rather than health (Partnership for Prevention, 2007; Schoen, Osborn, How, Doty, & Peugh, 2008; Wennberg, Fisher, Goodman, & Skinner, 2008). Consequently, it is much more difficult to envision a system focused on promoting and maintaining health and preventing and/or managing chronic illness. Nursing students and registered nurses who are engaged in hospital-based care may wonder how public health nurses design and deliver preventive services for entire populations because their practice is focused on the provision of care to individuals within a circumscribed inpatient unit. The very thought may be overwhelming and sometimes confusing. The public, condi-

tioned by prior experience, may wonder why they should see a nurse if they are not sick. The population-based interventions depicted in the blue wedge of the wheel—counseling, consultation, and health teaching—are critical processes for bridging these gaps and moving providers and the public into preventive care.

MINNESOTA DEPARTMENT OF HEALTH POPULATION-BASED PUBLIC HEALTH NURSING PRACTICE INTERVENTION WHEEL STRATEGIES

Counseling

The public health nursing intervention process begins with professional conversations between the nurse and the individual, family, and/or target population within the context of the community or system. **Counseling** "establishes an interpersonal relationship with a community, system, family or individual intended to increase or enhance their capacity for self-care and coping. Counseling engages the community, a system, family or individual at an emotional level" (Keller et al., 2008, p. 199). The counseling relationship helps the population to reflect, clarify views, identify alternatives, examine available resources, and explore options in a supportive context. The public health nurse encourages the individual/family and population to consider the consequences of potential courses of action and to formulate their own decisions.

Counseling relationships evolve as the public health nurse earns trust through continuing contact with the population. Deborah Antai-Otong (2007) notes "Trust is germane to therapeutic and authentic nurse-client relationships. . . . The client's capacity to trust is governed by early inter-actions with patients and caregivers. . . . However, trust evolves through nurse-client relationships that convey accept-ance, empathy, caring, and understanding" (p. 29). Truglio-Londrigan (2008) spoke about trust as a process that takes shape and forms first through a connection that unfolds over time, allowing for a working together that further builds the relation-ship. Previous negative experiences with "the system," cultural norms, and life stressors may contribute to lack of trust. In addition, as the sphere of communica-tion widens, from individuals/family, community, systems, and to populations, the possibility for miscommunication multiplies. Public health nurses as well as other public health practitioners need to be conscious of this as they seek to work "with" individuals/families and popula-tions, always practicing with intention those actions that build trust.

Although public health nurses often deal with sensitive issues such as inti-mate partner violence, addiction, or homelessness, it is important to keep discussions focused on "here and now" problem solving via counseling. Psy-chotherapy is not within the scope of practice for public health nurses, and referrals to prescreened sources should be facilitated when needed (Clark, 2008; Keller et al., 2008). The prescreening process takes place as the public health nurse locates organizations and agen-cies to serve as partners. These partners may assist the public health nurse in the provision of services such as psychother-apy. The prescreening process clarifies eligibility requirements, fees, and waiting lists, ensuring that those being served will not encounter bureaucratic barriers

to treatment. This prescreening process ensures a "place" where the needs of the individual/family or a population can be addressed. The public health nurse in this situation promotes trust by facilitat-ing access to care and following up on its efficacy.

The literature presents evidence of the importance of counseling as a population-based public health nurse intervention strategy. Edinburgh and Saewyc (2008) studied a home-visiting intervention that helped young (10- to 14-year-old) sexually assaulted adolescents who ran away. The authors noted that the teens in this study refused traditional counseling as an intervention. Traditional counseling was not culturally congruent with the needs of this specific age group. The authors noted "the solution was to offer all teens participation in a thera-peutic empowerment group, which met after school weekly under the guidance of a skilled therapist" (p. 45). Other inter-ventions in this home-visiting interven-tion program included mental health and screening referrals, health education, and daily living skills. Outcomes were positive in terms of reconnecting these young runaways to school and family. Hollen-beck (2008) advocated for universal new-born hearing screening and stressed the importance of providing emotional sup-port, counseling, and education through-out the process, particularly if the screening identified that further examina-tion was needed.

Frank and Grubbs (2008) studied the effectiveness of a faith-based screening and education program focusing on dia-betes, cardiovascular disease, and stroke. The study outcomes noted the impor-tance of conducting the programs in small groups that facilitated one-to-one counseling. Huang, Lin, and Li (2008) addressed the vulnerable population of older adults. These authors studied the service needs of residents in community-based long-term care and noted a need for psychological support and counseling pertaining to lifestyle change, role change, and environmental change. The importance of counseling as a population-based intervention is also noted among other public health practitioners. Olshtain-Mann and Auslander (2008) studied parents' stress and perceptions of competence 2 months after their preterm infant was discharged from a neonatal intensive care unit. These authors noted the importance of emotional support and counseling during the first year after discharge. Although this work comes out of the social work literature, many public health nurses work in early childhood programs supporting families during these first few years after discharge. Counseling is an intervention strategy that public health nurses in all settings "apply" and "do" daily in their practice.

Consultation

The complexity of public health practice may require a wide range of expertise. Public health nurses may therefore find themselves seeking the **consultation** of others in their practice. These consultation services may include health officers, sanitarians, health educators, area professionals, epidemiologists, environmentalists, and media experts. Public health nurses may consult with a media expert if they need assistance on how to reach out into the community and gain the attention of a targeted population. Or, the public health nurse may seek consultation services of many different types of pro-

fessionals or organizations. In this situation the development of a coalition may be the answer, and the public health nurse may be instrumental in the organization of this coalition and the development of a partnership between and among all involved.

Part of the success of partnerships and coalitions is that every organization involved in the coalition is actively seeking consultation from the other. Working together in these types of partnerships serves to facilitate discussion, a give and take of ideas, and information where everyone's expertise is honored and used in the decision-making process. The public health nurse works within coalitions to mediate power and to ensure that decision making remains within the target population. Consultation "seeks information and generates optimal solutions to perceived problems or issues through interactive problem solving with a community, system, family or individual. The community, system, family or individual selects and acts on the option best meeting the circumstances" (Keller et al., 2008, pp. 199 & 204). Just as the public health nurse draws upon multiple sources of information to assist populations to meet their needs, they may in turn be sought to provide nursing expertise within the community-at-large. Ideally, the coalition includes members of the targeted population.

Hopson and Steiker (2008) presented such a situation, noting that schools differ and that each and every school has its own culture and population of students. "Interventions that work well at one school may be a poor fit for others" (p. 116). To address this issue Hopson and Steiker (2008) used participatory action research as their foundational framework. The evidence-based drug abuse prevention program, Keepin' It REAL, was adapted to improve the "fit within a particular school" (p. 118). This was done via the application of a participatory action research. "PAR [participatory action research] is dialogical and proactive typically focusing on empowerment and with researchers' and participants' values both being central to the planning process" (Kidd & Kral, 2005, p, 187). Furthermore, Kidd and Kral (2005) note how this collaboration exists in every phase of the research project. The collaborative partnership of the students and staff of the schools is critical so that the researchers may collaborate and learn from these partners about interventions that are most likely to succeed at each school.

Health Teaching

Health teaching focuses on providing information needed by the individual/family or population so they may become more aware of the promotion of health, the prevention of disease and injury, health screenings, available community services, and how to access those services. Health teaching "communicates facts, ideas and skills that change knowledge, attitudes, values, beliefs, behaviors, and practices of individuals, families, systems, and/or communities" (Keller et al., 2008, p. 199). Health teaching engages participants at an intellectual level, whereas counseling engages participants emotionally. In practice, health teaching proceeds from the counseling relationship. For example, if a public health nurse is developing a mammography program for a particular population residing in a particular community, the nurse may first have to provide counseling services to

address barriers to participation such as fear. The public health nurse must carefully assess the population and structure information accordingly. Once this assessment is completed, the public health nurse can develop educational programs that provide information the individual/family or population sees as a priority and is ready to receive and to provide that information in a "user friendly" form and in measured amounts that can be absorbed. The goal for the public health nurse is to facilitate outcomes such as knowledge attainment and behavior change in the individual/family or population.

The public health nurse takes a flexible approach that facilitates the individual/family or population to progress gradually from nonthreatening topics to areas that may be more emotionally or culturally challenging. For example, a public health nurse who offers a support group for battered women may have minimal attendance. Offering instead a "mothers' group" may bring women who eventually, once trust is established, reveal abuse. These mothers may explain that if their partner caught them attending a group focused on domestic violence, their risk of battering would increase.

If we are to consider that public health is an interdisciplinary science, of which nursing is a critical participant, we may see the entire process of the development of health teaching programs in the following way. For example, multiple organizations in a particular community may form a coalition to promote health. The members of this coalition together have agreed to form a formal partnership and have identified one of the organizations as the lead agency. Methods of communication, formal and informal, have been developed to reduce miscommunication.

The coalition decides to collectively conduct an assessment of their community to identify issues and to organize these issues in order of priority. The coalition also has members of the community involved as key participants. All the data from the community assessment are compiled and an analysis reveals several issues. One of the issues is obesity in elementary school children. Once the key issue is decided on, the members of the coalition must collectively determine who the targeted individual/family or population will be, what content will be delivered, how the content will be delivered, where and when the content will be delivered, and by whom. **Table 10-1** identifies these areas with key questions that the members of the coalition and the public health nurse must ask in the development, implementation, and evaluation of the educational program.

Many of these areas noted in Table 10-1 correspond with the determinants of health noted in a "Systematic Approach to Health Improvement" as outlined in Healthy People 2010 (U.S. Department of Health and Human Services, 2000). The determinants of health depicted in the "Systematic Approach to Health Improvement" include policies and interventions, behavior, biology, social environment, physical environment, and access to quality health care. Each factor is considered here in great detail because many apply to health teaching and from here forward is referred to as a systematic approach to health teaching.

Biological determinants such as age, intellectual capacity, sensory function, and overall health impact the individual/family or population's ability to learn, as indicated earlier, and must be a considered when developing a health teaching program. Gender and ethnicity can

influence whether an individual seeks out new information, places relevance on the information, and puts that information to use. For example, Kaye, Crittenden, and Charland (2008) noted that "reaching and properly serving older men can be a challenge for practitioners" (p. 9). Older men may fail to participate in health education programs or to actively seek help because "many older men believe that a stigma is attached to seeking help" (p. 9). Age is associated with learning styles, sensory capacity, and familiarity with technological developments (Knowles, Holton, & Swanson, 2005). For example, the act of producing a pamphlet requires the public health nurse to be conscious of normal aging changes with regard to vision, requiring the production of pamphlets that have larger print and colors that are easily identifiable.

Working with children also brings challenges. The public health nurse must secure the cooperation of school or organizational officials in addition to obtaining each child's parental consent before any information is presented. Teaching about bodily functions, family life, and sexuality is likely to evoke worry and require extensive preliminary work with organizational officials and parent groups. Detailed consent and opt-out procedures must be agreed on before proceeding. Children's developmental level is also important. For example, the adolescent's sense of invincibility pairs poorly with information structured to startle or scare participants into compliance. Strategies that emphasize active participation and peer group values are more likely to catch the interest of adolescents.

Social determinants such as education and culture are critical considerations in health teaching. Individuals may be reticent to reveal language, educational, or

Table 10-1 Questions to Ask in the Development of Health Teaching Programs

Who: Individual/ Family/Population	What Is the Issue?	How Is the Program Delivered and by Whom?	When and Where?
Who is the targeted individual/targeted or population? What do we know about the targeted individual/ family or population? What is their age? What is the gender? What are their cultural ideas, values, and beliefs? What is their level of education? What is the primary language spoken? What is their income level? What are past health experiences? What are significant past experiences? What behaviors or lifestyle characteristics does the individual/family/ population exemplify? Are there any physical barriers to participating in the educational program, such as pain, hunger, or illness? Is the individual/family/ population ready to learn or is there an emotional barrier present? Or, does the individual/family/ population not see the issue as a priority at the present time? Are there marital issues or concerns? Child care issues or concerns? Transportation issues or safety issues that must be taken into consideration?	What is the content or the message that must be covered? How detailed is the content or message? Can the content or message be divided into sessions? How will the public health nurse know if the educational program is successful? In other words, what will be the evaluation process? What behavioral change is expected? Did the educational program connect with the individual/ family/population and get the message across?	What is the best way to deliver the content given the information pertaining to the individual/family/ population? What is the best channel that the message will be delivered given individual/family/ population age, gender, physical and behavioral characteristics, etc. For example: Will the educational program be delivered via lecture, one-to-one, small group discussion, demonstration, media such as billboards, television, or radio. Will the Internet be used as a channel, including text messaging, Facebook, etc.? What materials will be used to deliver the message? For example: Will there be pamphlets, books, songs, games, or toys? Are the materials appropriate? Is the message clear and to the point? Who is the best person to deliver the message? For example: If the issue involves adolescent boys who are involved in sports, perhaps an athlete is the best person to present the information.	When and where is the best time to conduct the educational program? When and where is the best place to connect with the individual/family/ population? For example: if the public health nurse wishes to conduct child car safety seat checks, it may be best to conduct this educational program at parks where young families may bring their children on the weekends.

literacy issues that can interfere with accurate interpretation of health information. Translating written material into the individuals/family or populations first language may be ineffective if limited education and health literacy are not also considered or if cultural mores render some topics taboo. When the public health nurse is working with an individual or family, discussion of written materials in private to solicit feedback and confirm comprehension while protecting self-esteem is essential. In other situations the enlisting of a culturally appropriate licensed medical translator is also a consideration.

Economic determinants overlap heavily with social determinants in terms of educational background, available income, and access to resources (Chang et al., 2004). Individual/family and populations with limited income may find it difficult to gain access to health education programs even if they are free. Transportation costs or costs affiliated with babysitting may make participation in these programs impossible. In addition, the implementation of health recommendations such as including fresh fruit and vegetables in the diet may not be an attainable goal. The public health nurse must adapt teaching materials to fit the needs and the economic resources of the target population, providing information on economical substitute sources of fiber, vitamins, and minerals.

Environmental determinants such as characteristics of the physical and structural environment may necessitate the tailoring of information or the way in which information is provided. For example, many clinics have environments that are not conducive to teaching given the constant interruptions and the noise, yet many clinic nurses make do with what they have and offer great health teaching programs. Examples of educational programming in waiting rooms include reading and math corners for young children to enhance literacy while at the same time modeling behavior for families, food corners with varying boxes and cans from grocery stores that can be used as props to teach clients how to read labels, and healthy menu guides that are culturally congruent for the targeted clinic population. **Box 10-1** illustrates this use of clinic waiting time for educational programming.

Finally, consider the psychological status of the target population to determine readiness for learning. Public health nurses frequently encounter individuals and family members in the community who have been discharged from the hospital after an episode of acute illness. Before hospital discharge these individuals and family members receive volumes of information, typically diet sheets, medication schedules, activity restrictions, and follow-up instructions—all during the stress of illness and compounded by anxiety related to going home. Short hospital stays make this pattern hard to avoid, but nevertheless the public health nurse must plan accordingly. Expect the newly discharged to be overwhelmed and confused. Allow time during early visits to contact providers, clarify instructions, and adapt the information to fit the client's circumstances (Drury, 2008). In addition, public health nurses find themselves working with **vulnerable populations** with complex needs such as people who are homeless or who have mental illnesses compounded by comorbid chronic diseases. These situations must also be accounted for in the development of teaching sessions and/or programs.

BOX **10-1**　**What To Do When Waiting: Example of Group Health Teaching Diabetes Education**

Anny M. Eusebio, RN, MSN, FNP-BC

I practice in an outpatient satellite clinic affiliated to a major hospital in the New York area. The population is about 75% Latino and has limited reading skills in either English or Spanish. There is a high rate of obesity and diabetes in this clinic population. Furthermore, the majority have uncontrolled diabetes despite the best efforts of health care providers.

In 2007 we attended an informational session where RNs and NPs were introduced to and taught how to use the U.S. Diabetes Conversation Map Kits created by Healthy in collaboration with the American Diabetes Association.

The concept was intriguing. It uses visually stimulating maps (in 5 topics) as teaching aides for individuals in group settings. They are appropriate for all educational levels and are available in English and Spanish. These maps provide the data needed for individuals to improve diabetes self-management in a fun and interactive manner. This easy and engaging method facilitates discussion and is appropriate to populations such as ours with limited formal education.

About a year ago the program was launched in our clinic in an effort to improve education via groups. The education included information such as diet modification and the expected health outcomes included improved fasting glucose and HbA_{lc} levels. We have one English-speaking diabetes educator who supervises the group meetings. A Spanish-speaking nurse was also educated in the use of the Conversation Maps.

Over the past 4 months this forum was extended to include the family members of the individual participants. This creates a further bond between spouses, children/parents, grandchildren/grandparents, and siblings. In particular, the family members that prepare meals for the individual clients are invited, but all family interested in expanding their knowledge of diabetes are welcome.

These Conversation Maps are an interesting way to teach about diabetes, not only to individuals but groups in a culturally sensitive and congruent way.

Source: Healthy Interactions, Inc. (2008).

Policy interventions and *access to care* must also be assessed. In situations where there is a law that has been developed and implemented to protect the public, such as bike helmet laws, the public health nurse must be aware of how the law is implemented and develop health teaching for the population to facilitate compliance. In addition, when developing health teaching, the coalition and its members must constantly ask if the targeted population will be able to access the program they are developing. This question involves discussion pertaining to time of the program, cost of the program, transportation to the program, location of the program, and how the content of the program addresses the targeted populations ideas, values, emotions, and beliefs pertaining to the topic. This particular discussion also demonstrates consideration of the seven A's outlined in Chapter 3.

What is of interest to note in the above description of counseling, consultation, and health education is how many of the population-based intervention strategies are closely intertwined with one another. For example, public health nurses find they must carry out counseling first to emotionally support individuals through their decision-making process and at the same time provide health teaching and seek consultation from others.

PUBLIC HEALTH ISSUES IN PRACTICE

In the other intervention chapters of this text, the authors present issues that public health nurses work with every day. Many of these issues and challenges are disease processes that are communicable, noncommunicable, and chronic ill-

nesses. For this chapter I describe a community as a system that presents with many issues and challenges. These issues and challenges have a profound effect on the individual/families and the population that reside within its borders. What follows is a description of this community in need.

Community in Need

The Henry Street Settlement (HSS) is a not-for-profit social service institution located on the lower east side of Manhattan in New York City. Since 1893 the settlement has focused on meeting the needs of vulnerable populations and has expanded to include 19 sites serving more than 100,000 clients from around the world and across the life span. Although HSS was founded by the early 20th century nursing leader Lillian Wald to address the health problems of impoverished immigrants, Wald's insights into the determinants of health led to the development of programs encompassing education, recreation, the arts, sociopolitical activism, and economic development in addition to home and agency-based nursing care (Lewenson, Keith, Kelleher, & Polansky, 2001).

Today's HSS programs reach clients in their homes, in day care centers, youth groups, workforce training, homeless shelters, mental health centers, summer camps, senior centers, and in the performing arts. Ironically, nursing did not remain among HSS's core services. As the settlement grew over the decades and professional specialization increased, nurses left HSS and formed the Visiting Nurse Service of New York in 1944. Following this separation, HSS referred clients to outside medical providers (Feld, 2008).

Like their predecessors for over 100 years, current HSS clients are at high risk for a wide range of physical and psychosocial health problems. Substantial populations at HSS today were born in China, Africa, Latin America, or Russia. Disenfranchised by language, culture, and economic barriers, the needs of today's clients are complex and interdependent. Meanwhile, constraints on health care spending have reduced providers' incentives to accept such patients. As a result, HSS found its referral sources dwindling and its clients poorly equipped to compete for increasingly scarce public health care.

THE COMMUNITY

In 1893 the lower east side was a neighborhood of impoverished immigrants geographically and socially isolated from the wealthy sections of Manhattan. Lillian Wald found families doubled and tripled up in small deteriorating apartments. Airless rooms, inadequate plumbing, and vermin joined with malnutrition and overwork to foster disease. Poverty and social isolation enforced by language and cultural differences contributed to despair. Turn of the century residents had few options for improvement (Wald, 1915).

Today, the lower east side is gentrifying. Luxury housing and business developments are replacing the tenements and attracting upscale residents (National Trust for Historic Preservation, 2008). The shrinking supply of affordable apartments has concentrated the HSS client population into dense blocks of New York City Housing Authority buildings and deteriorating rent-stabilized units. Immigrants still come to the area, and poor families repeat the pattern of previous centuries, doubling up or taking in boarders to meet

The Lower East Side of New York City, 1893. *Source:* Courtesy of the Visiting Nurse Service of New York.

rising rents in substandard accommodations. HSS clients share the geography of the lower east side but are isolated from their affluent neighbors by an unmarked economic boundary line.

POPULATION AND PROGRAMS

HSS clients range in age from newborns to centenarians. The population is outstandingly diverse, reflecting New York City in terms of race/ethnicity, culture, religion, and education/literacy. Specific programs target selected high-need groups. For example, the Parent Center provides drop-in support, education, and socialization to parents of infants and toddlers. The overwhelming majority of participants are African American or Spanish-speaking women of childbearing age, but there are no restrictions on attendance, and an occasional father or grandparent joins the program. Children in HSS

Head Start programs reflect the demographics of families within walking distance of the centers. At one HSS Head Start site, nearly all the children are monolingual Chinese. The Home Housekeeping program serves more than 2,000 elderly and/or disabled clients throughout the city. On a single day the caseload of that program includes 62 languages or dialects and an even larger number of cultures.

DETERMINANTS OF HEALTH: ECONOMIC

Clients across HSS programs have one characteristic in common, poverty. In addition, HSS grows its own employees by offering entry-level jobs to successful program participants. Consequently, HSS clients plus most of the rank and file employees represent vulnerable populations in terms of socioeconomic level, cognitive status, illness or disability, and life circumstances (Aday, 2001;

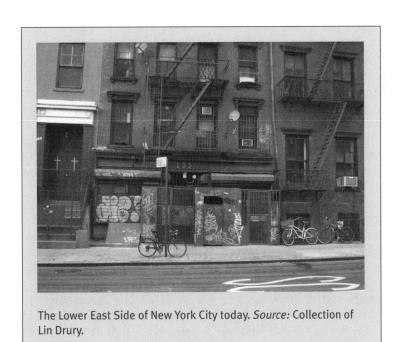

The Lower East Side of New York City today. *Source:* Collection of Lin Drury.

de Chesnay, 2005). City demographic data divide Manhattan into 10 clusters by zip codes. The HSS area cluster is combined with two more affluent zip codes in calculating the median household income, but it still ranks fourth from the bottom (Thompson, 2007).

Economic factors are strong determinants of population health in New York City. In September 2007 the city comptroller released a report on a 15-year study of the health of city residents. A key finding was the widening gap in illness rates between rich and poor New Yorkers. Since data collection began in 1990, preventable and manageable chronic disease has risen among low-income residents. For example, hospitalization of people with type 2 diabetes has increased 82% citywide, with poor individuals five times more likely to require hospital care than individuals from the city's wealthiest neighborhoods. The diabetes death rate was 125.2 per 100,000 people in the poorest neighborhoods but only 14.8 per 100,000 people in the richest neighborhoods.

The city comptroller summed up the report by stating that New York needs to do a better job of providing primary care and preventive care. He acknowledged that low Medicaid reimbursement rates for routine care and wellness visits contribute to providers' preference for emergency department services for their publicly insured clients (Thompson, 2007).

Low-income New Yorkers are at high risk for a wide range of preventable physical and psychological disorders. They are two to six times more likely to experience serious psychological distress than their counterparts with higher incomes, and they are four times more likely to be hospitalized for substance abuse and/or

mental health treatment instead of receiving outpatient care (Karpati et al., 2004; Thompson, 2007).

Determinants of Health: Social and Health System

In addition to the economic disparity, many HSS clients are recent immigrants who face documentation issues, language barriers, employment disparity, and cultural distance from healthcare workers. Long-term HSS clients therefore not only must deal with poverty but with social determinants that have an impact on their health. The HSS clients commonly suffer from congestive heart failure, diabetes, arthritis, emphysema, cancer, depression, and alcoholism. These individuals would benefit from case management and/or monitoring by a visiting nurse but most are not eligible for these services under current Medicare or Medicaid regulations. Limited coverage for hearing, vision, and dental care further restricts many clients' functional capacities.

Working poor clients and HSS front-line employees often hold jobs that do not provide paid sick days; thus they cannot afford to miss work while seeking care. If offered, their health insurance is high in cost and low in coverage; many cannot justify this expense amid conflicting budget priorities. Clients and employees alike seek health care only when they are acutely ill.

For both clients and front-line employees at HSS, contact with healthcare providers is often limited to emergency department treatment, and opportunities for preventive care are lacking. Both clients and employees need user-friendly services that are culturally appropriate and available in a context they trust. In response to this burgeoning need for health care, HSS opened an on-site medical office. A multilingual physician and a culturally diverse staff run the office, but appointments during the workday are required. Medicaid and Medicare are accepted, but no free services are available, even for HSS employees. Perhaps as a result, since it opened in 2002 the office has been underutilized (V. Stack, personal communication, 2007).

DETERMINANTS OF HEALTH: ENVIRONMENTAL

The unmarked economic boundary line separating low-income and upscale housing on the lower east side also determines the accessibility of shops and services for HSS clients. One subway line runs at the periphery of the area, and taxis do not cruise the streets as they do in middle class neighborhoods. The blocks within walking distance of HSS are dominated by retailers who aim for low-income customers: currency exchanges, bodegas (gritty urban convenience stores), 99 cent stores, and "greasy spoon" diners. At the local bodega clients on food stamps find it impossible to spread their entitlement across the month if they purchase the fruits, vegetables, and whole grains recommended for a healthy diet.

Retailers and professional offices targeting upscale customers have recently opened several blocks away but are inaccessible to most HSS clients due to economic disparity, distance, language, and culture. Clients seeking a bank, a supermarket, department store, gym, or restaurant must speak English, must have the agility to board a bus or have cash for a "gypsy" cab (informal and unregulated car service), and then muster up the energy to transport their purchases (and sometimes several children

as well) up unreliable elevators to their apartment. A common refrain among clients is "It's just all too much . . ."

MINNESOTA DEPARTMENT OF HEALTH POPULATION-BASED PUBLIC HEALTH NURSING PRACTICE INTERVENTION WHEEL: APPLICATION TO PRACTICE

The Intervention

The above presents a picture of a community with needs that have a profound health effect on the individual/families and the population who reside in that community. The proposed answer was to develop a university/community partnership to reintegrate public health nursing in a social service setting through a faculty/student public health nursing clinical practice.

The Partnership: Application of Consultation, Counseling, and Health Teaching

In the mid-1990s HSS administrators looked for healthcare resources for their clients while faculty from Pace University Lienhard School of Nursing sought community health experiences for their nursing students. They discovered a mutual opportunity. Consultations between the school of nursing and HSS led to an AmeriCorps grant in 1995. Ongoing faculty efforts plus internal funding from the school of nursing provided the groundwork for the current partnership between HSS and the school (Lewenson et al., 2001).

In 2004 a Lienhard School of Nursing faculty member, with a specialty in public health nursing, approached HSS with a proposal to develop a faculty practice and student clinical practicum in public health nursing on-site. HSS administrators recognized an opportunity to integrate preventive care, health teaching, and counseling activities into their social service delivery programs. The faculty member initiated the public health nursing practice and began planning for the current partnership.

The purpose of the partnership was to expand the breadth and depth of public health nursing practice at the HSS. The overall goal was to improve the health of an underserved population, HSS clients and employees, by engaging them in the process of community health planning with public health nursing faculty and students from the Lienhard School of Nursing. Thus the partnership incorporates the public health nursing faculty member, students from the school of nursing, clients and employees from HSS, and community residents and professionals who have interest or expertise on community issues. The partners decide what health issues should be addressed and suggest approaches. All members of the partnership jointly determine what evidence will be collected to assess the outcomes of its work. Members of the partnership continuously discuss where they are going and what process will work best to get them there.

This consultation approach is particularly appropriate at HSS, given the facility's history and current pattern of service delivery. The Settlement was founded on the wisdom of listening to its constituency and then acting on the information obtained (Wald, 1915). Most HSS programs go a step further in empowering the population by employing current or former service recipients to mentor new clients: Children are trained as peer counselors, teens run a retail bicycle shop, mental health clients operate a clothing boutique, vocational program graduates gain paid employment within the home care program, formerly homeless people work with shelter residents in preparation for permanent housing, and ambulatory senior citizens visit homebound elderly. The public health nurse faculty member continuously consults with all participants in the partnership to create interventions that provide learning opportunities for the students and positive outcomes for clients and employees. Many of these interventions take the form of health teaching and counseling.

How the Collaborative Partnership Works: Counseling, Consultation, and Health Teaching at the Individual/Family, Community, and Systems Levels

Public health nursing practice inclusive of health teaching, counseling, and consultation are often linked, particularly when working with vulnerable populations whose experiences with the healthcare and social services systems have inspired mistrust. In an attempt to engage a broad range of clients and employees, information, materials, and professional expertise from the school of nursing faculty and students are available at multiple HSS locations. The cultural diversity and life experiences of the school of nursing students make it possible to match the special skills and interests of students with particular populations at HSS. The public health nursing faculty member and students spend time at each location counseling clients and employees and offering nonthreatening health teaching sessions to build trust. As clients and employees share their interests and concerns, the school of nursing faculty member and students respond with information, hands-on interventions, and individualized counseling as needed. The partnership works collectively and collaboratively to design, implement, and evaluate health promotion, disease management, and prevention programs for the HSS population at large. The school of nursing students perform community health assessments, conduct group health educational programs, organize activity sessions, provide one-on-one health counseling, make home healthcare visits, and provide referrals and follow-up care. The school of nursing provides loaner and donor equipment and supplies to assist the population in self-monitoring of health or management of chronic illness.

For example, the HSS population is a high risk for a comorbidity pattern of obesity, diabetes, hypertension, and heart disease. A healthy diet is key to interrupting this pattern, but the economic and environmental disparities detailed above foster diets high in carbohydrates, sodium, and fat. Students intervene at the systems level by joining with advocacy groups to increase food stamp allocations, contacting the city council to permit the use of food stamps at farmers markets, and participating in a neighborhood coalition to obtain city-sponsored "green carts" for the area. At the community level, students canvass local bodegas and more distant grocery stores to counsel managers about the condition and price of perishable foods in an attempt to protect the public. They make reports to the department of health when needed and follow-up on results. In addition, students consult with food service administrators on menu planning and provide classes for the cooking staff in the day

care and senior centers. They work with the housekeepers and senior companions to select healthy foods when doing grocery shopping and light meal preparation for homebound seniors. On the individual and family level, students offer classes and cooking demonstrations throughout HSS that are focused on healthy eating on a budget.

Each counseling and health teaching activity leads to others, sometimes progressing from the individual or group out to a wider audience. Students discovered that homeless clients in residential shelter program had little experience in meal planning and preparation. They created a series of groups, including grocery shopping field trips, as a way to council and teach this vulnerable population. Clients found they could not stretch their food stamps across the month unless they bought in bulk, but their rooms came with individual-size refrigerators. The students organized their clients to meet with the shelter director and to begin a letter-writing campaign requesting larger refrigerators. The building has a complex funding stream, multiple layers of management, and subcontracted program operations. It was a challenge just to determine who should receive the letters, but working through the system has united the clients around a common goal. It may be a long time before the Department of Housing and Urban Development responds to the client's request, but they have developed a "voice" within the shelter program.

Outcomes

The partnership began with eight students during one semester in one HSS program serving one population. After 3 years 80 to 100 students deliver year-round care to clients and employees in

12 distinct HSS programs at multiple sites that serve populations across the organization. There is increased participation by clients and employees at each site as well as an increase in requests for further public health nursing services. Employees are taking an increasingly active role in urging nonparticipating clients and coworkers to obtain services. During the past 2 years, public health nurses have been hired for HSS programs that had not previously employed them, and recent graduates from the school of nursing with experience in the partnership have been hired to provide professional nursing assessments for clients in the home housekeeping program. A director of nursing was recently hired to launch a home health care service at HSS.

LESSONS LEARNED

A partnership between two organizations with multiple "players" is always a work in progress with multiple unknowns. The public health nursing faculty member has made a substantial commitment of time and energy to become a trusted figure within HSS. Changes in clients' circumstances, employee turnover, and school of nursing student rotations are constants that require continuous adjustment and modification. Organizational dynamics, funding issues, and political variables can dramatically alter the climate in which the partnership works.

Participation in all activities and programs is voluntary for all clients and employees who choose to be involved. Data collection is limited to what clients and employees are comfortable in providing. Risks to participants are limited to minor discomfort associated with some screening procedures and potential stress associated with discussing personal issues. Participants benefit, however, by obtaining free and convenient attention for health concerns and by having access to nursing students and a faculty member who provide health teaching and counseling within their own home community. Referrals and follow-up are available for any participant who needs additional care, but still some choose not to take advantage of the services offered. The partnership continues to reach out.

CONCLUSION

The HSS case study highlights the enormous impact of the determinants of health on the individual/family or population and demonstrates that the nursing interventions of counseling, consultation, and health teaching must address health disparities at the systems level while simultaneously providing direct care to people. The systematic approach to health teaching and the seven A's assist the public health nurse to synthesize information in a complex environment. The participatory action approach ensures that the population guides public health nurses in collaborative practice with the community.

References

Aday, L. A. (2001). *At risk in America: The health and health care needs of vulnerable populations in the United States*. San Francisco: Jossey-Bass.

Antai-Otong, D. (2007). *Nurse-client communication: A life span approach*. Sudbury, MA: Jones and Bartlett.

Chang, B. L., Bakken, S., Brown, S. S., Houston, T. K., Kreps, G. L., Kukafka, R., et al. (2004). Bridging the digital divide: Reaching vulnerable populations. *Journal of the American Informatics Association, 11*, 448–457.

Clark, M. J. (2008). *Community health nursing: Advocacy for population health*. Upper Saddle River, NJ: Pearson Education.

de Chesnay, M. (Ed.). (2005). *Caring for the vulnerable: Perspectives in nursing theory, practice, and research*. Sudbury, MA: Jones and Bartlett.

Drury, L. J. (2008). Transition from hospital to home care: What gets lost between the discharge plan and the real world? *Journal of Continuing Education in Nursing, 39*(5), 198–199.

Edinburgh, L. D., & Saewyc, E. M. (2008). A novel, intensive home-visiting intervention for runaway, sexually exploited girls. *Journal Compilation, 14*(1), 41–48.

Feld, M. N. (2008). *Lillian Wald: A biography*. Chapel Hill, NC: University of North Carolina Press.

Frank, D., & Grubbs, L. (2008). A faith-based screening/education program for diabetes, CVD, and stroke in rural African Americans. *ABNF Journal, 19*(3), 96–101.

Healthy Interactions, Inc. (Healthyi) in collaboration with the American Diabetes Association, (2008). U.S. D. conversation map program. Retrieved April 10, 2009, from http://healthyinteractions.com/us/en/diabetes/hcp/about/program

Hollenbeck, L. (2008). Advocating for universal newborn hearing screening. *Creative Nursing, 14*(2), 75–81.

Hopson, L. M., & Steiker, L. K. H. (2008). Methodology for evaluating an adaptation of evidence-based drug abuse prevention in alternative schools. *Children & Schools, 30*(2), 116–127.

Huang, J.-J., Lin, K.-C., & Li, I.-C. (2008). Service needs of residents in community-based long-term care facilities in northern Taiwan. *Journal of Clinical Nursing, 17*(1), 99–108.

Karpati, A., Kerker, B., Mostashari, F., Singh, T., Hajat, A., Thorpe, L., et al. (2004). *Health disparities in New York City*. New York: New York City Department of Health and Mental Hygiene.

Kaye, L. W., Crittenden, J. A., & Charland, J. (2008). Invisible older men: What we know about older men's use of heathcare and social service. *Generations, 32*(1), 9–14.

Keller, L. O., Strohschein, S., & Briske, L. (2008). Population-based public health nursing practice: The intervention wheel. In M. Stanhope & J. Lancaster (Eds.), *Public health nursing: Population-centered health care in the community* (pp. 199–205). St. Louis, MO: Mosby/Elsevier.

Kidd, S. A., & Kral, M. J. (2005). Practicing participatory research. *Journal of Counseling Psychology, 52*(2), 187–195.

Knowles, M. S., Holton, E. F., & Swanson, R. A. (2005). *The adult learner: The definitive classic in adult education and human resource development* (6th ed.). Boston: Elsevier.

Lewenson, S., Keith, K. A., Kelleher, C., & Polansky, E. (2001). Carrying on the legacy of Lillian Wald: Partnership with the Henry Street Settlement and the Leinhard School of Nursing at Pace University. *Nursing Leadership Forum, 5*(4), 116–121.

Minnesota Department of Health/Office of Public Health Practice. (2001). Public health interventions: Applications for public health nursing. Retrieved June 1, 2008, from www.health.state.mn.us/divs/cfh/ophp/resources/docs/ph-interventions_manual2001.pdf

Moore, E. J. (1900). Visiting nursing. *American Journal of Nursing, 1*(1), 17–21.

National Trust for Historic Preservation. (2008). National trust for historic preservation names: 2008 list of America's 11 most endangered historic places. Retrieved November 2, 2008, from www.nationaltrust.org

Olshtain-Mann, O., & Auslander, G. (2008). Parents of preterm infants two months after discharge from the hospital: Are they still at (parental) risk? *Health & Social Work, 33*(2), 299–308.

Partnership for Prevention. (2007). Preventative care: A national profile on use, disparities, and health benefits. Retrieved June 1, 2008, from www.prevent.org/NCPP

Schoen, C., Osborn, R., How, S. K. H., Doty, M. M., & Peugh, J. (2008). In chronic condition: Experiences of patients with complex health needs in eight countries. Retrieved November 18, 2008, from http://www.commonwealthfund.org/publications/publications_show.htm?doc_id=726496

Thompson, W. C. (2007). *Health and wealth: Assessing and addressing income disparities in the health of New Yorkers.* New York: Office of the New York City Comptroller.

Truglio-Londrigan, M. (2008). Flattening the field: Group decision-making. In S. B. Lewenson & M. T. Londrigan (Eds.), *Decision-making in nursing: Thoughtful approaches for practice* (pp. 131–144). Sudbury, MA: Jones and Bartlett.

U.S. Department of Health and Human Services. (2000). *Healthy people 2010* (Vol. 1). Washington, DC: U.S. Government Printing Office.

Wald, L. D. (1915). *The house on Henry Street.* New York: Henry Holt & Company.

Wennberg, J. E., Fisher, E. S., Goodman, D. C., & Skinner, J. S. (2008). Tracking the care of patients with severe chronic illness. Retrieved June 1, 2008, from www.dartmouthatlas.org

WORKING TOGETHER: COLLABORATION, COALITION BUILDING, AND COMMUNITY ORGANIZING

ADRIENNE WALD

Public health nursing, being closely related to the activities of several other professions and many community organizations, cannot be carried on successfully and productively as an isolated service. The more closely it is coordinated with the interests and activities of other related and cooperating agencies through a constant sharing and interchange of ideas and service, the more soundly and economically will it fulfill its purpose (National Organization for Public Health Nursing, 1939, p. 15).

LEARNING OBJECTIVES

At the completion of this chapter, the reader will be able to

- Define collaboration, coalition building, and community organizing.
- Apply collaboration, coalition building, and community organizing strategies at appropriate levels of practice.
- Explore evidence-based ways that public health nurses practice these strategies to impact public health outcomes.

KEY TERMS

- Coalition building
- Collaboration
- Community organizing

The interventions in the orange section of the Minnesota Department of Health Population-Based Public Health Nursing Practice Intervention Wheel are presented in this chapter. This orange section includes the three interventions of collaboration, coalition building, and community organizing as depicted in the wheel conceptual model (Minnesota Department of Health, 2001; Keller, Strohschein, & Briske, 2008). This chapter devotes a separate section to each of the three interventions. Section one is about *collaboration*, section two presents *coalition building*, and section three discusses *community organizing*. Together, these three interventions are considered types of "collective action" (Keller et al., 2008, p. 193). Each of these three interventions is discussed with examples of how they are applied at the appropriate level of intervention: individual/family, community, and system. Each of the following sections (collaboration, coalition building, and community organizing) describes evidence-based practices used to address the issue examined in depth in this chapter: *physical inactivity*. The application of these interventions to this important 21st century public health crisis illustrates aspects of how each intervention strategy works and reinforces key concepts.

ISSUE: PHYSICAL INACTIVITY IS A MAJOR 21ST CENTURY PUBLIC HEALTH CONCERN

Today, leading experts consider physical inactivity to be one of the most critically important public health problems of our times (Blair, 2009; Sallis, 2009). In 2003 physical inactivity was estimated to be responsible for over 200,000 deaths each year in the United States (Pate et al., 1995). Additionally, the World Health Organization (WHO, 2002) estimates that, worldwide, 2 million deaths per year can be attributed to physical inactivity, making it a global health crisis as well.

Substantial improvements in health and quality of life are possible by including moderate amounts of physical activity in daily life, according to evidence-based findings from a major report over a decade ago and updated in 2008 by the Surgeon General on physical activity and health (U.S. Department of Health and Human Services, 1996, 2008). The health benefits of physical activity and its importance in promoting good overall health and in reducing the risk of many chronic diseases, such as heart disease, type 2 diabetes, depression, and some cancers, and obesity are well known (Blair, 2009; Pollard, 2003). Strong evidence is emerging on the role of physical activity in brain health and the delay of cognitive decline (Blair, 2009).

In spite of this evidence that regular physical activity is necessary for health promotion and disease prevention for all populations, individuals in age groups from children to adolescents to older adults are not engaging in sufficient physical activity to achieve these benefits. According to the WHO (2002), 60% of the world's population does not get enough physical activity to achieve even the minimal recommendation of at least 30 minutes daily of moderate intensity activity. For those who do not follow the minimum recommendations for physical activity, the risk of getting a cardiovascular disease increases by 1.5 times.

Further, the costs associated with inactivity and obesity accounted for some 9.4% of the national U.S. health expenditure, whereas in Canada physical inactivity accounted for about 6% of total healthcare costs in 1995. Data from 1998 indicate that in the United States, individuals who are physically active save an estimated $500 per year in healthcare costs. It is reported that inactivity alone may have contributed as much as $75 billion to U.S. medical costs in the year 2000 (WHO, 2002). In the United States there has been no increase in the level of physical activity participation from 1986 through 2000 (**Figure 11-1**), implying that most of the strategies during this time period have been ineffective in increasing physical activity participation in Americans.

Experts suggest that new strategies and innovative approaches are needed to impact physical activity participation and health outcomes (Blair, 2009; Pollard, 2003). As discussed, interventions of collaboration, coalition building, and community organizing can be effective in accomplishing this goal.

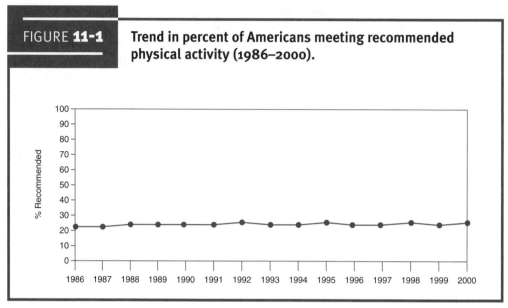

FIGURE 11-1 Trend in percent of Americans meeting recommended physical activity (1986–2000).

Source: Data from Centers for Disease Control and Prevention, 2000.

MINNESOTA DEPARTMENT OF HEALTH POPULATION-BASED PUBLIC HEALTH NURSING PRACTICE INTERVENTION WHEEL STRATEGIES AND LEVELS OF PRACTICE

Collaboration

A working definition of **collaboration** has been offered as:

> . . . a mutually beneficial and well-defined relationship entered into by 2 or more organizations (individuals) to achieve common goals. The relationship includes a commitment to: a definition of mutual relationships and goals; a jointly developed structure and shared responsibility; mutual authority and accountability for success; and a sharing of resources and rewards. (Mattessich & Monsey, 1992, p. 7)

Collaboration has been defined in the intervention wheel as an approach that "commits 2 or more persons or organizations to achieving a common goal through the enhancement of the ability of one or more of them to promote and protect health" (Keller et al., 2008, p. 204). We know that public health nursing may be practiced by one public health nurse or by a group of public health nurses working together or collaboratively.

Clearly, collaboration with other healthcare professionals or with those in other organizations working toward mutual goals is often part of the work of the public health nurse to promote the health of any population. Working in collaboration with others to achieve goals requires that public health professionals and practitioners possess or acquire skills that are applied to develop a shared vision and agree on an effective plan of action (Sullivan, 1998). However, although collaboration is often highly effective in increasing the quality of results and offers the potential of many benefits, including the opportunity for a more comprehensive evaluation and assessment of issues, collaborative projects may not always work (Gray, 1998). An understanding of how successful collaborations are formed is important in considering, or undertaking, a collaborative effort.

In 1992 the Wilder Research Center offered a theoretical understanding of what is needed for collaboration to succeed (Mattessich & Monsey, 1992). An initial review of 133 studies identified 18 relevant and valid studies, and the combined findings from these studies resulted in identification of 19 factors reported to influence whether or not a collaboration formed by government agencies and nonprofit organizations will succeed. These factors were grouped into six key categories: (1) environment, (2) membership, (3) process/structure, (4) communications, (5) purpose, and (6) resources. The 19 factors are listed in the category to which they belong and are described in **Box 11-1**.

This information can be useful in guiding the decision to enter into a partnership with potential collaborators by a careful evaluation of whether the important factors for success exist before undertaking an effort. However, not every collaboration is the same, and the exact combination of the factors for success may not always be identical. Consideration of these factors can assist those who work in public health in assessing the potential of a collaborative approach and in maximizing the impact of collaborative projects (Mattessich & Monsey, 1992).

Collaborative approaches to the problem of physical inactivity have taken on a new importance as the evidence base on physical activity has grown. New models of health behavior and health promotion, such as the social-ecological model, have been developed and are being applied to areas such as physical activity participation (Elder et al., 2007). These models offer new understanding of the many determinants of physical activity and suggest potential interventions at multiple levels of influence on behavior, with a growing emphasis on environmental and policy influences. These models are used to target behavior change beyond the individual level only. As a result, it is increasingly evident to those working in public health and prevention that the decisions and policies in sectors ranging from agriculture to transportation to education may have a huge impact on physical activity participation and health. Yet these groups have not traditionally understood the connections between them nor have they often sought opportunities to collaboratively engage in health promotion efforts.

Important environmental and policy approaches may be implemented by applying collaboration, coalition building, and community organizing interventions. These approaches can effect physical activity participation at the population-based level, complementing the individual-level focus of changing one person's behavior at a time (Heath et al., 2006).

Projects that involve the collaboration of those from multiple sectors are promising approaches to impact physical activity at the population level (Pollard, 2003). The impact of the built environment—the man-made physical structures and infrastructure of communities—(Prevention Institute, 2009) on health and the potential to alter aspects of the built environment to promote health are now being recognized by public health professionals

---

BOX **11-1**   **Six Categories of Factors That Influence the Success of Collaboration**

1. Environment
   A history of collaboration exists in the community.
   The collaborative group is seen as a community leader in the area in which it is focused.
   There is a favorable political/social climate.

2. Membership
   There is mutual respect, understanding, and trust.
   Cross-section of members in the group is appropriate.
   Collaboration is viewed as being in the self-interest of members.
   There is the ability to compromise.

3. Process/structure
   Members share a stake in both process and groups.
   There are multiple layers of decision making.
   There is flexibility and openness.
   Clear roles and policy guidelines are developed.
   There is adaptability in the face of changing conditions.

4. Communications
   There is open and frequent communication.
   Formal and informal communication links exist.

5. Purpose
   There is a concrete and unique purpose.
   There are clear, realistic, and attainable goals.
   There is a shared vision, with an agreed-on mission, objectives, and strategy.

6. Resources
   Funding is sufficient to support operations.
   The leader, or convener, of the collaborative group is skilled interpersonally and is fair and
      respected by partners.

Source: Adapted from Mattessich and Monsey (1992).

(Pollard, 2003). Offering opportunities for walking and cycling as a regular part of daily life, for example, are important to increasing physical activity and to improving health among a largely sedentary population in the United States. To promote healthier communities, multiple approaches directed at all levels of the government—local, state, and federal—are needed. The creation of communities and transportation systems that promote physical activity require the support of public health professionals working collaboratively with other disciplines such as architects, builders, public officials, bike and pedestrian advocates, and others on common concerns (Pollard, 2003).

The literature shows results of community-led initiatives to improve the built environment. For example, the Prevention Institute (2009) compiled a report that profiled 11 communities around the country to show how they were able to impact the built environment to positively affect the health of community residents. One community built a jogging path around a cemetery as a way to increase physical activity (Aboelata et al., 2004).

As another example of a collaborative effort to address physical activity, the American Heart Association Council on Nutrition, Physical Activity, and Metabolism (Physical Activity Committee) together with the Councils on Cardiovascular Disease in the Young and Cardiovascular Nursing issued a scientific statement (Pate et al., 2006) focused on this issue, specifically in youth. Evidence gathered from the 2003 Youth Risk Behavioral Surveillance System indicated that 37% of students (high school–aged youth) did not participate in adequate physical activity (20 minutes or more of vigorous physical activity on 3 or more of the previous 7 days). Also, Black, Hispanic and female students were less likely to participate in vigorous physical activity at the recommended levels (Pate et al., 2006). Nine key recommendations were made for improving policy and practice to impact physical activity participation at the population level. The statement called for U.S. schools to renew and expand their role in the offering and promotion of physical activity for youth by, for example, delivering evidence-based health-related physical education programs that meet national standards. Also recommended were policies and practices to ensure that all children and youth participate in a minimum of 30 minutes of moderate to vigorous physical activity during the school day as well as other recommendations that, if implemented on a national basis, would better provide U.S. youth with the physical activity needed for health (Pate et al., 2006). This report, the result of a large collaborative approach of bringing together key organizations with a common objective, illustrates how working together to share resources and information can be highly effective. Collaborative efforts such as this, to develop evidence-based guidelines, are an approach to inform practitioners about current best practices.

Another recent example of a collaborative effort to impact physical activity is the initiative spearheaded by the American College of Sports Medicine, working together with the American Medical Association to encourage the prescribing of exercise as medicine. Launched in 2007, *Exercise is Medicine* is a program that calls on U.S. physicians to prescribe exercise and encourage their patients to incorporate physical activity and exercise into their daily routine. It also encourages physicians and primary care providers to assess patients' physical activity level and record it as a vital sign. In addition, this initiative has called for greater collaboration between healthcare professionals and those in the fitness industry, including fitness and athletic trainers, to work together to get clients active and improve health outcomes (Sallis, 2009).

Evidence-based guidelines issued by organizations collaboratively may be more comprehensive than would otherwise be possible without the contribution of a range of perspectives brought together in a group effort. For example, as a result of the latest comprehensive review of the scientific research on physical activity, in October 2008 the U.S. Department of Health and Human Services released new guidelines for physical activity participation. These new guidelines, revised from a decade ago, provide current evidence-based recommendations to improve individuals' health through appropriate physical activity and are intended for use primarily by policymakers and health professionals.

In addition to the guidelines issued by the federal government, several other government agencies and health organizations also issued guidelines for physical activity based on their own scientific research and made recommendations for the public or for practitioners. These guidelines or recommendations each were written with a somewhat different emphasis or focus (i.e., to prevent chronic disease, to promote health, or to manage weight) and address a specific population (i.e., adults or children). The evidence-based recommendations from some of the major government and health organizations are summarized in **Box 11-2**.

INDIVIDUAL-FOCUSED LEVEL

At the individual level of practice, a public health nurse working in an agency may be caring for an older adult, female Hispanic client with early heart disease who has received an exercise prescription from her physician or nurse practitioner. The exercise prescription was based on evidence in the literature indicating that writing an exercise prescription has been shown to be more successful than if healthcare professionals merely discuss the benefits of physical activity with a patient (Sallis, 2009). The nurse may collaborate with other healthcare professionals, such as the prescribing physician or nurse practi-

tioner or perhaps an exercise physiologist or fitness specialist, to ensure that an appropriate program for this particular client is offered. In this case the common goal of this collaborative effort is to provide the most effective treatment plan as prescribed for the client.

Further, data from a study on the association of physical activity-related social support in a national U.S. sample of minority women ($N = 2,912$) indicate that social support from family and friends can impact an individual's participation in physical activity (Eyler et al., 1999). Of the determinants of physical activity that were studied, social support is one of the strongest correlates, and providing additional social support may be an important component of interventions that aim to increase physical-activity participation in a population of sedentary women of racially/ethnically diverse backgrounds (Eyler et al., 1999). Knowing this, the public health nurse may collaborate at the individual-focused level by working with a member of a family or a friend of the client who may be able to assist in meeting the care goal for this client by offering social support and encouragement for the client's physical activity program.

COMMUNITY-FOCUSED LEVEL

At the community level the public health nurse may collaborate with others such as staff in the local parks department or leaders in local fitness businesses to initiate a collaborative effort to identify the available resources in the local area for those at risk of cardiovascular disease seeking information on active lifestyles and physical activity. To help direct these members of the community to safe locations in which to engage in physical activity, they may work together to develop a list or brochure

---

BOX **11-2** Overview of Key National Guidelines and Recommendations
on Physical Activity

Population: Adults

American College of Sports Medicine/American Heart Association—jointly issued 2008

- A minimum of 30 minutes of moderate intensity aerobic physical activity 5 days per week (150 minutes) or 20 minutes of vigorous intensity aerobic physical activity 3 days per week—*to promote health and prevent chronic disease.*

American Cancer Society Guidelines on Nutrition and Physical Activity for Cancer Prevention 2006

- Balance caloric intake with physical activity—*to maintain a healthy weight throughout life.*
- Engage in at least 30 minutes of moderate to vigorous physical activity, above usual activities, on 5 or more days of the week; 45 to 60 minutes of intentional physical activity are preferable.

U.S. Department of Health and Human Services: 2008 Physical Activity Guidelines for Americans

- At least 2 hours and 30 minutes (150 minutes) of moderate aerobic exercise per week or 1 hour and 15 minutes of vigorous aerobic exercise per week, or an equivalent combination of moderate- and vigorous-intensity aerobic physical activity, performed in episodes of at least 10 minutes and should be spread throughout the week—*to promote health and prevent chronic disease.*
- Increase aerobic exercise to 300 minutes (5 hours) of moderate intensity per week or 150 minutes of vigorous aerobic exercise per week, or an equivalent combination of moderate- and vigorous-intensity aerobic physical activity—*to achieve additional and more extensive health benefits.*
- Do muscle-strengthening activities (that are moderate or high intensity and involve all major muscle groups) on at least 2 nonconsecutive days per week—*to achieve additional health benefits.*
- Avoid inactivity; some physical activity is better than none—*to achieve some health benefits.*

Population: Youth (Children and Adolescents)

U.S. Department of Health and Human Services: 2008 Physical Activity Guidelines for Americans

- Aerobic: most of the 60 minutes a day should be either moderate- or vigorous-intensity aerobic physical activity; it should include vigorous-intensity physical activity on at least 3 days a week.
- Muscle-strengthening: as part of their 60 minutes of daily physical activity, muscle-strengthening physical activity should be included on at least 3 days of the week.
- Bone-strengthening: as part of their 60 minutes of daily physical activity, bone-strengthening physical activity should be included on at least 3 days of the week.

Population: Older Adults

U.S. Department of Health and Human Services: 2008 Physical Activity Guidelines for Americans

- Older adults who cannot do 150 minutes of moderate-intensity aerobic activity a week due to chronic conditions should be as physically active as their abilities and conditions allow.
- Older adults should do exercises that maintain or improve balance if they are at risk of falling.
- Older adults should determine their level of effort for physical activity relative to their level of fitness.
- Older adults with chronic conditions should understand whether and how their conditions affect their ability to do regular physical activity safely.

Source: Haskell et al. (2007); Lawrence et al. (2006); Nelson et al. (2007); U.S. DHHS (2008).

of local resources such as parks and trails as well as gyms and community facilities that are available. They can then disseminate these materials to members of the community perhaps by using the social marketing intervention, discussed later in Chapter 12.

SYSTEM-FOCUSED LEVEL

At the systems level practice is focused on making a change in organizations, policies, laws, or power structures within a community, according to the assumptions of the intervention wheel (Keller et al., 2008, p. 192). A public health nurse may collaborate with leaders of other organizations that have a mutual interest in or concern with increasing physical activity, for example, in children who are at risk of being physical inactive. They may begin by gathering data on local and other policies that impact the issue of children who are not sufficiently physically active in their community and decide to work together to make a change by lobbying the state for a school-based state policy to increase physical activity by offering after-school programs. The nurse may identify local leaders of local organizations such as the Parent Teachers Association as well as religious or other community groups that are concerned about physical inactivity among local school children, or who serve children as part of their mission. This collaboration may lead to coalition building, the next intervention in the intervention wheel that also entails collective action.

Coalition Building

Whereas collaboration can occur at the individual-focused level, the other two interventions in the orange wedge of the intervention wheel, coalition building and community organizing, are not appli-

cable at the individual level. These two interventions most often take place at the community or systems level of practice. For the most part the interventions in the orange wedge are used most often by public health nurses who are focused on impacting community- and systems-level practice in their work rather than on individual-level practice (Keller et al., 2008). A coalition can be described as an alliance of individuals, groups, or organizations that come together or join forces for a specific or common purpose.

As defined in descriptions of this intervention in the intervention wheel model, **coalition building** "promotes and develops alliances among organizations or constituencies for a common purpose. It builds establishes linkages, solves problems, and/or enhances local leadership to address health concerns" (Keller et al., 2008, p. 204). Often, by forming a coalition the new organization or alliance or group becomes more effective in achieving a goal or goals. Usually, by bringing people or organizations together in pursuit of a common goal, resources can be maximized and more can be accomplished than could be by any individual person or organization alone.

Coalitions have been considered to be a foundation for creating successful change within a community. Because a range of local interests is represented and brought together, forming a coalition can build a powerful base of key individuals or organizations who can work to influence social change of a mutual concern. There are a number of types of coalitions that can be formed. Coalitions may be permanent or temporary; they can be formed to address a single issue or multiple issues. Typically, a coalition that is well organized and broad based will be more successful in effecting policy

---

| FIGURE **11-2** | **A mission statement should answer the question, "What are we doing here?"** |

A mission statement should:

- Include a program overview.
- Include a program aim.
- Incorporate a short narrative that describes the general focus of the program, including the intent and philosophy behind the program.
- Help to guide program planners in the development of program goals and objectives.

Misson Statement ➡➡➡ **Goals** ➡➡➡ **Objectives**

Source: Courtesy of the Minnesota Department of Health, Center for Health Promotion (n.d.).

---

change, increasing knowledge of the public, and creating innovative solutions to complex problems of concern (Wisconsin Clearinghouse for Prevention Resources, 2009).

A mission statement is important to provide direction and purpose for a group of people or organizations brought together in a coalition. In fact, this mission statement provides a common vision for all involved. It is developed collaboratively and typically contains specific components. **Figure 11-2** includes more information about the development of a mission statement.

In addition to the mission statement, eight key steps have also been identified as critically important to coalition building (Butterworth, 2009). These eight steps are listed in **Box 11-3**. Following these steps may help ensure the success of a coalition.

SYSTEM-FOCUSED LEVEL

Coalition building is an intervention used to address the problem of physical inactivity at the policy or system level. For exam-

> **BOX 11-3 Steps to Coalition Building**
>
> 1. Clarify/reaffirm coalition's vision and mission.
> 2. Create community ownership of the coalition.
> 3. Solidify coalition infrastructure and processes.
> 4. Recruit and retain an active, diverse membership.
> 5. Develop transformational leaders.
> 6. Market your coalition.
> 7. Evaluate your coalition.
> 8. Focus on action and advocacy.
>
> *Source*: Courtesy of CoalitionsWork. Butterworth (2009).

ple, there is currently an initiative underway that has built a coalition of organizations to develop a national physical activity plan to assist Americans in becoming more physically active (National Plan for

Physical Activity, 2008). The plan will be developed by a combination of efforts from researchers, educators, healthcare professionals, and mass media experts from across the country.

The coalition that will develop the plan was initially formed under the leadership of the Centers for Disease Control and Prevention and the Prevention Research Center at the University of South Carolina, who are providing the organizational infrastructure. The importance of having a strong organizational structure for a collaboration or coalition to succeed has been previously mentioned, and the strength of these two leading and reputable organizations can help ensure its success. Other organizations who are part of the coalition include the American Academy of Pediatrics; American Alliance for Health, Physical Education, Recreation and Dance; American Association of Retired Persons; American Cancer Society; American College of Sports Medicine; American Heart Association; Active Living Research, American Association for Cardiovascular and Pulmonary Rehabilitation; and the National Coalition for Promoting Physical Activity, itself a coalition with a clear mission statement (**Box 11-4**).

Community Organizing

Community organizing, as defined in the intervention wheel, "helps community groups to identify common problems or goals, mobilize resources, and develop and implement strategies for reaching the goals they collectively have set" (Minkler, 1997 as cited in Keller et al., 2008, p. 204).

BOX **11-4** **Example of a Coalition to Address Physical Activity in the United States and Its Mission Statement: National Coalition for Promoting Physical Activity (NCPPA)**

NCPPA is "an extraordinary group of national organizations that independently address a host of issues pertaining to physical activity including health/science, education, environments, population specific outreach, and activity behavior" (NCPPA, n.d., n.p.).

Mission: to "unite the strengths of public, private, and industry efforts into collaborative partnerships that inspire and empower all Americans to lead more physically active lifestyles" (NCPPA, n.d., n.p.).

Source: Courtesy of the National Coalition for Promoting Physical Activity.

Community-Focused Level

The Safe Routes to School (SRTS) program provides an example, or case study, of a framework for community organizing aimed at providing options that would allow children to walk and bicycle to school safely and thereby increase physical activity opportunities for school children. The program was first started in Denmark in the 1970s and was initiated in the United States in The Bronx and Florida in 1997. It has a grassroots history whereby the success of pilot community projects led to federal interest and funding. The national SRTS program is funded for $612 million from 2005 to 2009 by federal transportation legislation, and its success illustrates how collaboration and coalition building, along with local community organizing around an issue, can expand into further intervention actions such as advocacy and policy implementation (National Center for Safe Routes to School, 2009).

A framework that has been successfully used is available on the SRTS Web site (http://www.saferoutesinfo.org) to support the development of other programs in local communities and is illustrative of how a community-based approach can begin with a grassroots effort focused on a particular community concern. The framework suggested by SRTS is based on the evidence of what has worked in other communities starting a program. The steps are outlined for others who are interested in starting a program, and they are meant to provide guidance on a process that has worked. However, each community is unique, and using these steps in a different order may work better for some communities, or some communities may require different approaches than outlined in the steps suggested by SRTS. The seven steps are to (1) bring the right people together, (2) hold a kickoff meeting and set a vision, (3) gather information and identify issues, (4) identify solutions, (5) make a plan, (6) get the people and the plan moving, (7) evaluate,

adjust, and keep moving (National Center for Safe Routes to School, 2009).

COMMUNITY AND SYSTEM-FOCUSED LEVEL

Another effective community organizing approach to promoting physical activity among underserved older adults is the Southeast Senior Physical Activity Network (SESPAN) in southeast Seattle (Cheadle, Egger, LoGerfo, Walwick, & Schwartz, 2008). SESPAN is based on an organizing strategy that involved networking between several community-based organizations (including senior housing buildings and religious organizations) and senior centers and other organizations to meet two broad objectives. The first objective was to create new senior physical activity programs where there were no programs by making connections between two or more community-based organizations. Networking among organizations led to the creation of a number of potentially sustainable walking and exercise programs that are reaching previously underserved communities within southeast Seattle. A second objective was to build a broader coalition of groups and organizations to assist in making environmental and policy changes on a larger scale. After a health fair event, organizations involved in the event decided to continue to work together. A health coalition was established with the potential to continue to develop new programs and larger scale environmental changes (Cheadle et al., 2008).

Beaglehole and colleagues (2004) suggested that "a suitable definition of public health is collective action for sustained population-wide health improvement"

(Beaglehole et al., 2004, p. 2085). This definition of public health focuses attention on the importance of the interventions of collective action discussed in this chapter and highlights the key role they play in achieving public health goals.

MINNESOTA DEPARTMENT OF HEALTH POPULATION-BASED PUBLIC HEALTH NURSING PRACTICE INTERVENTION WHEEL: APPLICATION TO PRACTICE

The case study on page 281 illustrates how one nurse practices in a way that exemplified the "doing" of the intervention wheel strategies described in this chapter. Once you have read and discussed the case, collaborate with each other on the field exercise in **Box 11-5**.

CONCLUSION

This chapter presents the interventions of the orange section of intervention wheel aimed at collective action. The intervention wheel model considers that the three interventions in the orange section that were described in this chapter are all part of "collective action" (Keller et al., 2008, p. 193).

Collaboration, coalition building, and community organizing are the interventions aimed at harnessing the collective energy of more than one person or group. Perhaps Margaret Mead said it best when describing the power of collective action: "Never doubt that a small group of thoughtful, committed citizens can change the world: indeed it is the only thing that ever has" (Margaret Mead® Used with permission.).

As we have discussed in this chapter, when presenting a variety of approaches to the problem of physical inactivity, public health nursing can incorporate best practices and evidence-based interventions when engaging in or supporting collective action to address this concern effectively. The strategies used in public health nursing consist of the development of collaborative efforts that maximize the efforts of each individual or organization for a mutual goal. Further, this chapter shows how public health nursing strategies can be applied on the community, systems, and individual/family levels. Public health professionals are often key players in any community-based effort. They can support important initiatives whether on the issue of physical activity or any other health concern by applying the intervention wheel interventions.

BOX 11-5 Field Exercise

- Select an issue on your own campus.
- Who is the population of interest?
- In what way would you organize the college community and the surrounding community? How would you connect with each of these communities? Would you apply varying strategies to ensure these connections?
- On what types of interventions would you collaborate? How would you determine if they were based on evidence and what level of evidence?
- Would a coalition be helpful? If yes, who would be members of this coalition?

Case Study

Unfit University Gets Active—Interventions of Collective Action

An Ivy League university in the northeast, Unfit University (UU), is a member of the American College Health Association (ACHA), a national professional organization that serves college health professionals (http://www.acha.org/about_acha/history.cfm). A nurse (Ms. Fit, RN, MPH) who works at the University Health Services Center has a public health background, and part of her role is to work with the UU community and serve as a resource and to develop and implement evidence-based student health programs to meet the needs of the UU student population. UU participates in the ACHA-National College Health Assessment (NCHA) survey to collect data on the health behaviors of their student population, and they use these data to help inform decisions on priority needs and programs and to determine resource needs.

Ms. Fit has seen national data published from the ACHA-NCHA survey on the health behaviors of college students who participate in the assessment and from these data learns that inadequate physical activity participation in college students is a concern nationally (American College Health Association, 2009). Further, she read a review study published in the *Journal of American College Health* that reports high percentages of college students (about 40%–50%) who are not sufficiently physically active to achieve health benefits. Of note, it is reported that female students met the guidelines significantly less than male students (Keating, Guan, Pinero, & Bridges, 2005).

In addition, Ms. Fit knows that Healthy Campus 2010 has identified lead indicators for health, including physical activity, and has set targets for physical activity in college students by 2010. One target, objective 7-3b11, "is to increase the proportion of college students who have received information on physical activity and fitness from the baseline of 33.5% to the 2010 target of 55%" (American College Health Association, 2009). A second objective, 22-2/3, is "to increase the proportion of college students who engage in physical activity at least 3 days/week at moderate intensity for at least 30 minutes, or vigorous physical activity for 20 minutes or more minutes, from the baseline of 40.3% to the 2010 target of 55%" (American College Health Association, 2009, PowerPoint no. 26).

The population of interest is inactive students (i.e., those not meeting the Healthy Campus target at UU in Anytown, USA). The problem is that insufficiently active college students are at risk of chronic illness, including cardiovascular disease, obesity, depression, diabetes, and cancer (Blair, 2009). UU is an all-women's university and is concerned that, based on this national data, their students are at risk of not engaging in sufficient physical activity for acute health benefits and for long-term health outcomes.

Community Level
Ms. Fit of UU's Health Services Department brings together leaders of several key groups at the University, including the leaders of the student environmental committee, the student wellness committee, and student athletes (team captains) to conduct an audit to evaluate the University's environmental facilitators and barriers to physical activity on the UU campus and to make recommendations to the university administration on ways to increase physical activity for all students on campus.

Systems Level

Ms. Fit is invited by Administration to work with the architects and designers who are developing plans for expanding the campus at UU to collaborate on ways to improve environmental factors to encourage physical activity, such as expanding bike paths and adding more recreational facilities.

Individual/Family Level

Ms. Fit meets with the Student Health Services nurses to collaborate on how individual students can be better assessed for physical activity level and counseled on the importance of physical activity for their unique health and activity status. Ms Fit and the nurses decide that the Health Services nurses will screen for physical inactivity on all students who visit the clinic and offer a Fitness Challenge on a monthly basis, campus-wide to raise awareness of physical fitness levels.

References

Aboelata, M. J., Mikkelsen, L., Cohen, L., Fernandes, S., Silver, M., & Parks, L. F. (2004). *The built environment and health: Eleven profiles of neighborhood transformation*. Oakland, CA: Prevention Institute. Retrieved August 13, 2009, from http://www.preventioninstitute.org/pdf/BE_full_document_110304.pdf

American College Health Association. (2009). *Healthy campus 2010: Making it happen.* PowerPoint presentation Healthy People 2010, Healthy Campus 2020, slide no. 26, presented at the ACHA Annual 2002 meeting. Retrieved August 13, 2009, from http://www.acha.org/Info_resources/hc2010.cfm

Beaglehole, R., Bonita, R., Horton, R., Adams, O., & McKee, M. (2004). Public health in the new era: Improving health through collective action. *Lancet, 363*(9426), 2084–2086.

Blair, S. N. (2009). Physical inactivity: The biggest public health problem of the 21st century. *British Journal of Sports Medicine, 43*(1), 1–2.

Butterworth, F. D. (2009, May 9). *Strength in numbers: Building strategic partnerships to advocate for change.* New Orleans, LA: SOPHE State Health Policy Summit.

Centers for Disease Control and Prevention (CDC). (2000). *Behavioral Risk Factor Surveillance System Survey data.* Atlanta, GA: U.S. Department of Health and Human Services, Centers for Disease Control and Prevention.

Cheadle, A., Egger, R., LoGerfo, J. P., Walwick, J., & Schwartz, S. (2008). A community-organizing approach to promoting physical activity in older adults: The Southeast Senior Physical Activity Network. *Health Promotion and Practice, 0*, 1524839908318167v1.

Elder, J. P., Lytle, L., Sallis, J. F., Young, D. R., Steckler, A., Simons-Morton, D., et al. (2007). A description of the social-ecological framework used in the trial of activity for adolescent girls (TAAG). *Health Education and Research, 22*(2), 155–165.

Eyler, A. A., Brownson, R. C., Donatelle, R. J., King, A. C., Brown, D., & Sallis, J. F. (1999). Physical activity social support and middle- and older-aged minority women: Results from a US survey. *Social Science & Medicine, 49*(6), 781–789.

Gray, B. (1998). *Collaborating.* San Francisco: Jossey-Bass.

Haskell, W. L., Lee, I. M., Pate, R. R., Powell, K. E., Blair, S. N., et al. (2007). Physical activity and public health: Updated recommendation for adults from the American College of Sports Medicine and the American Heart Association. *Medicine & Science in Sports & Exercise, 39*, 1423–1434.

Heath, G. W., Brownson, R. C., Kruger, J., Miles, R., Powell, K. E., Ramsey, L. T., and the Task Force on Community Preventive Services. (2006). The effectiveness of urban design and land use and transport policies and practices to increase physical activity: A systematic review. *Journal of Physical Activity and Health, 3*(Suppl 1), S55–S76.

Keating, X. D., Guan, J., Pinero, J. C., & Bridges, D. M. (2005). A meta-analysis of college students' physical activity behaviors. *Journal of American College Health, 54*(2), 116–125.

Keller, L. O., Strohschein, S., & Briske, L. (2008). Population-based public health nursing practice: The intervention wheel. In M. Stanhope & J. Lancaster (Eds.), *Public health nursing: population-centered health care in the community* (pp. 187–214). St. Louis, MO: Mosby Elsevier.

Lawrence, H., Kushi, L. H., Byers, T., Doyle, C., Bandera, E. V., McCullough, M., et al. (2006). Nutrition and Physical Activity Guidelines Advisory Committee. American Cancer Society guidelines on nutrition and physical activity for cancer prevention: Reducing the risk of cancer with healthy food choices and physical activity. *CA Cancer Journal for Clinicians, 56,* 254–281.

Mattessich, P. W., & Monsey, B. R. (1992). *Collaboration: What makes it work.* St. Paul, MN: Amherst H. Wilder Foundation.

Minnesota Department of Health. (2001). *Public health interventions: Applications for public health nursing practice.* St. Paul, MN: Author.

Courtesy of the Minnesota Department of Health, Center for Health Promotion. (n.d.). Developing a mission statement. Retrieved December 18, 2009, from http://www.health.state.mn.us/divs/hpcd/chp/hpkit/text/tea_mission.htm

National Center for Safe Routes to School. (2009). Retrieved August 13, 2009, from http://www.saferoutesinfo.org

National Organization for Public Health Nursing (1939). *Manual of public health nursing* (3rd ed.). New York: MacMillan.

National Plan for Physical Activity. (2008). Retrieved August 13, 2009, from http://www.physicalactivityplan/org

National Coalition for Promoting Physical Activity. (nd). *NCPPA to manage implementation of national physical activity.* Retrieved August 13, 2009, from http://www.ncppa.org

Nelson, M. E., Rejeski, W. J., Blair, S. N., Duncan, P. W., Judge, J. O., King, A. C., et al. (2007). Physical activity and public health in older adults: Recommendation from the American College of Sports Medicine and the American Heart Association. *Medicine & Science in Sports & Exercise*, 39, 1435–1445.

Pate, R. R., Davis, M. G., Robinson, T. N., Stone, E. J., McKenzie, T. L., & Young, J. C. (2006). Promoting physical activity in children and youth: A leadership role for schools. A scientific statement from the American Heart Association Council on Nutrition, Physical Activity, and Metabolism (Physical Activity Committee) in collaboration with the Councils on Cardiovascular Disease in the Young and Cardiovascular Nursing. *Circulation, 114*(11), 1214–1224.

Pollard, T. (2003). Policy prescriptions for healthier communities. *American Journal of Health Promotion, 18*(1), 109–113.

Prevention Institute (2009). *The built environment and health: 11 profiles of neighborhood transformation.* Retrieved April 30, 2009, from http://www.preventioninstitute.org/builtenv.html

Sallis, R. E. (2009). Exercise is medicine and physicians need to prescribe it! *British Journal of Sports Medicine, 43*(1), 3–4.

Sullivan, T. J. (1998). *Collaboration: A health care imperative.* New York: McGraw-Hill.

U.S. Department of Health and Human Services. (1996). 2008 physical activity guidelines for Americans. Retrieved April 30, 2009, from http://www.health.gov/paguidelines

U.S. Department of Health and Human Services. (2008). 2008 Physical activity guidelines for Americans. Retrieved April 30, 2009, from http://www.health.gov/paguidelines

Wisconsin Clearinghouse for Prevention Resources. (2009). Prevention—Coalition building. Retrieved April 30, 2009, from http://wch.uhs.wisc.edu

World Health Organization [WHO]. (2002). *The World Health Report 2002—Reducing risks, promoting healthy life.* Geneva: Author.

Getting the Word Out: Advocacy, Social Marketing, and Policy Development and Enforcement

Susan Moscou

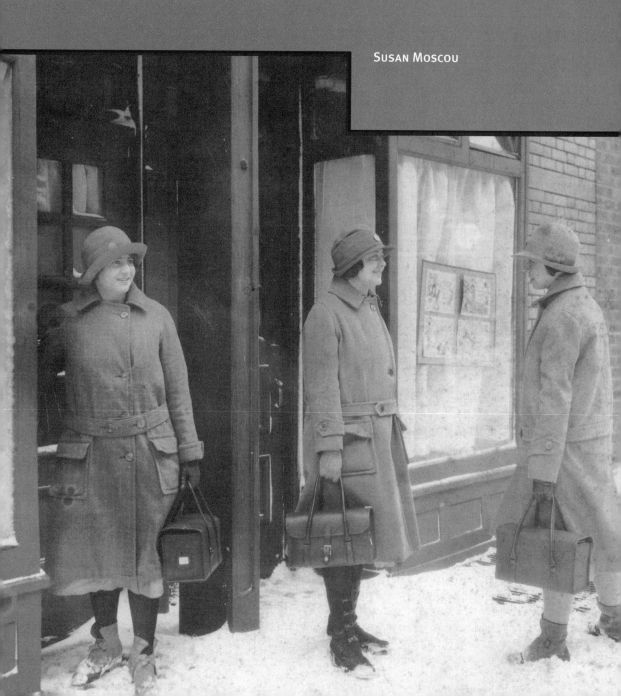

If people knew things—and "things" meant everything implied in the condition of this family—such horrors would cease to exist, and I rejoiced that I had had a training in the care of the sick that in itself would give me an organic relationship to the neighborhood in which this awakening had come (Wald, 1915, pp. 7–8).

LEARNING OBJECTIVES

At the completion of this chapter, the reader will be able to

- Describe social marketing, advocacy, and policy development and enforcement.
- Apply social marketing, advocacy, and policy development and enforcement to the levels of public health practice.

- Explore the ways that public health nursing may apply and do social marketing, advocacy, and policy development and enforcement.

KEY TERMS

- Advocacy
- Policy development

- Policy enforcement
- Social marketing

The Minnesota Department of Health Population-Based Public Health Nursing Practice Intervention Wheel Strategies describes public health interventions that are applicable to public health nursing. This chapter presents the yellow section of the intervention wheel, otherwise known as advocacy, social marketing, and policy development and enforcement of public health nursing interventions. Advocacy is considered the precursor to policy development, and social marketing is viewed as a strategy for carrying out advocacy (Minnesota Department of Health, 2001).

This chapter is divided into three sections. The first section provides a discussion about overweight and obesity in children. Overweight and obese children are a major public health issue. The section will focus primarily on overweight and obese children in junior high school. The second section is a case study that highlights this public health issue. Finally, the third section depicts how the public health nurse in the case study engages in the application of three interventions: advocacy, social marketing, and policy development and enforcement through the three levels of public health practice.

This chapter specifically addresses strategies to deal with the growing public health problem of overweight and obese children in the United States. For example, the case study provides a paradigm of how a public health nurse uses the intervention wheel to address the prevalence of overweight and obese junior high school children in a community. The nurse gathers the appropriate facts about the prevalence of overweight and obese children in the school by looking at the present school records pertaining to weight and comparing those data with standards as well as past school records to note trends. Once he or she has these data, the nurse applies the intervention wheel interventions of advocacy and social marketing to develop policy and enforcement strategies around the problem of overweight and obese children attending the school. Advocacy, social marketing, and policy development and enforcement strategies are applied at the community level, systems level, and individual/family levels.

ISSUE: OVERWEIGHT AND OBESITY ARE A MAJOR 21ST CENTURY PUBLIC HEALTH CONCERN

Overweight and obesity are considered an emerging public health problem in the United States. Within the last four decades the number of overweight adults, children, and adolescents has increased (Blair & Nichaman, 2002; Ogden et al., 2009). Approximately 9 million children aged 6 to 19 are overweight, and more than 80% of these adolescents will become obese

adults (Jordan & Robinson, 2008). The incidence of weight gain in children has become alarming to the public health community (Harbaugh, Jordan-Welch, Bounds, Blom, & Fisher, 2007). Furthermore, overweight and obesity contribute to various health complaints and chronic diseases (Patterson, Frank, Kristal, & White, 2004) such as diabetes (Yanovski & Yanovski, 2002), cardiovascular diseases such as high blood pressure (Kumanyika et al., 2008), and asthma (Chen, Dales, & Jiang, 2006). In addition, elevated body weights are also correlated with higher death rates.

Body mass index (BMI) determines if a person is underweight, normal weight, overweight, or obese. BMI is a number calculated from a person's weight and height and is a reliable indicator of body fatness for people (Centers for Disease Control and Prevention [CDC], 2009). BMI-defined categories for adults (CDC, 2009) are as follows:

- Underweight = <18.5
- Normal weight = 18.5–24.9
- Overweight = 25–29.9
- Obesity = 30 or greater

For children and adolescents the BMI is calculated the same way as adults, but the criteria to interpret meaning is different. For example, for children and teens BMI age- and sex-specific percentiles are used because the amount of fat changes with age and is also different between girls and boys (CDC, 2009). The prevalence of overweight female children and adolescents from 1999 to 2004 increased from approximately 13% to 16%, male children and adolescents increased from 14% to 18%, the prevalence of obesity in male adults went from 28% to 31%, and in women the prevalence remained the same, at about 33% (Ogden et al., 2009).

In 2003 to 2004, 32% of adults were considered obese, and about 17% of children and adolescents in the United States were thought to be overweight. Adults were obese if they had a BMI of 30 or higher, and children were considered overweight if they were at or above the 95th percentile of their BMI specific to age and gender (Ogden et al., 2009).

The prevalence of overweight American children in age groups 6 to 11 and 12 to 19 has tripled between 1980 and 2002. Furthermore, overweight and obesity in childhood often persist into adolescence and adulthood (Nader et al., 2006). Although the consequences of overweight children tend to be social rather than medical, many of these children become overweight or obese adults and develop health problems such as type 2 diabetes, high blood pressure, and asthma (de Onis & Blossner, 2000). As a result of this growing trend, many healthcare professionals are now seeing adult-onset diseases in children.

Globally, the prevalence of overweight children has also increased. Flynn et al. (2006) noted the following:

> Available estimates for the period between the 1980s and 1990s show the prevalence of overweight and obesity in children increased by a magnitude of two to five times in developed countries (e.g. from 11% to over 30% in boys in Canada), and up to almost four times in developing countries (e.g. from 4% to 14% in Brazil). (p. 7)

The World Health Organization found that childhood obesity is such a problem that obesity warrants consideration along with the continued attention to malnutrition. The World Health Organization (The Lancet, 2001) is developing population strategies that promote healthy diets and increase physical activity as public health interventions to reduce or reverse the alarming obesity trend.

Related Health Conditions of Overweight and Obesity

Chronic health conditions such as type 2 diabetes, hypertension, coronary heart disease (Kumanyika et al., 2008; Patterson et al., 2004), respiratory illnesses (Chen et al., 2006; Murugan & Sharma, 2008), and osteoarthritis are related to overweight and obesity (Yanovski & Yanovski, 2002). Since 1960 the percent prevalence of diabetes for all ages has increased by more than 400%. Major risk factors for diabetes are obesity, high-fat diet, and physical inactivity (CDC, 2001). Additionally, diabetes is the fifth leading cause of death and is responsible for new-onset blindness, kidney failure, and lower limb amputations (Hogan, Dall, Nikolov, & American Diabetes Association, 2003).

Diabetes has reached epidemic levels, and the prevalence of diabetes in the United States continues to increase. The National Health and Nutrition Survey found that 9.3% of Americans 20 years and older (approximately 19 million people) had diabetes; two-thirds had an actual diagnosis and one-third were not diagnosed (Sheehy, Coursin, & Gabbay, 2008). Further, it has been estimated that by 2050 about 43 million people will be diagnosed with diabetes (Narayan, Boyle, Geiss, Saaddine, & Thompson, 2006).

Coronary heart disease, used interchangeably with cardiovascular disease, occurs because the body builds plaque that clogs the inner walls of the arteries. Coronary heart disease is responsible for heart attacks, strokes, and chest pain and is the principal cause of death in the United States (Wallace, Fulwood, & Alvarado, 2008). Cardiovascular disease is associated with poor dietary practices, physical inactivity, overweight, obesity, and cigarette smoking (Lee & Cubbin, 2002).

Obesity is now recognized as a risk factor for developing respiratory diseases such as asthma, pneumonia, and sleep apnea, a condition in which a person will stop breathing several times during the sleep cycle. Weight reduction has been shown to reduce the possibility of developing these conditions or improving the episodes of these conditions (Murugan & Sharma, 2008).

Arthritis is responsible for physical disabilities in elders. Arthritis affects about 70 million Americans. Osteoarthritis is the most common form of arthritis and leads to muscle weakness, which in turn results in decreased physical activity and problems with balance. When this occurs, people are at increased risk for physical disability. Weight reduction and moderate exercise has been shown to improve mobility in overweight and obese adults diagnosed with knee osteoarthritis (Mes-sier et al., 2004). Considering the increasing prevalence of overweight children and adolescents in America, one questions what the future holds for these young individuals as they move into adulthood with regard to these chronic illnesses as well as the corresponding morbidity and mortality rates.

Mental Health and Overweight and Obesity

Individuals diagnosed with such mental illnesses as schizophrenia, depression, and bipolar disorder may be at a higher risk for becoming overweight and obese because of psychotropic medications, decreased physical activity, and inadequate attention paid to nutrition. The prevalence of obesity among people with diagnosed mental health disorders is more than the general population. Women schizophrenics had higher BMIs than nonschizophrenic women, whereas male schizophrenics and nonschizophrenics had comparable BMIs. Experiencing a depressed mood during adolescence may have a role in the prevalence of obesity in this group, but being obese in adolescence does not necessarily cause depression. Young women, however, who were overweight or obese were more likely to experience a depressed mood, which is defined as "feeling sad, blue, or depressed for at least 7 days during the previous month" (Allison et al., 2009).

The prevalence of metabolic syndrome is higher among individuals diagnosed with a mental health disorder than in the general population. Metabolic syndrome is a group of risk factors such as high blood pressure, obesity in the abdominal area, elevated blood sugar levels, elevated cholesterol, and lower levels of the good cholesterol (high-density-lipoprotein cholesterol). These conditions often occur together and increase one's risk of developing heart disease, stroke, and diabetes (Newcomer, 2007).

Reasons for the Increase in Overweight and Obese Individuals

The fattening of America is due to worsening diets, higher carbohydrate intakes, physical inactivity, genetics, sedentary lifestyles, food overproduction due to subsidies, increased portion sizes, and aggressive food marketing of snacks and fast foods (Seiders & Petty, 2004). Aggressive food marketing strategies have also resulted in Americans eating more fast foods, and the "super-sizing" trend has resulted in larger portion sizes. Another example of this excessive eating is noted as follows. U.S. food companies produce about 3,800 calories/day per person, whereas food production in 1970 was 3,300 calories/day per person. Further, Americans have vast amounts of food choices in supermarkets, and approximately 12,000 new food products are developed yearly (Blair & Nichaman, 2002). Family-prepared meals have become less frequent due to work schedules, and this has contributed to poorer dietary habits (CDC, 2000). As family-prepared meals have decreased, eating outside the home has increased, resulting in meals that are 20% higher in fat (Ward & Martens, 2000).

Urban sprawl has also contributed to increased rates of overweight and obesity in Americans. Urban sprawl is defined as patterns of housing development that are considered low-density residential areas; therefore people residing in these areas live in larger houses and commute longer distances to their jobs, often relying on automobiles because of inadequate public transportation (Lopez, 2004). Because these areas lack pedestrian amenities such as walking to school, shopping locally, and socializing with friends within walking distances, urban sprawl is considered a risk factor of overweight and obesity for those residing in those communities.

The composition of a neighborhood can contribute to the overweight and obesity of the residents. Lower BMIs have been associated with neighborhoods that have higher population density, access to public transportation, and mixed land uses that included houses, apartments, parks, green spaces, access to healthy foods, and private and public resources that encourage healthier lifestyles

(Lovasi, Neckerman, Quinn, Weiss, & Rundle, 2009).

Contribution of Schools to Overweight and Obese Children

Children spend a large portion of their day in educational institutions. In 2000 approximately 53 million children attended public and private schools in the United States. Further, schools serve as the location for preschool, after-school, and child-care programs (Koplan, Liverman, & Kraak, 2005). Additionally, many children receive their meals at their schools. Schools, because of loss of monies, may sell foods that are not part of federally reimbursable lunches. Additionally, many schools have become distributors of vending machines that carry candy, beverages, and chips. Vending machines are found in about 43% of elementary schools, 74% of middle schools, and most high schools. These vending machines provide schools with about 50% of the profits from the machines (Seiders & Petty, 2004). On the surface, these profits may appear very attractive to financially struggling schools.

Foods sold outside of federally reimbursed school meals are widely available in educational institutions. These food items sold to students are high in saturated fats and calories, higher in salt content, higher levels of sugar, and of little nutritional value. Additionally, the meals served at these schools often do not meet the lower standards for total fat and saturated fat, 42% do not provide fresh foods and vegetables in their reimbursable lunches, and whole grain breads and rolls accounted for only 5% (Story, Nanney, & Schwartz, 2009).

Fast-food consumption in 2- to 18-year-olds has increased fivefold from 1977 to 1995. Further, fast food was eaten in 9% of all eating situations, and 12% of the required caloric intake came from fast food. Because most fast-food places are located within walking distances from schools, it is thought there is a correlation between the poorer quality diets and weight status (Davis & Carpenter, 2009).

Physical Activity Improves Health

Regular physical activity during childhood and adolescence is related to physical and psychological benefits. Further, it has been found that for youths to start physical activity and maintain regular levels of physical activity, success occurs more often when friends are involved (Salvy et al., 2009).

Moderate physical activity has been shown to reduce or delay chronic health conditions. The Diabetes Prevention Program clinical trial found that walking 2½ hours a week and eating a low-fat diet resulted in a 58% reduction in the development of type 2 diabetes, and seniors age 60 and older saw a 71% reduction in type 2 diabetes. Participants entered the clinical trial with BMIs of 34 and a medical diagnosis of impaired glucose intolerance, a precursor to diabetes. Individuals who were randomized to modest physical activity saw greater reductions in disease prevention than participants randomized to drug therapy alone (Diabetes Prevention Program Research Group, 2002).

Healthy People 2010 selected physical activity, overweight, and obesity as important leading health indicators for the next 10 years because physical activity reduces preventable chronic diseases (U.S. Department of Health and Human Services, 2000). Lifestyle modifications such as diet and exercise offer enormous benefits to the individual and play a role in the prevention and reduction of many diseases associated with overweight and obesity (Peterson, 2007; Reiser & Schlenk, 2009).

So important is physical activity that in 2008 the federal government issued the first comprehensive guidelines on physical activity (U.S. Department of Health and Human Services, 2008):

> We clearly know enough now to recommend that all Americans should engage in regular physical activity to improve overall health and to reduce risk of many health problems. Physical activity is a leading example of how lifestyle choices have a profound effect on health. The choices we make about other lifestyle factors, such as diet, smoking, and alcohol use, also have important and independent effects on our health. (p. 1)

Box 12-1 provides information on the *Physical Activity Guidelines for Americans* and describes the major research findings.

People, however, need assistance in developing routines to maximize adherence to their desired goals. Getting children and adolescents to increase physical activity levels requires multiple approaches, specific community interventions, advocacy strategies, social marketing, and social policy and enforcement.

BOX **12-1** **Physical Activity Guidelines for Americans**
— **Major Research Findings**

1. Regular physical activity reduces the risk of many adverse health outcomes.
2. Some physical activity is better than none.
3. For most health outcomes, additional benefits occur as the amount of physical activity increases through higher intensity, greater frequency, and/or longer duration.
4. Most health benefits occur with at least 150 minutes (2 hours and 30 minutes) a week of moderate intensity physical activity.
5. Both aerobic (endurance) and muscle-strengthening (resistance) physical activity are beneficial.
6. Health benefits occur for children and adolescents, young and middle-aged adults, older adults, and those in every studied racial and ethnic group.
7. The health benefits of physical activity occur for people with disabilities.
8. The benefits of physical activity far outweigh the possibility of adverse outcomes.

Source: U.S. Department of Health and Human Services (2008, pp. vi–vii).

Case Study

Ms. Jones, a public health nurse, has worked at Greene Junior High School (GJHS) school-based clinic for 10 years. Children come to the healthcare clinic for acute medical problems such as colds and sore throats and chronic medical problems such as asthma and diabetes. In the last several years Ms. Jones has noticed that children coming to the school-based clinic seem to be more overweight and obese.

During her time at this school Ms. Jones has seen gym classes reduced and children participate in very little physical activity. Ms. Jones also noted that the school cafeteria offers processed foods that are high in saturated fats, such as fries and chicken nuggets, and the range of nutritious healthy foods are limited. Further, the cafeteria contains several soda and snack machines.

Ms. Jones recently obtained a Master's in Public Health. Armed with knowledge about public health, epidemiology, social epidemiology, and health policy, Ms. Jones decided to examine the prevalence of overweight and obese children at GJHS and determine the average calories of the typical lunch served and if the soda and snack machines contributed to children becoming overweight and obese. Ms. Jones recognizes that obesity is considered an emerging public health problem not only in the United States but worldwide and that children are not immune from the overweight and obesity epidemic.

The following sections (advocacy, social marketing, and social policy and enforcement) describe the strategies Ms. Jones can use to address the issue of overweight and obese children at GJHS.

MINNESOTA DEPARTMENT OF HEALTH POPULATION-BASED PUBLIC HEALTH NURSING PRACTICE INTERVENTION WHEEL STRATEGIES AND LEVELS OF PRACTICE

Advocacy

What is **advocacy** and why is it important to the public health nurse? Advocacy can be defined in several ways depending on one's perspective. Cohen, de la Vega, and Watson (2001) presented a value-neutral view of advocacy and spoke to this concept as action oriented. They noted how advocacy influenced decisions on the political, economic, and social system front that affects people. The public health nurse is participating in advocacy when he or she ". . . pleads someone's cause or acts on someone's behalf, with a focus on developing the capacity of the community, system, individual, or family to plead their own cause or act on their own behalf" (Keller, Strohschein, & Briske, 2008, p. 204).

Advocates support a particular cause or issue to get individuals and communities involved in influencing the public and policymakers about their particular issue. Using the above case study, Ms. Jones has identified the presiding problem to be overweight and obesity in a particular population of interest—GJHS children.

The first step in advocacy is to introduce the problem to those who can assist Ms. Jones in reducing the prevalence of overweight and obesity at GJHS.

Ms. Jones knows that successful advocacy requires that people are informed and educated about the issue she wants to address. Ms. Jones requests to speak at the next Parent-Teacher Association (PTA) meeting. Ms. Jones prepared fact sheets about the emerging problem of overweight and obesity in the United States and in particular the growing problem of children who are overweight and obese. Ms. Jones knows that when parents and teachers have information about the problem, they will be more likely to participate in advocacy activities that can influence decision makers to make changes at GJHS that could lead to lower rates of overweight and obesity. **Box 12-2** provides examples of how Ms. Jones uses advocacy interventions at community level, systems level, and individual or family level. Of note, there is quite a bit of strategic overlap in each of these levels. Ms. Jones can utilize many of the same strategies at the other levels.

COMMUNITY-FOCUSED LEVEL

At the community-focused level, Ms. Jones must identify the different community groups that can play an advocacy role in dealing with this problem. Before Ms. Jones meets with the PTA, Board of Education, and Community School Board, she must have the information needed to educate these groups about the problem. Ms. Jones uses epidemiological and social epidemiological approaches to gather information about children who are overweight and obese (see Chapter 4).

Ms. Jones examined the environmental, social, and personal factors that have contributed to the phenomenon of overweight and obese children. Examples of

---

BOX **12-2** Advocacy Intervention Applied at the Community, System, and Individual/Family Levels

Advocacy Case Management

- *Population of interest*: overweight and obese children at GJHS
- *Problem*: Overweight and obese children
- *Community example*: Ms. Jones, RN, MPH, works with the GJHS Parent-Teacher Association to increase physical activity, modify cafeteria offerings, and remove snack and vending machines from the school.
- *Systems example*: Ms. Jones works with the Board of Education and local farmers to bring healthy and nutritious foods to the children at GJHS.
- *Individual/family example*: Ms. Jones meets with individual parents of overweight and obese children enrolled in the school-based clinic to discuss the importance of weight reduction, healthy foods, and physical activity.

---

environmental factors are the cafeteria meals, an overabundance of vending machines in the school, and the decrease in gym classes. Examples of social factors are poverty (family and neighborhood of the children), socioeconomic status (family and neighborhood), and discrimination experienced by children growing up in their particular neighborhood. When

Ms. Jones completed her study, she then prepared fact sheets for the PTA and a research issue brief for the Board of Education and Community School Board.

Ms. Jones approached the PTA to advocate for a healthier dietary intake and an increase in physical activity levels for the children at GJHS. Ms. Jones and the PTA advocated their cause to the Board of Education and the local Community School Board. The Board of Education agrees to meet with the U.S. Department of Agriculture to develop and implement nutritional standards for food and beverages sold or served in GJHS. Additionally, the Board of Education and the local Community School Board agree that the school-based clinic should develop strategies and interventions that would play a role in preventing as well as reducing overweight and obese students at GJHS.

SYSTEM-FOCUSED LEVEL

At the systems level Ms. Jones works with the Board of Education, the local Community School Boards, and local farmers to bring healthy and nutritious foods to GJHS. Further, the local Community School Board decides to investigate if setting up a farmer's market in the communities they serve is doable as well as sustainable. Ms. Jones contacts the Culinary Institute of America, a culinary college located in Hyde Park, New York, to discuss the possibility of partnering with them to teach school cooks and parents how to prepare healthy meals with local farm produce and to establish student internships at GJHS. In addition, Ms. Jones knows that developing policies that both facilitate and sustain the integration of healthy meals and local produce into the school system meals needs specific mandates to ensure system-level changes.

INDIVIDUAL/FAMILY-FOCUSED LEVEL

On the individual/family level, Ms. Jones contacts her public high school and makes arrangements for educational workshops for parents to be held at the school-based clinic. The workshops will address understanding and preventing obesity, nutritional information, and promoting healthy lifestyles.

Ms. Jones identified a problem at GJHS and then developed and implemented advocacy strategies to reduce the prevalence of overweight and obese students at GJHS. Problem identification and developing strategic interventions required an understanding of the role of advocacy as outlined in the intervention wheel.

Social Marketing

Social marketing is defined as the utilization of ". . . commercial marketing principles and technologies for programs designed to influence the knowledge, attitudes, values, beliefs, behaviors, and practices of the population-of-interest" (Keller et al., 2008, p. 204). Social marketing makes use of "commercial marketing strategies to promote public health" (Evans, 2006, p. 1207) on the population level. Social marketing is used to influence health behavior. What follows is Ms. Jones' strategy for social marketing at the various practice levels.

Ms. Jones recognizes that using social marketing has the potential to bring about an understanding of social problems such as childhood obesity and getting people involved to make changes necessary to reduce overweight and obesity in children. Ms. Jones must use a myriad of communication strategies to ensure that the message not only gets out but is received in such a way

that change is possible. Communication strategies are based on mass media and mediated communication such as information from the healthcare clinician, message placements in the school-based clinic, and community-level outreach to the PTA, Community School Board, Board of Education, Department of Health, and the children/population involved.

Before Ms. Jones begins to engage in aspects of social marketing, she must approach the situation with a working knowledge of behavioral theory. An example of behavioral theory is the health promotion model developed by nurse theorist Pender in 1987 (Sakraida, 2005). The health promotion model is widely used by nursing to identify how well an individual may adhere to preventive health recommendations such as exercise, smoking cessation, and diet modifications. Making changes to existing health behaviors are largely based on how the person perceives his or her risk or susceptibility to a particular disease (Sakraida, 2005). Ms. Jones knows that mass media campaigns will have an effect if the person perceives and believes he or she is at risk for becoming overweight or obese. However, because the population in question is children, the families and community must also buy into the notion that overweight and obese children are being seen in epidemic proportions in their communities. The application of the health promotion model may assist Ms. Jones as she makes decisions pertaining to the intervention of social marketing.

To assist her with the intervention of social marketing, Ms. Jones creates a social marketing wheel to visualize the steps needed to accomplish a public health education campaign around the problem of overweight and obese children in GJHS (**Figure 12-1**). Social marketing is

FIGURE **12-1**   **Obesity campaign social marketing wheel.**

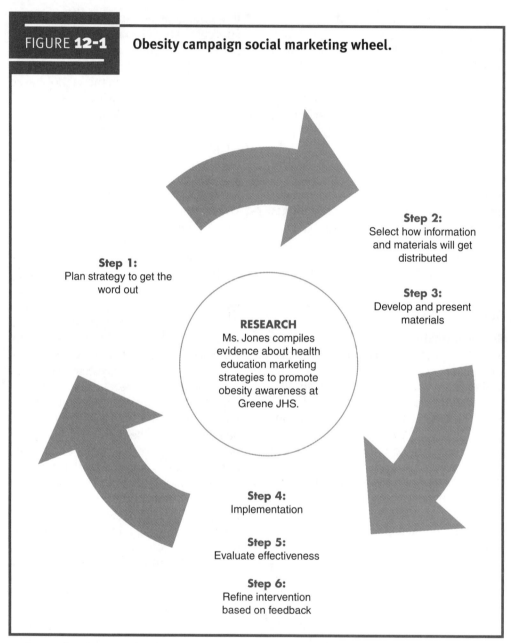

Source: Adapted from Evans (2006).

similar to health teaching because they both call for social campaigns to change public attitudes and behavior to solve a particular problem (Kotler & Roberto, 1989). Social marketing overlaps with advocacy and often is implemented at the same time a mass media strategy is organized.

Effective social marketing consists of six steps. Ms. Jones starts with the planning phase (step I). During this phase Ms. Jones assesses the level of knowledge each group has about the problem of overweight and obese children at GJHS using focus groups. The focus groups also serve to elicit suggestions about crafting a health promotion campaign to increase physical activity in GJHS as well as out of school and develop healthy eating strategies in school, home, and the neighborhood. Additionally, Ms. Jones works with each of the focus groups to create a health promotion slogan. These strategies are needed to ensure that an effective social marketing message will be understood by students, parents, teachers, Board of Education, and Community School Board. Further, Ms. Jones recognizes that by holding several focus groups, she is able to reach out to many different constituents, which is needed to understand each group's unique perspective about how to approach and address this problem. For a breakdown of the specific actions that Ms. Jones may enact within step I of the social marketing wheel for this particular situation, see **Figure 12-2**.

After the focus groups, Ms. Jones addresses how the information will be presented and distributed (step II) and pretested within select groups (step III). Based on focus group results, Ms. Jones works with teachers in the art department and media services to create posters,

brochures, and a public service announcement. The teachers decide that this will be a school-wide project so that all students will participate. The Board of Education decides to present awards for the most innovative and creative poster, brochure, and public service announcement. The Community School Board works with the local businesses and community centers to place the posters, brochures, and public service announcement. A review of Figure 12-2 provides a breakdown of the specific actions that Ms. Jones may take during steps II and III of the social marketing wheel.

The implementation phase is next (step IV) followed by ongoing evaluation (step V) and refinement of the process based on feedback (step VI). During these phases Ms. Jones continually assesses knowledge, attitudes, and beliefs of the stakeholders (those participating in this process). Examples of successful outcomes on the systems-focused level are the Board of Education removing vending machines from school cafeterias or replacing juice and soda drinks with water. Further, the Board of Education hires more physical education teachers and mandates daily gym classes for all students. Examples of successful outcomes on the community-focused level are the Community School Board in concert with the local community center's work with local farmers to set up a weekly farmer's market. Examples demonstrating individuals/families-focused level outcomes are behavioral change as evidenced by attendance of families at the weekly shopping and cooking classes at the local churches and community centers. For a breakdown of the specific actions that may be taken in steps IV, V, and VI of the social marketing wheel, review Figure 12-2. Ms. Jones will assess

| FIGURE **12-2** | **Social marketing conceptual model actions.** |

1. Social marketing initiatives (plan strategy)
   a. Convene several focus groups to assess knowledge about the obesity problem at Green JHS:
      i. Junior high school students
      ii. Parent-teacher association (PTA)
      iii. Board of Education
      iv. Community school board
   b. Develop a health promotion campaign that addresses:
      i. Increasing physical activity at school and within neighborhood
      ii. Healthy eating in school, home, and in the neighborhood
   c. Create a health promotion campaign slogan to be used by the children, PTA, Board of Education, and community school board.

2. Exposure to the message—awareness and receptivity (select information modalities; develop and pretest materials)
   a. Based on focus groups results
      i. Design posters
      ii. Design brochures
      iii. Develop public service announcement (PSA)
   b. Decide on placement of posters
      i. School-based clinic
      ii. Supermarkets, bodegas
      iii. Community centers
      iv. Local cable company
   c. Mail brochures to interested parties

3. Knowledge, attitudes, and beliefs (implementation)
   a. Belief in health promotion value of diet modification and physical activity
      i. Board of Education removes vending machines from cafeteria
      ii. Board of Education mandates daily gym classes for all students
      iii. Community school board set up
   b. Attitudes about diet modification and physical activity
      i. School-based clinic begins weight loss program for parents and children
   c. Intent to modify one's diet and participate in physical activity
      i. Parents attend weekly shopping and cooking seminars at their community centers
      ii. Begin local farmer's market

4. Behavior modifications
   a. Collect feedback to refine the program and strategies

Source: Adapted from Minnesota Department of Health Division of Community Health Services Public Health Nursing Section. (2001). Public health interventions: Application to public health nursing practice. St. Paul: Minnesota Department of Health.

the effectiveness of the behavior modifications by developing a population-based database that keeps track of children and families participating in the programs developed to address overweight and obese children at GJHS as well as their BMIs.

Policy Development and Enforcement

Policy development is the final resolution of what comes out of advocacy and social marketing. **Policy development**, in fact, is often unsuccessful unless it is carried out in conjunction with advocacy. "Policy development places health issues on decision-makers' agendas, acquires a plan of resolution, and determines needed resources. Policy development results in laws, rules and regulations, ordinances, and policies. **Policy enforcement** compels others to comply with the laws, rules, regulations, ordinances, and policies created in conjunction with policy development" (Keller et al., 2008, p. 204). The application of this strategy to the various levels of practice is highlighted below.

Ms. Jones has been successful in bringing together all the stakeholders in her school and the surrounding communities to deal with the problem of overweight and obese children. Ms. Jones has seen that the programs addressing healthy eating in schools were developed and that partnerships with local farmers, the Culinary Institute of America, and the school-based clinic were formed to ensure that the community has access to healthy and nutritious foods as well as learning about the nutritional value of food. Additionally, the local Community School Board established walking programs within the

neighborhood, and the Board of Education was committed to increasing physical activity in GJHS.

Ms. Jones knows that she wants the programs started at GJHS and within the community to be sustainable and thus needs to ensure that the interested parties, such as students, teachers, parents, community partners, and Board of Education, continue their involvement. Ms. Jones is charged with making sure that decision makers are informed about the problem of overweight and obese children so that laws, rules, regulations, ordinances, and policies can be enacted to address this issue. Further, Ms. Jones needs to make certain that the programs and interventions developed are effective, funding is available, surveillance systems are set in place to monitor health statistics, and school-based clinics become a model for addressing overweight and obesity at the community-focused, systems-focused, and individual/family-focused levels. The basic steps needed for policy development and enforcement are illustrated in **Figure 12-3**.

Step 1 requires that Ms. Jones identify the issue (increased numbers of overweight and obese children at GJHS) and the relevance of the issue locally and nationally. By identifying the problem and the target population, Ms. Jones decides what can be done about this issue. During this phase Ms. Jones set a policy agenda and identified the local, state, and federal policymakers who would have authority to develop and mandate policies.

Step 2 requires that Ms. Jones begin to formulate policy and establish goals and objectives to resolve this problem. Because Ms. Jones had already started the advocacy and social marketing

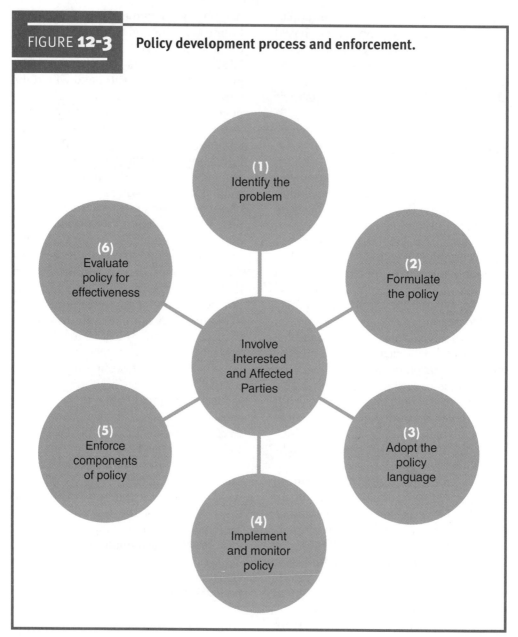

FIGURE **12-3**   **Policy development process and enforcement.**

Source: Adapted from Minnesota Department of Health Division of Community Health Services Public Health Nursing Section (2001).

process earlier, many of the key stakeholders have already been identified and involved in resolving the problem.

Step 3 requires that Ms. Jones draft a policy to address the issue. The policy should consist of a budget and funding and arrange for public hearings as necessary to bring this problem to the attention of additional stakeholders.

Step 4 requires that Ms. Jones develop rules and guidelines needed to sustain the suggested programs, such as mandating daily gym classes, changing the food choices at the school cafeteria, and setting up local farmers markets in the community. Ms. Jones has to also decide how these programs will be monitored and who will be responsible for monitoring these programs.

Step 5 requires that Ms. Jones knows how the enforcement of any policy will take place. Strategies for policy enforcement can take many forms such as negotiation, education, and legal repercussions.

Step 6 requires that Ms. Jones evaluate the effectiveness of all policy implemented. This phase is an ongoing process and is necessary to assess the effectiveness of a strategy, intervention, or program. This phase provides policy developers with knowledge about the program and is the basis for improvement.

Ms. Jones knows that policy development and enforcement can also be achieved by legislation or regulation. Legislation provides a legal framework that embodies the principles of a program and the policy basics are unlikely to change. Enacting policy legislatively requires approval by a governing body such as congress, state assembly, and so forth. The laws are promulgated and passed by a legislative branch and then,

after passage, implemented by local, state, or federal administrative agencies. Legislation provides the basis for the regulatory process; therefore regulations have the force and the effect of the law that are issued by an executive authority of the government (Milstead, 2008).

Even though Ms. Jones' advocacy, social marketing, and policy development and enforcement strategies were mostly developed on the local level, many of the interventions put into place can lead to government action. The success of enacting legislation and regulations will largely depend on how involved Ms. Jones can get the interested parties and ongoing evaluation of the programs. Ms. Jones knows that public health nurses have a responsibility to identify health problems that affect the larger community/population and that policy development and enforcement comes out of the principles of public health nursing.

CONCLUSION

This chapter discusses the advocacy, social marketing, and policy development and enforcement sections of the intervention wheel. The growing public health problem of overweight and obesity in children and adolescents was used to discuss how public health nursing could bring this issue to the attention of interested parties. The strategies used by public health nursing consist of advocacy, which then leads to social marketing, and culminating with policy development and enforcement. Further, this chapter discusses how public health nursing strategies can be applied on the community level, systems level, and individual/family level.

References

Allison, D. B., Newcomer, J. W., Dunn, A. L., Blumenthal, J. A., Fabricatore, A. N., Daumit, G. L., et al. (2009). Obesity among those with mental disorders: A National Institute of Mental Health Meeting Report. *American Journal of Preventive Medicine, 36*(4), 341–350.

Blair, S. N., & Nichaman, M. Z. (2002). The public health problem of increasing prevalence rates of obesity and what should be done about it. *Mayo Clinical Procedures, 77*(2), 109–113.

Centers for Disease Control and Prevention [CDC]. (2000). Prevalence of overweight and obesity among adults: United States, 1999. Retrieved April 12, 2009, from http:/www.cdc.gov/nchs/nhanes.htm

Centers for Disease Control and Prevention [CDC]. (2001). Diabetes. CDC [On-line]. Retrieved April 12, 2009, from http://www.cdc.gov/diabetes/statistics

Centers for Disease Control and Prevention [CDC]. (2009). Health weight. Retrieved April 12, 2009, from http://www.cdc.gov/healthyweight/assessing/bmi/adult_BMI/index.html

Chen, Y., Dales, R., & Jiang, Y. (2006). The association between obesity and asthma is stronger in nonallergic than allergic adults. *Chest, 130,* 890–895.

Cohen, D., de la Vega, R., & Watson, G. (2001). *Advocacy for social justice: A global action and reflection guide.* Sterling, VA: Kumarian Press.

Davis, B., & Carpenter, C. (2009). Proximity of fast-food restaurants to schools and adolescent obesity. *American Journal of Public Health, 99*(3), 505–510.

de Onis, M. & Blossner, M. (2000). Prevalence and trends of overweight among preschool children in developing countries. *American Journal of Clinical Nutrition, 72,* 1032–1039.

Diabetes Prevention Program Research Group. (2002). Reduction in the incidence of type 2 diabetes with lifestyle intervention or metformin. *New England Journal of Medicine, 346*(6), 393–403.

Evans, W. D. (2006). How social marketing works in health care. *British Medical Journal, 332,* 1207–1210.

Flynn, M. A., McNeil, D. A., Maloff, B., Mutasingwa, D., Wu, M., Ford, C., et al. (2006). Reducing obesity and related chronic disease risk in children and youth: A synthesis of evidence with "best practice" recommendations. *Obesity Reviews, 7*(Suppl. 1), 7–66.

Harbaugh, B. L., Jordan-Welch, M., Bounds, W., Blom, L., & Fisher, W. (2007). Nurses and families rising to the challenge of overweight children. *Nurse Practitioner, 32*(3), 30–35.

Hogan, P., Dall, T., Nikolov, P., & the American Diabetes Association. (2003). Economic costs of diabetes in the US in 2002. *Diabetes Care, 26*(3), 917–932.

Jordan, A. B., & Robinson, T. N. (2008). Children, television viewing, and weight status: Summary and recommendations from an expert panel meeting. *Annals of the American Academy, 615,* 119–132.

Keller, L. O., Strohschein, S., & Briske, L. (2008). Population-based public health nursing practice: The intervention wheel. In M. Stanhope & J. Lancaster (Eds.), *Public health nursing: Population-centered health care in the community* (pp. 199–205). St. Louis, MO: Mosby Elsevier.

Koplan, J. P., Liverman, C. T., & Kraak, V. A. (Eds.). (2005). *Preventing childhood obesity: Health in the balance.* Washington, DC: National Academies Press.

Kotler, P., & Roberto, E. L. (1989). *Social marketing: Strategies for changing public behavior.* New York: New York Free Press.

Kumanyika, S. K., Obarzanek, E., Stettler, N., Bell, R., Field, A. E., Fortmann, S. P., et al. (2008). Population-based prevention of obesity: The need for comprehensive promotion of healthful eating, physical activity, and energy balance. *Circulation, 118,* 428–464.

The Lancet. (2001). Editorial: Childhood obesity: An emerging public-health problem. *Lancet, 357*(9273),1989.

Lee, R. E., & Cubbin, C. (2002). Neighborhood context and youth cardiovascular health behaviors. *American Journal of Public Health, 92,* 428–436.

Lopez, R. (2004). Urban sprawl and risk for being overweight and obese. *American Journal of Public Health, 94*(9), 1574–1579.

Lovasi, G. S., Neckerman, K. M., Quinn, J. W., Weiss, C. C., & Rundle, A. (2009). Effects of individual neighborhood disadvantage on the association between neighborhood walkability and body mass index. *American Journal of Public Health, 99*(2), 279–284.

Messier, S. P., Loeser, R. F., Miller, G. D., Morgan, T. M., Rejeski, W. J., Sevick, M. A., et al. (2004). Exercise and dietary weight loss in overweight and obese adults with knee osteoarthritis: The arthritis, diet, and activity promotion trial. *Arthritis & Rheumatism, 50*(5), 1501–1510.

Milstead, J. A. (2008). *Health policy and politics: A nurse's guide* (3rd ed.). Sudbury, MA: Jones and Bartlett.

Minnesota Department of Health Division of Community Health Services Public Health Nursing Section. (2001). *Public health interventions: Application for public health nursing practice.* St. Paul: Minnesota Department of Health.

Murugan, A. T., & Sharma, G. (2008). Obesity and respiratory diseases. *Chronic Respiratory Disease, 5*, 233–242.

Nader, P. R., O'Brien, M., Houts, R., Bradley, R., Belsky, J., Crosnoe, R., et al. (2006). Identifying risk for obesity in early childhood. *Pediatrics, 118*(3), e594–e601.

Narayan, K. M., Boyle, J. P., Geiss, L. S., Saaddine, J. B., & Thompson, T. L. (2006). Impact of recent increase in incidence on future diabetes burden: U.S., 2005–2050. *Diabetes Care, 29*(9), 2114–2116.

Newcomer, J. W. (2007). Metabolic syndrome and mental illness. *American Journal of Managed Care, 13*, S170–S177.

Ogden, C. L., Carroll, M. D., Curtin, L. R., McDowell, M. A., Tabak, C. J., & Flegal, K. M. (2009). Prevalence of overweight and obesity in the United States, 1999–2004. *Journal of the American Medical Association, 295*(13), 1549–1555.

Patterson, R. E., Frank, L. L., Kristal, A. R., & White, E. (2004). A comprehensive examination of health conditions associated with obesity in older adults. *American Journal of Preventive Medicine, 27*(5), 385–390.

Peterson, J. A. (2007). Get moving! Physical activity counseling in primary care. *Journal of the American Academy of Nurse Practitioners, 19*, 349–357.

Reiser, L. M., & Schlenk, E. A. (2009). Clinical use of physical activity measures. *Journal of the American Academy of Nurse Practitioners, 21*, 87–94.

Sakraida T. (2005). Nola J. Pender: The health promotion model. In T. A. Marriner-Tomey & A. M. Raile-Aligood (Eds.), *Nursing theorists and their work* (5th ed., pp. 624–639). St Louis, MO: Mosby.

Salvy, S. J., Roemmich, J. N., Bowker, J. C., Romero, N. D., Stadler, P. J., & Epstein, L. H. (2009). Effects of peers and friends on youth physical activity and motivation to be physically active. *Journal of Pediatric Psychology, 34*(2), 217–225.

Seiders, K., & Petty, R. D. (2004). Obesity and the role of food marketing: A policy analysis of issues and remedies. *Journal of Public Policy & Marketing, 23*(2), 153–169.

Sheehy, A. M., Coursin, D. B., & Gabbay, R. A. (2008). Back to Wilson and Jungner: 10 good reasons to screen for type 2 diabetes mellitus. *Mayo Clinic Procedures, 84*(1), 38–42.

Story, M., Nanney, M. S., & Schwartz, M. B. (2009). Schools and obesity prevention: Creating school environments and policies to promote healthy eating and physical activity. *Milbank Quarterly, 87*(1), 71–100.

U.S. Department of Health and Human Services. (2000). *Healthy people 2010: National health promotion and disease prevention objectives.* Washington, DC: Author.

U.S. Department of Health and Human Services. (2008). *2008 Physical activity guidelines for Americans.* Washington, DC: Author.

Wald, L. (1915). *The house on Henry Street.* New York: Henry Holt & Company.

Wallace, M. F., Fulwood, R., & Alvarado, M. (2008). NHLBI step-by-step approach to adapting cardiovascular training and education curricula for diverse audiences. *Preventing Chronic Disease, 5*(2), 1–7.

Ward, A., & Martens, L. (2000). *Eating out: Social differentiation, consumption, and pleasure.* London: Cambridge University Press.

Yanovski, S. Z., & Yanovski, J. A. (2002). Drug therapy: Obesity. *New England Journal of Medicine, 346*(8), 591–602.

PROTECTING, SUSTAINING, AND EMPOWERING: A HISTORICAL PERSPECTIVE ON THE CONTROL OF EPIDEMICS

CHRISTINE E. HALLETT

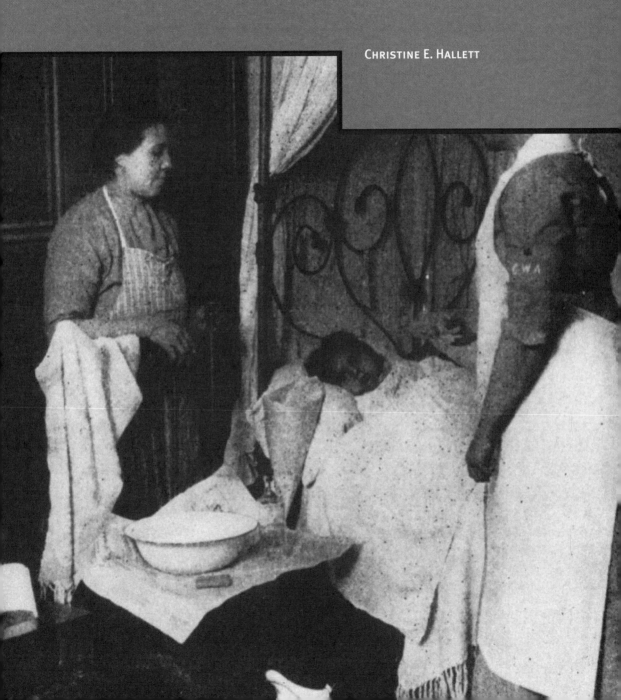

Does not the popular idea of "infection" involve that people should take greater care of themselves than of the patient? That, for instance, it is safer not to be too much with the patient, not to attend too much to his wants? Perhaps the best illustration of the utter absurdity of this view of duty in attending on "infectious" diseases is afforded by what was very recently the practice, if it is not so even now, in some of the European lazarets—in which the plague-patient used to be condemned to the horrors of filth, overcrowding, and want of ventilation, while the medical attendant was ordered to examine the patient's tongue through an opera-glass and to toss him a lancet to open his abscess with! True nursing ignores infection, except to prevent it. Cleanliness and fresh air from open windows, with unremitting attention to the patient, are the only defense a true nurse either asks or needs. Wise and humane management of the patient is the best safeguard against infection (Florence Nightingale, 1980 edition, pp. 23–24).

LEARNING OBJECTIVES

At the completion of this chapter, the reader will be able to

- Explore the ways in which human societies have attempted to combat global epidemics.
- Appreciate the role of the nurse, working alongside governments, doctors, and scientists, in the prevention of epidemic diseases.
- Explore the role of the nurse in the treatment and care of patients with life-threatening infectious diseases at different historical moments and in different places.

KEY TERMS

- Epidemic disease
- Infection control
- Pandemic

From its beginnings the human race has shared its habitats with infective microparasites. Harmless—even beneficial—microbes inhabited our planet long before we emerged as a species. They began the long evolutionary process that would enable them to live alongside—often in parasitic or symbiotic relationships to—their neighbors before the antecedents of the human species had even emerged from the primeval ocean. Catalyzing vital processes, such as the decomposition of the planet's toxic organic waste, microbes have long existed in a precarious, yet often positive, relationship with other organic life. Yet human beings notice their presence only when they fail to adapt quietly and harmlessly to the changing patterns of human life.

Of the many microparasites that inhabit our environment, it is the most inefficient—the least well adapted—that cause recognized infections. A "bug" that fails to live symbiotically with its host may expect to limit its own lifespan. If it kills its host it will die. If it keeps the host alive yet in a weakened state, it can expect that its host will eventually find a way to eradicate it. The purpose of this chapter is to trace the means by which humans have attempted to eradicate certain of those "bugs" they consider harmful: the bacteria and viruses that cause epidemic and endemic infections. The chapter focuses on three case studies of specific diseases appearing at specific historical moments: bubonic plague, as it appeared in the Early Modern Italian city states during the 16th and 17th centuries, "Spanish influenza" as it appeared in the cities of the United States in 1918 and 1919, and AIDS as it appeared in the United Kingdom during the 1980s.

The bubonic plague bacillus and the influenza virus caused **epidemic diseases** that affected such large sections of the world's population that they came to be seen as "global epidemics" or, more correctly, as **pandemics**. HIV exists on the cusp between endemic and epidemic disease, affecting large numbers of people worldwide; it is often spoken of as an epidemic because of its capacity to spread rapidly in certain populations and geographical areas of the world at certain times.

Humans have taken a range of measures to protect themselves against or to destroy pathogenic microorganisms. Through its case studies, this chapter considers four different approaches to disease: state-sanctioned control measures, medical interventions, nursing care and support, and individual empowerment. It traces the means by which human societies, more or less effectively, learned to protect themselves against, overcome, and survive severe life-threatening infection on a large scale. It focuses, in particular, on how societies mobilized and used nurses as "front-line" agents in combating infection.

PROTECTING THE PEOPLE AGAINST GOD'S WRATH: BUBONIC PLAGUE IN EARLY MODERN ITALY

The Black Death—the second recorded pandemic of the disease known as "bubonic plague"—swept across Europe from Central Asia in the 14th century, causing millions of deaths and devastating entire villages. It spread through Europe between 1348 and 1353 (Alexander, 1980; Hirst, 1953; Preto, 1978; Slack, 1985; Zinsser, 1935). Caused by the bacterium later to be named *Yersinia pestis*, the disease was carried in the body of a particular species of flea known as *Xenopsylla cheopis*, which in turn inhabited a particular species of black rat, known as *Rattus rattus*. It may seem extraordinary that a disease carried by one species of microbe in the bloodstream of one species of flea on the back of one species of rat could destroy so many communities, yet the lifestyle of the Middle Ages created an ideal ecological niche for these species. The black rat could live easily in the thatched roofs and grain stores of the largely agrarian communities of the 14th century, and the frequent overcrowding and lack of opportunities for good hygiene practices meant that flea and lice infestations were commonplace. Once the opening-up of trade routes to the East transported the plague to Western Europe, it rapidly gained a foothold there.

The first case study considers one small corner of the world two centuries after the plague caused its first great wave of devastation. The case-fatality rate of bubonic plague was probably around 30%, and its associated form, pneumonic plague, was even more lethal, with an 80% case-fatality rate. Having burned itself out by killing a large proportion of its host population, the Black Death remained endemic in the European rodent population, literally hovering at the gates of the towns and cities of Early Modern Europe. At particular risk were the inhabitants of the Italian city states such as Venice, Florence, Naples, and Rome that traded with the East, bringing within their borders goods likely to be infested with the black rat. Although they did not realize the disease was carried by rat fleas, the populations of these cities nevertheless recognized that it was somehow "imported" from outside. These states were the first to introduce systematic measures to protect their populations from plague (Christensen, 2003).

When confronted by plague, the magistrates of the city states had three aims: to avoid allowing the disease to arise in or to enter the city, to prevent its spread, and to maintain social order while, as much as possible, caring for the sick. Health magistrates, known as "Provveditori alla Sanita," appeared to have thought in terms of a complex relationship between plague and disorder. Plague was itself a form of physical disorder that could most easily arise in a disorderly environment that exuded disease-forming "miasmas" (or "pestilential" states of the air). Once plague had taken hold of a community, the relationship between the disease and social disorder was mutually reinforcing. The effect was perceived to be a spiral one in which the health—both physical and moral—of the community grew increasingly out of control. The work of the magistrates was to arrest this process. To properly coordinate their efforts during epidemics, the governments of Italian city states appointed specialist Health Boards, known as "Sanita," with wide-reaching powers, which became permanent in many Italian city states during the course of the 15th century (Campbell, 1931; Carmichael, 1983, 1986; Palmer, 1978).

Arising from a disorder within nature, plague threatened to create chaos within the community. Italian sanitary legislation aimed to prevent such chaos. Many of the measures in force during the Renaissance were introduced by legislation of the early 13th century, which preceded even experience of the Black Death (Carmichael, 1986). There were numerous attempts to legislate for cleanliness within city states. Unpleasant smells were believed to be particularly dangerous, because they were associated with noxious harmful vapors of which miasma was composed. By the end of the 14th century, there was already legislation against the keeping of animals such as pigs and ducks in Florence and against the selling of manure inside the city (Carmichael, 1986). The health authorities came to regard it as their responsibility to control the release of offensive smells associated with industrial activities such as tanning, butchery, and the retting of hemp (Cipolla, 1992; Palmer, 1978).

In taking responsibility for the eradication of plague, the patriciates (nobilities) of early modern cities fulfilled their roles as guardians of order and protectors of the state. King (1986) has identified the main preoccupations of Venetian patricians as evident in their humanistic writings. Noblemen such as Gasparo Contarini, Daniele Barbaro, Paolo Paruta, and Nicolo Contarini promoted the myth of a Venetian republic that was ordered and harmonious and in which the nobility conformed to the principle of "unanimitas." The Venetian patriciate presented itself as the personification of

order within the state. Furthermore, its members also saw themselves as the state's defense—as "moenia civitatis," or the "walls of the city" (King, 1986; Pastore, 1988; Ulvioni, 1989). The Italian Health Boards were the most effective and efficient organizations for controlling plague in Western Europe, and their measures became models for the establishment of health controls in other states (Cipolla, 1979, 1992).

Calvi (1989) examined the efforts of magistrates to maintain stability in Florence during the epidemic of 1630–1631. Through a close examination of the criminal trial records of the Health Magistracy and a reading of Francesco Rondinelli's contemporary account of the plague, she discovered that the regulations imposed during the "virtual dictatorship" of the public health officials reflected the desire for order and uniformity. Most of the 300 trials she examined dealt with violations against property, crimes committed by public health workers, and the unlawful hiding of the ill (Calvi, 1989).

It had been recognized since the Black Death that some diseases could be transmitted between individuals (Biraben, 1975; Campbell, 1931). An idea of contagion was part of the general stock of knowledge in early modern Europe. In Thomas More's *Utopia* (1516), the hospitals were situated outside the town so that people with diseases "such as be wont by infection to creep from one to another" (p. 35) might be separated from the rest of the population (Ficino, 1989). However, a theory of contagion was not articulated effectively until the mid-16th century when it formed the basis of a work by Girolamo Fracastoro (1930). His *De Contagione et Contagiosis Morbis et Eorum Curatione, Libri III,* first published in Venice in 1546, has interested historians because its theories bear some superficial resemblance to a germ theory of disease (Fracostoro, 1930 edition; Nutton, 1990).

Fracastoro emphasized that where plague was concerned, the most frequent means of transmission was contagion between individuals. He distinguished between diseases that were merely common to communities and those that were also contagious (Fracastoro, 1930 edition). The dominant theme in his work was the idea that plague was caused by invasion. It could be passed on from person to person rather than simply arising spontaneously from a disordered environment. It could also be carried in fomites—porous objects such as cloth and wood—and thus be transported between one community and the next. These ideas had immense influence in the Italian city states where plague came to be seen as an invading force against which siege measures must be adopted.

During the early modern period, as plague came to be identified more as an invasion from outside the state, measures taken by city state magistrates to preserve order were increasingly reinforced by a range of defensive strategies, many of which were already quite old, dating from the time of the Black Death, but all of which appear to have been imposed with increasing rigor and determination during the 16th and 17th centuries. In the late 16th century Gasparo Contarini (1599) commented on the work of the Provveditore alla Sanita, the city's health magistrate:

> His chiefest office is to forsee that there come not into the citie an contagious infection, which if at any time it happen to creepe in (as sometimes it chanceth) then to take such diligent and carefull order that in as much as

maybe the same come not to spread any further.

Throughout the early modern period, when it became known to its neighbors that a state was affected by plague, it was usual for commerce with that state to be banned. This meant the cessation of all forms of communication, including trade, with the plague-infested region, against whose inhabitants frontiers were closely guarded (Carmichael, 1983). Banning was controlled by means of a system of health passes that permitted only those who were well or who came from healthy areas to enter a territory. Passes were introduced by Milan during the 15th century and were then used by other states in the first half of the 16th century (Brozzi, 1982; Cipolla, 1973, 1979; Modena, 1988; Palmer, 1978; Petraccone, 1978). Centorio degli Hortensii (1631) described a series of measures introduced by the health deputies of Modena during the plague of 1575–1577:

> Besides unpaid officials at the gates, paid officials will be posted at the pass of the Fossa Alta, at the pass of the Marzoia at the high bridge and the low bridge . . . at Buon Porto, on the bank of the River Secchia, at San Marino, on the border with Mirandola. (p. 17)

They added that guards at these posts must be able to read and write and must be in possession of an official seal to stamp the passes of those allowed through (Hortensii, 1631). The defensive nature of these measures is striking: They illustrate the extent to which plague came to be associated with invasion.

All ships coming to the early modern state from any area suspected of plague were made to undergo a quarantine. Crew members were not permitted to enter the city or unload goods during the quarantine period, which usually lasted 40 days. This measure was originally designed to provide an early warning system for diseases on ships, but became one of the most enduring measures against contagion (Campbell, 1931; Carmichael, 1983; Palmer, 1978). It also became a measure for isolating entire communities of people: During a general quarantine only doctors and members of the government were allowed to leave their homes (Petraccone, 1978; Ulvioni, 1989).

When plague was diagnosed in an Italian city state, the victims were quickly segregated from the rest of the population. The sick were examined, and persons discovered to be suffering from the plague were taken to the "lazzaretto," or "pest house." The Lazzaretto Vecchio of Venice, founded by decree of the Senate on August 28, 1423, was the first permanent pest house in Europe (Campbell, 1931; Palmer, 1978). It was situated about 2 miles from the city on a small island off the Lido that had previously been the home of the Eremite Monastery of Santa Maria di Nazareth (Chambers & Pullan, 1992). A decree of the Venetian Senate on April 17, 1464, provided for "two suitable and competent citizens not of noble rank" (Chambers & Pullan, 1992, p. 114) to be appointed for each sestiere of the city to ensure that all infected persons were taken to the Lazzaretto Vecchio and all infected houses evacuated. The notary, Rocco Benedetti, described the horrors of the Venetian Lazzaretto Vecchio, which seemed to him like "Hell itself" (Chambers & Pullan, 1992):

> From every side their came foul odors, indeed a stench that none could endure; groans and sighs were heard without ceasing; and at all hours, clouds of smoke from the burning of corpses was seen to rise far into the air. Some who miraculously returned from that place alive reported, among other things, that at the height of that great influx of infected people there were three or four of them to a bed. Since a great number of servants had died and there was no one to take care of them, they had to get themselves up to take food and attend to other things. Nobody did anything but lift the dead from the beds and throw them into the pits. . . . And many, driven to frenzy by the disease, especially at night, leapt from their beds, and, shouting with fearful voices of damned souls, went here and there, colliding with one another, and suddenly falling to the ground dead. Some who rushed in frenzy out of the wards threw themselves into the water, or ran madly through the gardens, and were then found dead among the thornbushes, all covered with blood. (pp. 118–119)

A sufferer who died at the pest house was buried there or in a cemetery apart from the city. Survivors were usually sent to a convalescent hospital to undergo a 40-day quarantine before being returned home (Chambers & Pullan, 1992). The lazzaretti were also centers for the disinfection of fomites. In the Venetian lazzaretti, goods from infected homes and ships were aired for 40 days and, during that time, were constantly turned and moved to release any infection they might have absorbed (Brozzi, 1982; Castellacci, 1897; Pastore, 1988).

The monitoring and control of the poor were closely associated with the prevention of plague: It was a means of propitiating God, a measure for promoting order, and a defensive strategy. Indeed, the development of organized systems of poor relief was probably stimulated by the experience of plague, a disease associated with poverty at an early stage in its history (Preto, 1978; Pullan, 1971, 1992). Governments and physicians observed that the poor were affected in greater numbers than the rich. Theorists devised explanations for this pattern: The poor lived disorderly lives, their inadequate diets were a source of corruption that could spread through the community, and they did not dispose of waste properly and hence lived among filth that might create a poisonous miasma (Anselment, 1989; Biraben, 1975; Carmichael, 1986; Grell, 1990).

During the plague of 1575–1577, physicians expressed the view that the poor were a threat to the health of the community. Nicolo Massa and Girolamo Mercuriale both went so far as to argue that the poor should be removed from towns when there was a threat of plague. Mercuriale referred to them as "fomes" for the disease (Palmer, 1978, p. 144). In August 1576 the state—perhaps acting on such advice—decided that the link between poverty and plague was related to poor housing conditions and chose a site at Zaffusina at which to relocate the poor from plague-affected areas. It was said that the site could have accommodated over 10,000 people, and provision was made for the supply of tents and huts, but the plan was never put into effect (Preto, 1978).

Hospitals originated as hostels for the poor rather than as specialist centers for the cure of disease, and as such they were centers for the isolation of those likely to disrupt the social order (Cartwright, 1977; Pullan, 1992). The poor could be seen as plague in microcosm. The Mendicanti

hospitals established in many Italian states from the 1560s onward were designated to remove beggars from public places (Park & Henderson, 1991). By building hospitals magistrates responded to plague in three ways. First, by caring for its poor, the state obeyed God's commands and might thereby deflect his anger and prevent disease. Second, by housing beggars the state avoided the problems associated with squalor, dirt, filth, and bad smells that could give rise to miasma. Third, if the poor were seen as carriers of plague in a contagious sense, the state, by isolating them in hospitals, protected healthy citizens from the disease they carried.

Measures adopted by states from the second half of the 15th century illustrate their recognition that plague could easily be brought into cities by immigrants whose origins were uncertain (Carmichael, 1983). In 1498 in Venice it was decreed that all lodging housekeepers must have licenses (Pullan, 1971). The tendency to associate plague with invasion through theories of contagion is apparent in the way in which particular individuals were blamed for bringing plague into a city. It was believed, for example, that during October 1629 a soldier from Lecco brought the disease into Milan in a bundle of clothing obtained from German troops (Calvi, 1989; Cipolla, 1973; Galassi, 1966–1970).

A decree of the Venetian Council of Ten and Zonta of September 12, 1539 described how orders had been given to the Provveditori alla Sanita (Chambers & Pullan, 1992):

To bar from this city many poor persons suspected of carrying the plague, who, as we had heard by letters from Milan, had been expelled from the Milanese state and from Piedmont, and it was thought that they were certain to come here. Not only did the Provveditori carry out these orders both wisely and thoroughly, but they also expelled from Venice some 4000–5000 beggars and other kinds of persons who had recently come to live in this city. (p. 126)

The approaches of the Italian city states to the prevention and control of bubonic plague were thus a mixture of the pragmatic and the ideological. By closing their gates to anyone who might carry the disease and removing from their homes all those who were believed to be infected, states protected their healthy citizens. In holding masses and processions and in establishing hospitals for the poor, they worked to propitiate divine wrath. Most did not, however, have the capacity to provide adequate care and attention to those who succumbed to the disease. Early modern pest houses were places of dread—from which one had a poor chance of emerging alive.

SERVING AND SUSTAINING A DESPERATE POPULATION: INFLUENZA IN THE MODERN UNITED STATES

Modern sensibilities may identify a degree of ruthlessness in the approaches to plague prevention of the Early Modern Italian city states. If the beleaguered "Provveditori alla Sanita" took harsh and desperate measures, this can only have been because of their fundamental sense of helplessness when confronted by infectious disease. They had no cure. Keeping their options open, they worked hard to propitiate God; epidemics might, after all, as the Bible suggested, be visita-

tions of divine wrath. Yet, they also directed their energies toward protecting the healthy in their communities. The sick they condemned to the overcrowded pest houses where desperate and overwhelmed nursing attendants struggled to offer rudimentary support.

Perhaps no greater contrast can therefore be imagined than between the frantic efforts of the early modern pest house attendants and the home care offered by the confident district nurses of modern cities in the early 20th century. The influenza pandemic of 1918–1919 threatened to overwhelm much of Europe, the European colonies, and North America, yet one of the most striking findings of historians is that although medical science stood by helpless before this deadly disease, nursing care seemed effective in reducing death rates. Although no efforts have ever been made to quantify the successes of early 20th century district nurses (it is impossible to prove definitively that they actually saved lives), the writings of contemporaries indicate that there was a strong belief that good nursing care had made a real difference to survival rates.

This phenomenon of "good nursing care" appears frequently in the writings of late 19th century physicians and nurses but is rarely accompanied by a definition. It appears to refer to those nursing actions that enabled the patient's physiological system to survive best while his or her immune system fought the infectious disease. Thus the maintenance of a steady temperature by the judicious use of blankets and the warming of "sick rooms," the provision of copious fluids and nourishing food (usually in the form of nutritious soup), and the maintenance of patient hygiene, rest, and sleep acted both to stabilize the system and to prevent the development of new complications. Providing these prerequisites for recovery seems deceptively simple. In reality, providing core nursing care for a very ill individual required great artistry, skill, and patience, whereas going into a home to care for a person with a known deadly—and incurable—disease required more than a little courage.

The so-called Spanish influenza epidemic of 1918–1919 (caused by the virus H_1N_1) is estimated to have caused a global mortality of between 50 and 100 million (Johnson & Mueller, 2002; Quinn, 2008). It developed toward the end of the World War I and probably killed at least twice as many people as the war itself (Crosby, 1989; Johnson, 2006; Patterson & Pyle, 1991; Phillips & Killingray, 2003). Reid (2005) observed that accurate figures are difficult to obtain, partly because influenza was not made a notifiable disease until 1918 and partly because early cases were often labeled as bronchitic pneumonia or just pneumonia (Reid, 2005). It appears to have originated in China and then may have been spread throughout the United States via the mobilization and movement of troops who were housed in overcrowded barracks. From the American military camps it spread rapidly to Europe, where war-weary populations succumbed rapidly (Byerly, 2005; Quinn, 2008). Its most puzzling and unusual feature was its tendency to attack young, apparently healthy adults: Its mortality rate was very high within this group and was lower among the elderly (possibly because of acquired immunity) and the very young (Barry, 2005; Reid, 2005).

A devastating disease, Spanish influenza caused severe headache, cough, breathing difficulties, nosebleeds, aching joints, and intense fatigue. A characteristic symptom was the severe cyanosis that could rapidly turn the faces of sufferers blue or even black. The disease was often extremely rapid in its onset. An apparently healthy individual might suddenly collapse in the street, with blood pouring from his nose, and then die before there was time to get him to hospital. Already severe in its respiratory symptoms, the disease was frequently complicated by acute and severe bronchopneumonic symptoms, and death was frequently from these complications rather than from the more systemic effects of the virus. Victims of this terrifying disease became feverish to the point of delirium, cyanosed until their skin was black, and weak to the point of utter helplessness (Quinn, 2008).

Joyce Sapwell, a British volunteer-nurse, wrote the following in her diary:

> The terrible flu pneumonia epidemic broke out. About one-third of the staff were down with it, and the hospital was full. We had had one hundred and eight deaths in eight weeks. I was put on night duty in charge of four huts at the bottom of the hospital, the main part was full, each hut had 20 beds. Three of them flu pneumonia and one with convalescent colonials. I had not even one orderly to help. Several patients became delirious, and if they got out of bed they usually died. (n.d., n.p.)

Quinn (2008) argued that political leaders were slow to respond to the threat of the influenza outbreak, prioritizing the war effort over the fight against the disease. American President Woodrow Wilson, for example, at first ignored the advice of doctors to publicize details of the outbreak and to halt troop movements (Quinn, 2008). Doctors themselves were helpless against the disease. Just as in the

Italian city states there had been no cure for bubonic plague, similarly, 20th century medical science was unable to discover a "magic bullet" that would kill the influenza virus. And yet the perspective on disease of 20th century North Americans was very different from that of 16th century Italians. The emergence of germ theory in the late 19th century, prompted largely by the research of scientists such as Louis Pasteur and Robert Koch, had revolutionized medicine and given both physicians and the societies they served a sense of mastery over disease (Gradmann, 2001; Latour, 1988). If cures could not be found immediately, they would, nevertheless, eventually become available. The early 20th century's faith in science gave its people a belief that they could, collectively, control their own destiny. In the meantime, a range of remedies was attempted, from the use of opium and quinine to traditional herbal cures and bloodletting. "Heroic" remedies such as strychnine and steam baths, along with smallpox, diphtheria, and antitetanus serum, were also tried without success (Quinn, 2008).

The nurses of the United States were also very different from the largely untrained sick-room attendants or "servants" of the Early Modern period. The rapid development of medical science in the second half of the 19th century meant that the character of nursing had changed beyond recognition. Retaining their core functions of the care and nurturing of the sick, nurses were now also carefully trained technicians who administered the new, scientific, and often heroic remedies devised by medical science with dexterity and intelligence. It was their fundamental nursing skills, however, that came to the fore when they nursed thousands of influenza patients in the years 1918–1919. Many of those who died did so from exhaustion and starvation. Nurses could prevent these deaths. They took soup and hot drinks to the houses of sufferers and offered care and comfort that enabled the absolute rest that might help the body more effectively fight the disease (Keen-Payne, 2000). Quinn (2008) cites the Australian nurse in the outback town of Byrock, Australia, who delivered food and medicines "single-handedly" to a town of 27 families (Quinn, 2008).

Keeling (in press), using New York as a case study, showed that community-based nursing organizations could have a profound effect on both the well-being and probably the survival rates of whole communities of individuals (Keeling, in press). Keeling focused on the efforts of the Henry Street Settlement, a group of public health nurses founded in 1893 and working under the directorship of Lillian Wald. These nurses had, for decades, been working with the poorest communities in the city, basing most of their activities in the Lower East Side, where immigrant families lived in destitution. They were no strangers to epidemic disease and had at their disposal an armory of measures to improve the health, hygiene, and nutritional status and to promote the comfort of their severely ill patients (Buhler-Wilkerson, 2001; Keeling, 2007).

Wald and her nurses worked in cooperation with the American Red Cross, the U.S. Public Health Service, volunteer organizations, and city health officials. They used warm blankets, baths, and fresh air to both comfort patients and promote their capacities to fight the infection. Perhaps most importantly, they enabled their patients to obtain complete rest, so enabling their immune systems the best chance of destroying the virus without also overwhelming the body itself. City authorities provided automobiles for their use, and they were able to transport pneumonia jackets and quarts of soup to the homes of the sick, offering warmth and nourishment to patients. They were able to keep large numbers of sufferers at home, thus relieving the desperately overcrowded hospitals, preventing unnecessary journeys for already severely weakened patients, and containing the spread of the disease (Keeling, in press).

The influenza epidemic of the early 20th century was poorly controlled and contained. It is possible to argue that the governments of Western developed nations had learned nothing from the stringent isolation and quarantine regulations of their forebearers in the Early Modern city states. Yet it can also be argued that the nursing services of the early 20th century were able to ensure that influenza—although just as horrific as bubonic plague in its effects—was not a disease that left its victims totally helpless. Nursing care offered hope, not just to sufferers themselves but to whole societies.

EMPOWERING THE VULNERABLE: AIDS IN CONTEMPORARY BRITAIN

The AIDS virus, it can be argued, is a much more efficient microparasite than that which caused Spanish influenza. The reaction of the human body to influenza was rapid and devastating. Death or recovery followed infection within days; both outcomes ultimately destroyed the virus. HIV has a much more hidden effect on the body and can live within its host's cells for several years before the destruction of body systems begins, symptoms emerge, and treatment is sought. This subtle infection has demanded a subtle response—and one, again, in which nurses have been among the active agents in the fight against the spread of the disease.

The third case study focuses on the responses to AIDS within the large cities of the United Kingdom in the 1980s. London, Manchester, Liverpool, Edinburgh, Dundee, and Glasgow were the epicenters of HIV's spread within Britain. It quickly became well known that the AIDS virus thrived within body fluids and was spread by direct contact with those fluids. It was recognized that the virus could live outside the human body only for short periods of time and that it could not survive desiccation or extremes of temperature. Soon after the development of the first cases of HIV, it was recognized that its three main methods of transmission from host to host were via sexual intercourse, through blood transfusion, and through the sharing of hypodermic needles. It was, furthermore, fairly rapidly realized that the virus was spreading through the homosexual communities of large cities throughout the world.

The disease appears to have originated in Africa, where its prevalence was—and still remains—very high. Speculation as to the origin of the disease in medical experimentation soon gave way to efforts to combat it and to find a cure. Scientists achieved some success in developing therapies for **infection control** within a human host and transformed the condition from a rapidly fatal disease to one that can be survived as a long-term chronic condition. This moderate success of medical science has, however, been more than matched by the efforts of public health professionals, including nurses, to educate and empower populations to collectively control the disease.

The first cases of AIDS probably developed in the mid to late 1970s. The disease, however, was not recognized as a distinct entity until large numbers of cases of its associated conditions, Kaposi's sarcoma and *Pneumocystis carinii* pneumonia, began to appear in large U.S. cities in 1981 (AVERT, 2009; Hymes, Green & Mann, 1989). Centers for the control of communicable diseases throughout the developed world began to study what was being recognized as a new disease. The first case of AIDS to be documented in the United Kingdom appeared in December 1981 (Dubois, Braitwaite, Mikhail, & Batten, 1981). Because the earliest recorded symptoms affected gay men and because the disease was, at first, so closely associated with the gay community, some believed it could only be transmitted through homosexual contact. The disease was even, for a time, referred to as "gay compromise syndrome" (Brennan & Durak, 1981). Then a rapid increase in cases among hemophiliacs (who ac-quired the virus through blood transfusion) led to a dawning recognition that the disease could be transmitted in body fluids through both sexual contact and transfusion (Bateman, 1994). The recording of the first cases of the disease in women in January 1983 along with a rapid rise in the incidence among hemophiliacs also drew more public attention to a disease that could no longer be dismissed by the majority of the population as a "gay plague" (Anonymous, 1983). Amid widespread fear and uncertainty, the name acquired immune deficiency syndrome was coined and the disease clearly defined in September 1982 (Connor & Kingman, 1988). In May 1983 the AIDS virus (at first referred to as the lymphadenopathy-associated virus) was first isolated by scientists at the Pasteur Institute in Paris (Barre-Sinoussi et al, 1983; Harden, 1992).

One of the earliest voluntary organizations for the prevention and control of AIDS was formed in the United Kingdom in 1982 and came to be known as the Terence Higgins Trust—named after one of the disease's earliest victims (Berridge, 1996). Similar organizations developed in other western European countries and in the United States, and it was through these independent, well-organized, and proactive voluntary organizations that AIDS first became a disease that was controlled through individual education and empowerment. By conveying clear messages about how to protect oneself through safe sex, activists within the gay community probably prevented many potential cases of the disease.

By 1985 messages about AIDS prevention were spreading beyond the gay community. Clear statements were being made about which groups were most at risk. These included heroin addicts who shared needles, and the first needle exchanges were established in the Netherlands, soon to be followed by large numbers of other similar projects. In the United Kingdom the first needle exchange was established in Dundee in February 1986 (Robertson, Bucknall, & Welsby, 1986). Later that year the Kaleidoscope needle exchange in London and the Maryland Street needle exchange in Liverpool were established and a national campaign was launched, based on the message "don't inject AIDS" (AVERT, 2009).

As data became available from parts of Africa where AIDS was a much more established disease, it became clear that heterosexuals were at serious risk. The disease was clearly spreading through the heterosexual community, and vaginal transmission came to be recognized as an important cause of this spread. The first international conference on AIDS, held in Atlanta, Georgia, in April 1985, recognized that the disease was now a global pandemic (Mann, 1989). Irresponsible media reporting fueled public panic during the mid-1980s. Widespread fear led initially to widespread homophobia and created a scenario of moral panic that damaged the earliest health education campaigns by distorting their message. It also isolated sufferers, limiting the support they obtained (Fowler, 1991; Gronfors & Stalstrom, 1987; Tester, 1994; Wolf & Kielwasswe, 1991). Nevertheless, even amid the mass media–fueled panic of the mid-1980s, clear messages were beginning to reach those at risk and deliberate actions such as safer sex, the use of clean hypodermic needles, and the abstention of those at risk from blood donation were already beginning to have an effect (Arno & Feiden, 1992).

The history of the containment and control of HIV can be interpreted in part as a history of successful self-help. Voluntary organizations, often established by individuals whose friends or family members had died of AIDS, often led the way in developing campaigns that would both raise awareness of the disease and its transmission and overcome prejudice—thus promoting respect and compassion for sufferers. The Cardiff AIDS helpline grew out of an existing telephone service for gay men, and "body positive" groups throughout the country developed centers and helplines to support sufferers and those anxious about the disease. "Body Positive London" was established in 1985 and provided vital help and support for what was really the epicenter of the AIDS epidemic in the

United Kingdom (Berridge, 1996). The charity AVERT was founded in 1986 to campaign against AIDS-related prejudice and injustice, and the National Union of Journalists issued a leaflet advising journalists to offer more positive and respectful reporting of those with HIV (Berridge, 1996). In the same year the London Lighthouse, a care center for AIDS sufferers, was planned in the face of opposition from a small faction of hostile local residents and won widespread support (Cantacuzino, 1993).

In September 1986 the recognition that the drug azidothymidine could slow the progress of the disease led to the development of the first successful drug therapies for AIDS sufferers. Eventually, highly active antiretroviral therapy came to be widely used and dramatically lengthened the lifespans of those who obtained treatment early. Yet it was still successful health education that had the greatest impact on bringing the disease under control and preventing the escalation of the pandemic.

In 1987 the British government developed its prevention campaign through the newly formed Health Education Authority, using the mass media to promulgate the message "don't die of ignorance." Advertising on prime-time television used hard-hitting slogans and visually arresting images, such as an iceberg and a tombstone, the Authority reached millions of viewers. A televised "AIDS week" was held from February 27 to March 8 in which rival television stations simultaneously showed a film entitled "AIDS—The Facts" and advertised an AIDS helpline number. In the same year the National AIDS Trust was established to coordinate the activities of self-help and voluntary organizations (Berridge, 1996). That year, Princess Diana opened the first specialist ward for AIDS at the Middlesex Hospital, making the point, by shaking hands with HIV-positive patients, that the virus could not be transmitted by skin contact. In 1988 health education campaigns gained ground throughout the world, and in that year the first annual World AIDS Day was organized by the World Health Organization (1988).

From the discovery of the first cases of AIDS in 1981 to the launch of successful awareness campaigns in the mid-decade, rapid progress was made in developing projects that would combat the spread of the disease. Health education campaigns are difficult to evaluate, and some of the early attempts to measure the effectiveness of government campaigns in the mid-1980s produced inconclusive or disappointing results (Baggaley, 1988; Sherr, 1987). Nevertheless, it was possible, by the early 21st century, to demonstrate that reductions in the incidence of a range of sexually transmitted infections (among them HIV) had followed—and were probably the result of these campaigns (Nicholl et al., 2001). Nicholl and Hamers (2002) showed that incidences of a range of sexually transmitted diseases (not just AIDS) reduced significantly after the campaigns of the mid-1980s. They further argued that, as memory of those campaigns faded, there was a resurgence of HIV, gonorrhea, and syphilis throughout Europe (Nicholl & Hamers, 2002).

Furthermore, awareness-raising campaigns have, at times, had beneficial and unforeseen knock-on effects. The AIDS-awareness campaigns carried benefits on a global scale. Laurie Garrett argued that donations of public and private funds to third world countries increased dramatically because of the awareness-raising campaigns of HIV activists. Though the effects of this philanthropy have been patchy, because of the poor coordination of health promotion programs, the tendency of awareness-raising campaigns to arouse the compassion of individuals in the developed world can be seen as a positive development (Garrett, 2007; Leclerc-Madlala, 2005). These developments should not, however, give rise to complacency. African nations in particular have struggled in recent years to obtain the drug therapies they require and to develop effective health-promotion strategies in line with the World Health Organization's global program on AIDS (Friedman and Mottiar, 2005; VanderVliet, 2001).

CONCLUSION

The study of past epidemics offers us perspective on the ways we tackle the threats posed by our own era. It also teaches us that although new threats arise constantly and present new challenges, these threats and challenges are not so different from those faced by our ancestors. What *does* differ over time are the resources at our disposal to tackle new epidemic diseases. Among the most vital resources at the disposal of modern governments are the skilled workforces that combat epidemics, and among the largest—but least well recognized—of these are the nurses who care for the sick, empower the vulnerable, and undertake much of the work (in terms of data collection and treatment implementation) that makes it possible for medical science to destroy the causative organisms of disease.

The three case studies presented here were chosen because each demonstrates a distinct response—or more often, reaction—to an epidemic. All three of the diseases presented, bubonic plague, influenza, and AIDS, took their host populations by surprise. A study of the collective responses of some of those populations can offer insight into how humans perceive and combat disease. In the Early Modern Italian city states, magistrates adopted a "protective" approach to outbreaks of bubonic plague. They quarantined their cities, they moved the sick and their belongings to pest houses, and they imposed controls aimed at both preventing the spread of disease within their walls and propitiating "divine wrath." Their approach was a classic containment strategy.

In New York and other U.S. cities during the early 20th century, the movement of the sick was not controlled (in fact, troop movements probably exacerbated the epidemic), quarantines were not strictly imposed, and, although antisocial and obviously dangerous behaviors like spitting in public were outlawed, controls on public behavior were relatively mild. The American (and European) approach to Spanish influenza was one in which compassion overrode protectionism and enlightened self-interest ensured both negative consequences (the spread of the disease throughout the world) and, ultimately, positive outcomes (the support of individual sufferers).

The response to the AIDS epidemic in the United Kingdom was one in which self-help groups—often supported by local health professionals—led the way, offering information and support to vulnerable groups and demonstrating how clear messages could be conveyed to those at risk. The awareness and education campaigns of the mid-1980s in the United Kingdom were interesting and valuable because of their audacity (in the context of their time) and because of the commitment they demonstrated. Against

a backdrop of mass media–induced fear and negative, stereotypical attitudes to sufferers, self-help groups were able to develop awareness-programs that probably saved lives. The government followed swiftly, launching some of the most effective mass media campaigns ever devised for health education purposes. One of the problems with such campaigns was the difficulty of evaluating their effectiveness. It was only in retrospect that researchers were able to demonstrate epidemiological patterns that pointed to their success.

These differences in approach to disease highlight the differences between societies and their cultural norms. In Early Modern Italy even though some city states were nominally republics, the power of state and church was paramount; by contrast the modern, liberal society of early 20th century New York was one in which every individual life was considered more important than the power of the state. In the United Kingdom during the 1980s an open society with a free press and a highly active National Health Service at first distorted and later promoted a health promotion strategy that depended on the conveying of clear messages to vulnerable and often ostracized communities.

In each of these scenarios nurses—however independently they defined their roles and however determinedly they pursued their health-promoting strategies—were highly dependent on states and local authorities to sanction and enable their work. The pest-house attendants of Early Modern cities struggled in the face of hopelessness and lack of resources. The nurses of early 20th century New York, by contrast—supported as they were by local authorities, the Red Cross, and numerous voluntary agencies—were able to move rapidly into effective action. In the British cities of the 1980s, nursing personnel in a range of scenarios, such as genitourinary medicine clinics, specialist AIDS units, community health centers, and public health departments, were, after some initial delay, assisted by effective mass media campaigns to offer clear health-promoting messages to their client groups.

It would be all too easy to present this story as one of progress, one in which governments and societies became increasingly compassionate and effective. Such a perspective would be both complacent and distorting. States and societies have never been capable of doing more than the virulence of disease and the limitations of resources have permitted. As our own societies confront the advent of new and terrifying diseases, such as severe acute respiratory syndrome and Ebola, we can learn from the struggles of those past societies that confronted similar terrors and stood and fought then with all the means they had at their disposal. But the lessons are not simple ones. We should also be heartened by the knowledge that states and societies—with nurses among their vanguards—have survived epidemic diseases.

Perhaps, ultimately, societies will only completely escape the ravages of epidemics when they have learned to fully understand the nature of their cohabitants on this planet—the vast range of microorganisms that cause both harm and good to human populations. All too often it seems that the spread of disease can be traced to human behavior: the opening up of trade routes, troop movements, lifestyle changes, and possibly even the direct scientific manipulation of existing microorganisms. Perhaps only when human societies have learned to recognize quickly the consequences of their collective actions and have gained the skills required to launch concerted efforts that override vested interest will they cease to encounter the devastation caused by epidemic disease.

References

Alexander, J. T. (1980). *Bubonic plague in early modern Russia*. Baltimore, MD: Johns Hopkins University Press.

Anonymous. (1983). "Gay Plague" may lead to blood ban on homosexuals. *Daily Telegraph*, May 2.

Anselment, R. A. (1989). Smallpox in seventeenth-century English literature: Reality and the metamorphosis of wit. *Medical History, 33*, 72–95.

Arno, P. S., & Feiden, K. L. (1992). *Against the odds: The story of AIDS development, politics and profits*. London: HarperCollins.

AVERT. (2009). Retrieved December 9, 2009, from www.avert.org.

Baggaley, J. P. (1988). Perceived effectiveness of international AIDS campaigns. *Health Education Research, 3*(1), 7–17.

Barre-Sinoussi, F., Chermann, J., Rey, F., Nugeyre, M. T., Chamaret, S., Gruest, J., et al. (1983). Isolation of a T-lymphotrophic retrovirus from a patient at risk for acquired immune deficiency syndrome (AIDS). *Science, 220*(4599), 868–871.

Barry, J. (2005). *The great influenza: The epic story of the deadliest plague in history*. New York: Viking Press.

Bateman, D. (1994). The good bleed guide: A patient's story. *Social History of Medicine, 7*(1), 115–133.

Berridge, V. (1996). *AIDS in the UK. The making of a policy, 1981–1994*. Oxford: Oxford University Press.

Biraben, J. (1975). *Les Hommes et la Peste en France dans les pays europeens et mediterraneens*. Two volumes. Paris: Mouton.

Brennan, R. O., & Durak, D. T. (1981). Gay compromise syndrome. *Lancet, 2*, 1338–1339.

Brozzi, M. (Ed.). (1982). *Peste Fede e Sanita in una Cronaca Cividalese del 1598*. Milan: Giuffre.

Buhler-Wilkerson, K. (2001). *No place like home: A history of nursing and home care in the United States*. Baltimore: Johns Hopkins University Press.

Byerly, C. (2005). *Fever of war: The influenza epidemic in the US Army during World War I*. New York: New York University Press.

Calvi, G. (1989). *Histories of a plague year. The social and the imaginary in baroque Florence*. Translated by D. Biocca & B. T. Ragan. Berkeley, CA: California University Press, Berkeley.

Campbell, A. (1931). *The Black Death and men of learning*. New York: Columbia University Press.

Cantacuzino, M. (1993). *Till break of day*. London: Heinemann.

Carmichael, A. G. (1983). Legislation in the Italian Renaissance. *Bulletin of the History of Medicine, 57*, 516–536.

Carmichael, A. G. (1986). *Plague and the poor in renaissance Florence*. Cambridge: Cambridge University Press.

Cartwright, F. F. (1977). *A social history of medicine*. London: Longman.

Castellacci, D. (Ed.). (1897). Curiosi ricordi del Contagio Di Firenze nel 1630. *Archivio Storico Italiano* (5th series). Anno XX.

Chambers, D., & Pullan, B. (1992). *Venice. A documentary history*. Oxford: Blackwell.

Christensen, P. (2003). "In these perilous times": Plague and plague policies in early modern Denmark. *Medical History, 47*, 413–450.

Cipolla, C. M. (1973). *Cristofano and the plague*. London: Collins.

Cipolla, C. M. (1979). *Faith, reason and the plague*. Brighton: Harvester Press.

Cipolla, C. M. (1992). *Miasmas and disease*. Translated by E. Potter. New Haven: Yale University Press.

Connor, S., & Kingman, S. (1988). *The search for the virus. The scientific discovery of AIDS and the quest for a cure*. London: Penguin Books.

Contarini, G. (1599). *The commonwealth and government of Venice*. Translated by Lewes Lewkenor. London: John Windet.

Crosby, A. W. (1989). *America's forgotten pandemic: The influenza of 1918*. Cambridge: Cambridge University Press.

Dubois, R. M., Braitwaite, M. A., Mikhail, J. R., & Batten, J. C. (1981). Primary *Pneumocystis carinii* and cytomegalovirus infections. *Lancet, ii*, 1339.

Ficino, M. (1989). *Three books on life*. Translated by C. V. Kaske & J. R. Clark Binghamton. New York: Medieval and Renaissance Text and Studies.

Fowler, R. (1991). *Language in the news: Discourse and ideology in the press*. London: Routledge.

Fracastoro, H. (1930). *De Contagione et Contagiosis Morbis et Eorum Curatione, Libri III*. Edited and translated by W. C. Wright. New York: G. P. Putnam and Sons.

Friedman, S., & Mottiar, S. (2005). A rewarding engagement? The treatment action campaign and the politics of HIV/AIDS. *Politics and Society, 33*(4), 511–565.

Galasssi, N. (1966–1970). *Dieci Secoli di Storia Ospedaleria a Imola*. Vol. II. Imola: Galeati.

Garrett, L. (2007). The challenge of global health. *Foreign Affairs, 86*(1), 14–38.

Gradmann, C. (2001). Robert Koch and the pressures of scientific research: Tuberculosis and tuberculin. *Medical History, 45*, 1–32.

Grell, O. P. (1990). Plague in Elizabethan and Stuart London: The Dutch response. *Medical History, 34*(4), 424–439.

Gronfors, M., & Stalstrom, O. (1987). Power, prestige, profit: AIDS and the oppression of homosexual people. *Acta Sociological, 30*(1), 53–66.

Harden, V. A. (1992). Koch's postulates and the etiology of AIDS: An historical perspective. *History and Philosophy of the Life Sciences, 14*(2), 249–269.

Hirst, L. F. (1953). *The conquest of plague*. Oxford: Clarendon Press.

Hortensii, Centorio degli. (1631). *I cinque libri de gli avvertimenti, ordini, gride et editti: fatti et osservati in Milano, ne'tempi sospetosi della peste de gli anni MDLXXVI & LXXVII*. Milano: Bidelli.

Hymes, K. B., Green, J. B., & Mann, J. M. (1989). AIDS: A worldwide pandemic. In M. S. Gottlieb, D. J. Jeffries, D. Mildvan, A. J. Pinching, & T. C. Quinn (Eds.), *Current topics in AIDS* (Vol. 2). London: John Wiley & Sons.

Johnson, N. (2006). *Britain and the 1918–19 influenza pandemic*. London: Routledge.

Johnson, N. P. A. S., & Mueller, J. (2002). Updating the accounts: Global mortality of the 1918–1920 "Spanish influenza" pandemic. *Bulletin of the History of Medicine, 76*, 105–115.

Keeling, A. (2007). *Nursing and the privilege of prescription, 1893–2000*. Columbus, OH: Ohio State University Press.

Keeling, A. (in press). "When the City Is a Great Field Hospital": The influenza pandemic of 1918 and the New York City nursing response. *Journal of Clinical Nursing, 18*(19), 2732–2738.

Keen-Payne, R. (2000). "We must have nurses": Spanish influenza in America, 1918–1919. *Nursing History Review, 8*, 143–156.

King, M. L. (1986). *Venetian humanism in an age of patrician dominance*, Princeton, NJ: Princeton University Press.

Latour, B. (1988). *The pasteurization of France*. Translated by Alan Sheridan and John Law. Cambridge, MA and London: Harvard University Press.

Leclerc-Madlala, S. (2005). Popular responses to HIV/AIDS and policy. *Journal of Southern African Studies, 31*(4), 845–856.

Mann, J. M. (1989). AIDS: A worldwide pandemic. In M. S. Gottlieb, D. J. Jeffries, D. Mildvan, A. J. Pinching, & T. C. Quinn (Eds.), *Current topics in AIDS* (Vol. 2). London: John Wiley & Sons.

Modena, L. (1988). *Life of Judah*. Edited and translated by M. R. Cohen. Princeton, NJ: Princeton University Press.

More, T. (first published 1516). *Utopia*. Translated by R. Robinson. Ashgate Publishing Ltd.

Nicholl, A., & Hamers, F. (2002). Are trends in HIV, gonorrhoea, and syphilis worsening in western Europe? *British Medical Journal, 324*, 1324–1327.

Nicholl, A., Hughes, G., Donnelly, M., Livingstone, S., De Angelis, D., Fenton, K., et al. (2001). Assessing the impact of national anti-HIV sexual health campaigns: Trends in the transmission of HIV and other sexually transmitted infections in England. *Sexually Transmitted Infections, 77*, 242–247.

Nightingale, F. (1980/1860). *Notes on nursing. What it is and what it is not*. Edinburgh: Churchill Livingstone.

Nutton, V. (1990). The reception of Fracastoro's theory of contagion. *Osiris*. Second Series, 6.

Palmer, R. J. (1978). The control of plague in Venice and Northern Italy, 1348–1600. Unpublished PhD thesis, The University of Kent at Canterbury.

Park, K., & Henderson, J. (1991). The first hospital among christians: The Ospedale di Santa Maria Nuova in early sixteenth century Florence. *Medical History, 35*, 164–188.

Pastore, A. (1988). Tra Giustizia e Politico: Il Governo della Peste a Genova e Roma nel 1656/7, *Rivista Storica Italiana. Anno 100*, 126–154.

Patterson, D. K., & Pyle, G. F. (1991). The geography and mortality of the 1918 influenza pandemic. *Bulletin of the History of Medicine, 65*, 4–21.

Petraccone, C. (1978). La Difesa Contro la Peste, *Archivio Storico per le Province Napoletane*. Third Series, Anno XVI, pp. 253–280.

Phillips, H., & Killingray, D. (2003). *The Spanish influenza pandemic of 1918–19. New perspectives*. London: Routledge.

Preto, P. (1978). *Peste e Societa a Venezia nel 1576*. Vicenza: Neri Pozza.

Pullan, B. (1971). *Rich and poor in renaissance Venice*. Oxford: Basil Blackwood.

Pullan, B. (1992). Plague and perceptions of the poor in early modern Italy. In T. Ranger & P. Slack (Eds.), *Epidemics and ideas* (pp. 101–123). Cambridge: Cambridge University Press.

Quinn, T. (2008). *Flu: A social history of influenza*. London: New Holland.

Reid, A. (2005). The effects of the 1918–1919 influenza pandemic on infant and child health in Derbyshire. *Medical History, 49*(1), 29–54.

Robertson, J. R., Bucknall, A. B. V., & Welsby, P. D. (1986). An epidemic of AIDS-related virus (HTLV III/LAV) infection among intravenous drug abusers in Scottish General practice. *British Medical Journal, 292*, 527–530.

Sapwell, J. (n.d.). *The reminiscences of a VAD in two world wars*. London: The Red Cross Archives.

Sherr, L. (1987). An evaluation of the UK government health education campaign on AIDS. *Psychology and Health, 1*, 61–72.

Slack, P. (1985). *The impact of plague in Tudor and Stuart England*. London: Clarendon Press.

Tester, K. (1994). *Media, culture and morality*. London: Routledge.

Ulvioni, P. (1989). *Il Gran Castigo di Dio*. Milan: F. Angeli.

VanderVliet, V. (2001). AIDS: Losing "the new struggle"? *Daedalus, 130*(1), 151–184.

Wolf, M. A., & Kielwasswe, A. P. (Eds.). (1991). *Gay people, sex and the media*. London: The Haworth Press.

World Health Organization. (1988). *AIDS prevention and control: Invited presentations and papers from the World Summit of ministers of health on programmes for AIDS prevention*. London: World Health Organization.

Zinsser, H. (1935). *Rats, lice and history*. Boston: Little, Brown and Co.

HISTORICAL HIGHLIGHTS IN DISASTER NURSING

BARBARA MANN WALL
ARLENE KEELING

Out into pitchy darkness, leaped three men and seven women from a puffing, unsteady train, no physician with them, and no instructions save the charge of their leader as the last leap was made, and the train pushed on. "Nurses, you know what to do, go and do your best. . . ."

—Clara Barton (1904, p. 150), writing about Red Cross Nurses during the 1888 yellow fever epidemic in Florida

LEARNING OBJECTIVES

At the completion of this chapter, the reader will be able to

- Explore historical roots of disaster nursing through the lens of past disasters in the late 19th and 20th centuries.

- Describe the activities of public health nurses as they responded to past disasters.
- Relate past experiences of disaster nursing to present-day problems.

KEY TERMS

- American Red Cross
- Disasters

- Emergency preparedness
- Nursing history

This chapter examines specific instances of disaster nursing through the lens of **nursing history** to illustrate the important role nurses have had in providing prompt, efficient care to the ill or injured. In her classic text, *Disaster Nursing and Emergency Preparedness for Chemical, Biological and Radiological Terrorism and Other Hazards*, Tener Veenema (2007) argues for the importance of disaster responses that are evidenced based. Evidence for practice for disaster management logically comes from history—understanding what worked and did not work in the past. Although others have recorded the Red Cross and medical responses to disasters, the nursing response and **emergency preparedness** is often overlooked, accepted as "routine" or merely as following doctor's orders.

Nurses' work is highlighted during three late 19th century **disasters**, the yellow fever epidemic of 1888 and the Johnstown flood of 1889, and the turn of the century 1900 Galveston hurricane. These disasters are historically significant because they mark the first **American Red Cross** response, resulting in the federal government giving it a formal charter to provide disaster relief. In addition, the chapter focuses on three 20th century disasters: the 1918 influenza pandemic, the 1947 Texas City ship explosion, and the 1964 Alaska earthquake.

The causes of each disaster varied, and the response was tailored for the problem. In 1888, for example, mosquitoes caused the yellow fever epidemic in Jacksonville, Florida, and in 1889 catastrophic rains caused the Johnstown flood in Pennsylvania. As in Johnstown, the devastation from the 1900 Galveston hurricane—the most deadly hurricane of the 20th century—resulted from a largely uncontrollable force of nature. Death came from drowning or injury, as buildings collapsed and the unexpected and vicious storm surge devastated the coastal city. By contrast, the flu was a biological event—the rapid and overwhelming spread of a deadly virus. The Texas City disaster related to the consequences of increasing industrialization and the growth of the oil industry in the state and demonstrates what happens when hazardous materials are not properly contained. At that time it was the worst industrial accident in the country's history, killing over 500 people. The Alaska earthquake demonstrated the problems that can occur from seismic risks. In 1964 it was the second largest earthquake ever recorded, after the 1960 earthquake in Chile.

Although the disasters resulted from different causes, some related to weather, others to industrialization, and others to the spread of disease, in other ways these disasters reveal similarities. They occurred suddenly and without warning, they devastated communities, and they demanded a nursing and medical response. After each disaster nurses organized and provided care in both hospitals and the community.

YELLOW FEVER AND THE JOHNSTOWN FLOOD

Before World War II there was no permanent program of federal disaster relief in the United States, and private voluntary agencies such as the American National Red Cross and the Salvation Army took primary responsibility for disaster response (Kreps, 1990; Rubin, 2007). The International Committee of the Red Cross was founded in Geneva, Switzerland in 1863 by Henry Dunant. Today, national Red Cross societies exist in nearly every country in the world. Clara Barton was instrumental in the organization of the American National Red Cross in 1881 (Moorehead, 1998).

During the 1888 yellow fever epidemic in Jacksonville, Florida, the Red Cross recruited nurses to the danger zone. Barton turned to New Orleans for help; there many people had already had the disease and thus were immune. She recruited 30 nurses, both white and black, to travel with her by train to Jacksonville. On arrival in Jacksonville, however, the train's engineer refused to stop in the epidemic area. Thus, in the midst of a torrential rain, 10 nurses jumped off the moving train so they could assist the sick. Earning $3.00 a day, they worked 72-hour shifts for 79 days. A scandal developed, however, when several men and women refused to work for the $3.00 a day wage in hospitals and instead went into private nursing where they could make more money. Other nurses were accused of immoral conduct (Kernodle, 1949). Barton provided an explanation. She admitted that many of the volunteers she recruited were untrained, and clashes developed between them and the local boards of health who employed federal and municipal health officers who used newer scientific methods. In addition, many adventurers responded and called themselves Red Cross nurses even though they were not. Consequently, the local health board deported them (Barton, 1904; Dock & Pickett, 1922). Barton believed it was unfair to judge the status of Red Cross nurses by these latter individuals (Barton, 1904).

Consequently, the director of Sandhills Fever Hospital did not rely on Red Cross nurses. Rather, he recruited trained nurses and students, a new type of nurse that he had witnessed as an intern at the Bellevue Hospital in New York City. At Sandhills his chief nurse was Jane Delano, a graduate of Bellevue who later became president of the American Nurses Association and director of the Red Cross Nursing Service (D'Antonio & Whelan, 2004; Kernodle, 1949). One of Delano's classmates, Lavinia Dock, followed her there. As a trained public health nurse, Dock and the other nurses brought improved care to patients through their emphasis on order, cleanliness, ventilation, and nutrition, and they demonstrated the critical importance of what this new nursing profession could offer (D'Antonio & Whelan, 2004; Dock & Pickett, 1922).

A year later the Red Cross was called on to help at the site of the Johnstown Flood. On the afternoon of May 31, 1889, heavy rains had been pouring down on central Pennsylvania when the decaying South Fork Dam broke. Millions of tons of water and debris came crushing down into the valley in what became the worst flood in the nation's history. Within 10 minutes over 2,200 people were killed and tens of thousands more were injured or made homeless. Nurses and physicians from Mercy Hospital in Pittsburgh were among the first to respond both at the scene and in their hospital (Rafferty, 1974). Clara Barton and her relief team arrived 5 days later, on June 5. They distributed supplies to thousands of survivors and provided warm meals, medical care, and shelter to many in buildings that became known as "Red Cross Hotels" (Kernodle, 1949; National Park Service, 2006). Most of the nursing, however, was handled by a branch of the American Red Cross from Philadelphia not associated with Barton. Led by Lavinia Dock, graduate nurses trained in hospitals and public health worked in tent hospitals set up for the ill and injured. Their nursing proved invaluable as they worked with Barton and other Red Cross relief workers to carry out sanitation measures to prevent disease (Barton, 1904; Dock & Pickett, 1922).

THE GALVESTON HURRICANE, 1900

On September 10, 1900, meteorologist and eyewitness John D. Blagden wrote the following to his family (2000):

> There is not a building in town that is uninjured. Hundreds are busy day and night clearing away the debris and

recovering the dead. It is awful. Every few minutes a wagon load of corpses passes by on the street. . . . The more fortunate are doing all they can to aid the sufferers but it is impossible to care for all. (pp. 17–18)

Two days before, on September 8, a hurricane had hit Galveston, Texas, leaving approximately 8,000 people dead. The image of death pervaded the accounts of the Galveston storm, and by September 12 newspapers were filled with stories about recovering the dead. Eventually, the bodies had to be burned en masse in bonfires throughout the city. During the storm both blacks and whites took refuge in two local hospitals, John Sealy and St. Mary's Infirmary. Both suffered damage but were able to take patients again within a few days (Bixel & Turner, 2000).

Clara Barton and her staff arrived on September 17 and found an impromptu local relief committee that was tending to disaster recovery needs and collecting supplies. Barton was 78 years old at the time, and this would be her last trip to the scene of a disaster. She had presided over many disasters, and with each one her fame grew (Barton, 1900; Moorehead, 1998). Her arrival in Galveston was met with great fanfare, as one assistant recalled, "When Miss Barton's train got in the guards were ready, soldiers at present arms, everything in very martial style, in fact it was the only spice of the theatrical that there was in the whole business" (Fayling, 2000, p. 91).

Although the Red Cross had recruited nurses during the yellow fever epidemic and the Johnstown Flood in the 1880s, in Galveston it was primarily responsible for obtaining supplies. Rather than assuming total control, Barton and her staff worked with the local relief committee supplying food, clothing, and shelter. Galveston women had formed a new Red Cross Auxiliary, and Barton ensured they would provide greater leadership at the distribution stations. The Red Cross also worked with volunteers from various charitable and patriotic societies, including the Women's Relief Corps, the Women's Christian Temperance Union, and the Grand Army of the Republic. Blacks had formed their own relief committees, and Barton also set up a special fund for them (Barton, 1900). Barton stayed in Texas for 2 months. In addition to providing help in Galveston, she and her staff distributed supplies to people in towns and villages over a thousand-square-mile area that had suffered severe damage. Barton had a policy of restarting local work. When the hurricane washed away strawberry plants of farmers in six storm-swept counties and no money was available to buy more, she helped secure over a million plants.

After Barton's retirement, the Red Cross reorganized in 1905 and created state and territorial branches. One of the organization's newly assigned responsibilities included nursing during peacetime emergencies such as fire, floods, pestilence, and other national disasters. The state and local committees of enrolled Red Cross nurses served as volunteer recruiters of other nurses when the need arose. The new structure would be critical to the nursing response to the influenza pandemic when it hit the United States in the autumn of 1918.

THE FLU PANDEMIC, 1918–1919

The influenza epidemic of 1918, killing over 40 million people worldwide and causing over 675,000 deaths in the United

States (Hilleman, 2002; Johnson & Mueller, 2002), challenged the nation's public health service, the American Red Cross, the medical and nursing professions, and the U.S. federal government in much the same way it challenged other nations around the world. In 1918 the extremely high death rate—particularly among young adults—from a rare and highly contagious form of influenza was mysterious and frightening. According to one historian (Byerly, 2005):

> The influenza and pneumonia of 1918 shocked medical officers and soldiers alike. It rendered strong, healthy men powerless and struggling for breath; it distorted and saturated the lungs of those it killed; it rendered helpless professional physicians of great skill and knowledge; it consumed an enormous amount of army resources; and it killed in such great numbers that images of sick and dead bodies and coffins stayed with the survivors for the rest of their lives. (p. 87)

When the flu hit the cities of the United States and killed citizens, not soldiers, the country was unprepared for the magnitude of the crisis. Reflecting on the events of that year, nurse leader Janet Geister (1957) later wrote: "We weren't ready in plans and resources, nor were we ready in our thinking. A country-wide epidemic was utterly inconceivable" (p. 583). To complicate the situation, the United States had only recently entered the war in Europe and thousands of physicians and nurses had just been deployed. Few were left to cope with a major epidemic at home.

In the United States influenza first broke out in Kansas at a crowded military recruit camp. It then traveled with the soldiers to the cities of the East Coast, notably Boston, Philadelphia, and New York, where it also arrived on ships from Europe. Within a matter of days it raced south and westward across the country along transportation lines (Crosby, 2003; Markel et al., 2007).

On September 6, 1918, *The Boston Globe* reported an outbreak of "old fashioned grippe" among the sailors on the Commonwealth Pier (Fayling, 2000). By September 17 influenza reports were front page news. Within the next 24 hours health authorities recorded 41 more deaths, and the Boston health commissioner issued a warning against public hysteria. On September 18, only 12 days after the explosion of the epidemic in Boston, the flu spread through Philadelphia, the center of the war industry. Within days hundreds of sailors were ill; civilians were also succumbing to flu. Almost simultaneously, the epidemic erupted in New York City.

Meanwhile, in Boston, where they had been dealing with the flu for over 2 weeks, health officials were alarmed, enough in fact to send a telegram to the American Red Cross headquarters in Washington, DC, to ask for nurses. In Washington it was becoming increasingly clear that this was no ordinary flu epidemic. Reports were coming to the Red Cross from cities up and down the East Coast. The new strain had devastated Boston and was now sweeping through New York, Philadelphia, and Washington. It was also racing south and west. The Red Cross had to take action. As a result, on September 24 members of the American Red Cross National Committee assembled in Washington to discuss the federal response. Their plan was to implement the decentralized response they had adopted for home defense a year earlier. The U.S. Public Health Service would manage the medical response and distribute posters and pamphlets educating the public about the illness. The Red Cross National Committee would communicate with its local organizations and direct the nursing response. The major response would have to be done at the *local* level (Fieser, 1941). Thus, immediately after the meeting, Director of the Red Cross Bureau of Nursing Services Clara Noyes telegraphed all Red Cross Divisions with a directive: "Suggest you organize Home Defense nurses . . . to meet present epidemic . . . Provide nurses with masks" (Noyes, 1918, p. 2).

In New York City Lillian Wald, director of the Henry Street Settlement, did not need to be told to organize the nurses. In fact, she was all too aware of the alarming rapidity with which the flu was affecting the city's residents: her staff had already been working around the clock. In the slums of the Lower East Side, epidemics of infectious diseases were commonplace, and in September of 1918 it seemed this was just another bad flu epidemic. Only this time the intensity of the disease and the devastation it caused was remarkable. Finally, on October 10 the Atlantic Division of the Red Cross assembled New York City nursing leaders to plan their response. At that meeting the nurses organized the Nurses' Emergency Council to organize a city-wide response. The Red Cross also inserted a "quarter page advertisement in all the Sunday papers, calling for service from the women of the city" (Doty, 1919, p. 951).

In Philadelphia the situation was becoming increasingly serious, in part because on September 28, despite the fact that 123 civilians had been admitted to hospitals with flu just the day before, the city proceeded with its scheduled Liberty Loan parade to raise money for the war effort. Pandemic then exploded. By October 3 a doctor estimated that the city had seen 75,000 cases since September 11. Finally, the city government allocated $100,000 from its emergency war defense fund "to combat the disease" (Visiting Nurse Society, 1918, n.p.). It also coordinated all relief organizations under the direction of a central office and notified citizens struck with flu to call "Filbert 100" to obtain "a nurse, a doctor, an ambulance or an automobile" (Visiting Nurse Society, 1918, n.p.).

Under the direction of Katherine Tucker, RN, the Philadelphia Visiting Nurse Society handled thousands of influenza cases. In many of the families more than one member was ill; when both parents succumbed, the nurses had to supply food for the entire family. Soup kitchens were set up where the nurses could obtain soup, bread, and milk for such cases. And, as family after family was affected, the city's social infrastructure crumbled. Thousands of city workers were out sick, including streetcar drivers, telephone receptionists, shopkeepers, and garbage collectors. When the few nurses there also became sick, the situation became critical. There were simply not enough nurses. According to Health Director Kreusen (Visiting Nurse Society, 1918):

> If you would ask me the three things Philadelphia most needs to conquer the epidemic, I would tell you "Nurses, more nurses, and yet more nurses." (n.p.)

The flu then spread south and west, affecting cities and towns across the nation. Many of the cities suffered extremely high mortality rates, and as the dead piled up, health boards and emergency councils closed theaters, schools, and churches (Barry, 2005). By late

November 1918, the virus had made its way around the world. The second wave was over. However, the virus mutated again and a third wave struck in December and then in January 1919. Of all the major cities hit, San Francisco confronted the wave most efficiently, using both masks and vaccines to prevent its spread (Barry, 2005). Local chapters did their best to cooperate with the American Red Cross. According to one report, "Every chapter in Idaho, Oregon and Washington has appointed a committee on influenza . . ." (Kilpatrick, 1919, p. 1). The same was true for coal mining camps in Kentucky, logging camps in Michigan, and in small towns across the United States. In every area nurses were key to the response, and they responded promptly, without regard to race, class, or color.

1947 TEXAS CITY SHIP EXPLOSION

In 1947 the Dean of the University of Texas School of Nursing at Galveston wrote about healthcare workers' responses after a ship explosion in Texas City, Texas (Bartholf, 1947):

> We were proud of the performance of the whole organization, and particularly of the nurses and doctors—they just clicked and came up to par in a wonderful fashion. I had never seen morale quite so high in this institution. (p. 558)

Indeed, nurses and other healthcare personnel often experience a sense of camaraderie after working in a disaster. But this event also shows a more complicated story of competition among healthcare personnel.

In the late 19th and early 20th centuries, disasters mainly resulted from natural events such as hurricanes, disease, tornadoes, earthquakes, and floods. But as industry expanded in the 20th century, industrial accidents increased, with similar devastating results. On April 16 and 17, 1947, what was called the worst industrial catastrophe in U.S. history occurred when ammonium nitrate fertilizer on two merchant ships exploded in the Texas City, Texas docks, killing 405 people, with another 63 unidentified dead (Minutaglio, 2003; Stephens, 1997; Wall, 2008). When the first of the ships, the *Grandcamp*, exploded in the harbor, it caused smoke to rise 2,000 feet in the air and flaming cargo to fly over a 1-mile radius. The nearby Monsanto Chemical Plant caught fire from flying steel and burning debris, killing 145 workers. Every fireman who initially responded died, decimating the local fire department. Two planes flying over the docks at the time of the explosion fell from the sky, and windows shattered in Houston, Galveston, and other Texas cities. In addition to the many deaths, 3,000 injuries occurred, a third of all city dwellings were demolished, and 2,500 people lost their homes (Boyle, 1947; "1200 Feared Dead in Texas Blasts," 1947; Stephens, 1993).

A major priority after any disaster is the establishment of order out of chaos. With no disaster plan in place, the mayor and police chief had to recruit volunteers, and the disaster response initially was piecemeal. Without a local hospital, Texas City physicians and nurses organized a clearing station where casualties were triaged and the most serious moved to hospitals in surrounding cities and towns. Texas City clinics were full as well, and physicians and nurses worked with no water or electricity. A nurse's aide at one of the local clinics remembered that men from one of the plants came to help, and they worked "like Trojans" (Wheaton, 1948, p. 18).

The resources of other healthcare teams quickly organized and converged on the scene. Alerted by smoke columns across Galveston Bay, orthopedic surgeons, residents, senior medical students, nurses, and nursing students from John Sealy Hospital immediately left for Texas City with plasma, blood, and other supplies. Within an hour after the initial explosion, local American Red Cross chapters began mobilizing. Late on the evening of the first explosion, the Director of Nursing Service from the Red Cross Midwestern Area arrived from St. Louis and started recruiting more than 500 nurses from Texas and nearby states. As in every disaster since Clara Barton's day, many untrained women offered their services, so that it became necessary to weed them out by checking credentials (Kernodle, 1949).

In all, 3,000 persons required sudden medical assistance, and after emergency first aid, casualties went to 21 area hospitals. Many were hospitalized at the University of Texas Medical Branch (UTMB) facilities. Survivors began arriving within an hour, and all medical and nursing personnel were placed on 24-hour call. A nurse came in from her vacation and worked in a dispensary set up in the jail. Other nurses, both registered nurses and licensed practical nurses, worked at this dispensary and at the morgue. Soon, several bus loads of nurses, under motorcycle escort, came to Texas City and eventually went on to Galveston hospitals (Wheaton, 1948).

John Sealy Hospital handled a total of 498 casualties. Within the first 5 hours nurses and physicians classified 362

patients in the emergency department, gave them preliminary treatment, and hospitalized them. While physicians performed minor surgery in hallways, volunteer military medical and nursing personnel enabled 10 rooms to be outfitted for surgery. Doctors and nurses operated nonstop over the next 2 days. Multiple puncture wounds, contusions, cuts from shards of glass, compound fractures, and head, eye, and ear injuries (especially ruptured eardrums) were common. Sixteen patients died from severe head injuries (Blocker & Blocker, 1949; Leake, 1947).

In 1948 the Sisters of Charity of the Incarnate Word told the story of the response of Galveston's St. Mary's Hospital to the Texas City disaster to a writer for *Hospital Progress*, the official journal of the Catholic Hospital Association. St. Mary's benefited from nurses and nurse anesthetists flown in from San Antonio. Sixteen operating rooms were set up, and the sisters opened an unfinished wing to take in 96 patients. During that time 186 patients were detained in the hospital, whereas 8 died (McLeod, 1948). The Red Cross provided 2 billion units of penicillin, 5 million units of tetanus antitoxin, large quantities of whole blood and plasma, streptomycin, sulfa drugs, gas gangrene antitoxin, and tetanus antitoxin (Girardeau, 1947).

In 1958 a research associate in the Disaster Research Group of the National Academy of Sciences interviewed several nurses after another disaster and found they were apt to feel insecure when physicians were not around. At the time most nurses were still trained in hospital diploma programs, and they were task oriented. The data from the Texas City explosion both support and refute this conclusion. Although nurses indeed concentrated on tasks, they also developed a sense of pride when they were able to perform new assessments and expand their nursing roles, both dependent and independent of physicians.

As examples, students from the Schools of Nursing at John Sealy and St. Mary's Hospitals, part of UTMB, worked with teams to care for casualties, both at the scene and in hospitals. Stories from two students reveal they did more than merely assist the physician. One, who constructed her story in the *American Journal of Nursing* (Molsbee, 1947), worked on the pediatric ward at John Sealy Hospital and helped transfer children to other sites to make room for 40 injured adults. Patients came in ambulances, private automobiles, trucks, and milk wagons. Many activities by the nurses who suddenly found themselves in the midst of a disaster were improvised. Although it is not standard practice today, this student learned to fill 20-, 30-, and 50-cc syringes with morphine and give it by changing needles between patients. Nurses did not have regular charts, so they pinned tags on patients' clothes with dose and time they gave the medications (Molsbee, 1947).

A year after the explosion, another student from John Sealy composed a memoir of the events. An operating room supervisor had recruited her to Texas City as the student walked down the steps of the hospital. She was still in her nursing uniform, and, in the first part of the narrative, the form of her language conformed to the image of the compliant student she was taught to be. She said she "didn't have permission from the nursing office" (Givin, 1948, n.p.) to go. The supervisor cried, "It doesn't matter. I give you permission!" This group was one of the first from UTMB to arrive on the scene. Nurses' training in organiza-

tion and carrying out specific tasks helped them maintain order. The student was able to adapt to the situation and administer first aid to severely burned patients, including giving morphine for pain. In fact, she had an "open order to administer hypodermics of pain relievers as I saw the need . . . . In a situation like this," she wrote, "you are oblivious to anything except doing the job at hand. Somehow, everything you have ever learned in this area comes to the surface and you do the best you can." She worked there for several hours and accompanied a patient back to the hospital in a station wagon, guiding the driver while she held the patient's intravenous infusion. By that time, the hospital grounds were covered with tents, and the Red Cross had arrived (Givin, 1948).

In the above nurse's memoir, her image of a compliant nurse who had to follow orders and adhere to set routines was altered. She wrote, "I later realized there was no way that you could take a holistic view of a patient in a situation like this; it's only the immediate needs that are met. I will never forget that day from the time I felt the vibrations of the explosion coming down those steps of the main building to now when I realize what a confident twenty year old nurse I was." She was amazed at how, when she was at the scene of the disaster, "everything began to fall into place and regardless of rank or race we were a team. . . ." (Givin, 1948, n.p.). Thus, as the nursing student reconstructed her story, she moved herself from a peripheral position as a student with little power to a central position, where her words and deeds proclaimed her as equal with the other responders. These included those with higher "rank" such as physicians and people of a different race. Her opportunity to nurse during this disaster led her to repudiate her perceived limitations as a nursing student.

Although the people worked together initially, tensions quickly developed over who would get credit for the rescue work. Regular units of the armed forces arrived on the afternoon of April 16, but they worked independently of the Red Cross. This led the mayor to publicly criticize the Red Cross in the newspaper. He expressed his concern to an official that the Red Cross was "taking credit for everything that is being done in the way of relief" (Givin, 1948, n.p.). For one thing, its workers "went down to the gymnasium morgue and took it over from our people . . . after they had worked there ever since the explosion" (Givin, 1948, n.p.). Furthermore, the Red Cross had called a press conference that featured physicians it had brought in from the outside. "What about 10 of our local doctors that worked night and day?" the mayor retorted. "What is being said about them to those reporters?" (*Houston Chronicle*, 1947, n.p.). No mention was made of the nurses.

African American and Mexican American residents from El Barrio and The Bottom, neighborhoods closest to the docks, suffered most from the disaster. Many were left homeless after these areas were utterly destroyed. On April 19 the African American newspaper, the *Informer*, described the disaster, provided photographs, and told stories of dramatic escapes and heroic rescues on the part of African Americans. Black physicians and nurses from Houston cared for African American survivors at John Sealy Hospital, and they also rendered aid at the scene. African American morticians and embalmers came to help, and two ministers from local black

churches carried the injured and dying in their cars to hospitals in Galveston (*Informer*, 1947, pp. 1 and 10).

Red Cross nurses worked at the disaster site and in hospitals, and many stayed for 2 months until the regular nursing staff could take over. Red Cross and local public health nurses participated in case-finding activities by making home visits to care for the injured, seeing 2,231 patients in their homes (American National Red Cross, 1947). One of the most difficult tasks was to work with grieving families. City officials set up a temporary morgue in the local high school gymnasium, but they had no system for identifying the dead. Trained nurses accompanied families attempting to locate their missing relatives as they pulled back blankets and viewed the bodies, some so mangled they were never identified (Johnston, 1947).

Even though there were problems with communication and transportation, several groups responded quite well to the disaster, including medical and nursing personnel, because they had the skills and discipline needed for emergencies (Stephens, 1997). Writing after the disaster, Chauncey Leake, Vice-President and Dean of UTMB, noted that the successful responses were due to the application of military medical principles by a team of skilled specialists in a specialty hospital center. This included first aid by trained rescue personnel; preliminary dressings by general practitioners; rapid diagnosis and sorting by a team of specialty physicians; surgery with careful anesthesia and adequate wound drainage; generous administration of plasma and whole blood; use of penicillin, tetanus, and gas gangrene antitoxins; fluid control; and careful recordkeeping (Leake, 1947). Although this account risks overestimating physicians' importance at the expense of others, nurses no doubt participated in these activities.

Between 1900 and 1947 new research had occurred in blood types, the treatment of gas gangrene, and the use of penicillin and other antibiotics, and Texas City survivors benefited from these discoveries. Emergency medical techniques used in World War II were also put to good use and accounted for a more organized response. At the same time, skill and discipline proved essential to successful disaster relief responses. Particularly for nurses and other healthcare personnel, their jobs required them to deal with emergencies on a day-to-day basis. Although the disaster was new to them, the response process was familiar.

Finally, by 1947 changes were beginning to be seen in nurses' model identities that reflected those of skilled professionals. The writings of nurses who cared for victims in the aftermath of the Texas City disaster revealed self-images of skilled, hard-working, and often exhausted professionals who had opportunities to expand their healthcare roles in new ways. One student nurse chose to remember her experience in the 1947 disaster as a change in how she perceived herself as a nurse, no longer as a novice but as a competent and decisive professional.

After the Texas City disaster, on May 5, 1947, the Central Committee of the American National Red Cross approved a plan for the enrollment of nurses in the Red Cross Nursing for service to local communities through chapter programs. This plan replaced the type of enrollment in operation from 1905 to 1946, which served primarily as a reserve for the Army and Navy. This would prove beneficial to survivors of disasters in the future.

THE ALASKA EARTHQUAKE OF 1964

On March 27, 1964, at 5:36 p.m., the strongest earthquake ever recorded on the North American continent struck Alaska. In Anchorage the chronicler of Providence Hospital, which became the chief receiving agency of the injured in that city, wrote, "Everyone seemed to sense the need for immediate action and responsibility" (Chronicles of the Sisters of Providence, 1964, n.p.).

Known as the Good Friday Earthquake, it had a tremor that lasted approximately 4 minutes, measured 8.6 on the Richter scale, and caused damages estimated at $750 million. It was so powerful that tremors could be felt over a 500,000-square mile area, with shock waves tearing boats from moorings as far away as the Gulf of Mexico. Tsunamis struck all along the western coast of North America from the Arctic to as far south as Crescent City, California. In addition to Anchorage, a number of Alaskan communities such as Seward, Kodiak, and Valdez were affected, as well as several coastal native villages.

The 2-year-old Providence Hospital was the largest private hospital in the state. Owned and operated by the Sisters of Providence, it became the primary medical emergency center for the entire region. The fact that Providence Hospital received minimal damage was extremely important in its response to the disaster. It quickly shifted to emergency power, and its lights drew supplies and personnel from all over the city to its facilities. Two hospitals in the area, the 40-bed Presbyterian and 300-bed U.S. Air Force hospital at Elmendorf, suffered extensive structural damage. Although the Air

Force facility evacuated to nearby barracks and the 395-bed U.S. Public Health Service's Alaska Native Hospital, Presbyterian's patients went to Providence Hospital. As it became obvious that Providence would be the center of medical and nursing attention, there was little need for further coordination of medical care (Haas, 1964).

Hospital staff members mobilized quickly to care for survivors. Sister Barbara Ellen was administrator of Providence, and she and her five sister assistants coordinated the task of keeping the hospital in operation. They had to deal with lack of water and elevator use, no effective sanitation, and no sterilizers. Pharmacy medications had spilled all over the floor, and all phone links were dead (Special Report, 1964). Within a few minutes an emergency generator restored electricity and heat to vital areas such as the emergency department, surgery areas, nursing stations, and main halls. The U.S. Army provided a generator for the kitchen, and firemen pumped water from a nearby spring into the hospital (Chronicles of the Sisters of Providence, 1964).

No nurse left her unit to go to a safer place, and none of the 75 patients in the hospital at the time received injuries from the quake (Chronicles of the Sisters of Providence, 1964). Indeed, a survey team of sociologists from the Disaster Research Center, who arrived within 28 hours after the quake, stated, "Few if any persons actually abandoned an ongoing organizational responsibility" (Haas, 1964, p. 26). The physicians responded with their own action plan, and some brought their families. Key people were pulled to the emergency department, and within a half hour the first survivors arrived. Calmness was maintained throughout the hospital, led by Sister Barbara Ellen, who never lost control of the situation (Chronicles of the Sisters of Providence, 1964). Indeed, her authority and her maintenance of control in the crisis helped maintain stability throughout the emergency (Fortier, 1964). As the radio broadcasted a need for registered nurses, off-duty Providence personnel came as well as nurses from the evacuated Presbyterian Hospital. Military personnel from Elmendorf Air Force Base and Fort Richardson delivered a 200-bed civil defense hospital to Providence with beds and cots that were set up in the cafeteria, halls, and business office (Langston, 1964; Sister Philias, 1964). Eventually, Providence did not fill to capacity, however, and not all these supplies were needed (Haas, 1964).

The damage to the American Red Cross headquarters in downtown Anchorage delayed its response, but within 24 hours it had mobilized. Sigrid Bullard from Redwood City, California, the Red Cross Nursing Director for the Alaska disaster, put out a call for volunteers, and 45 registered nurses and 27 trained Red Cross nurses aides responded. All the aides and many of the nurses cared for survivors at Providence Hospital throughout the emergency period (Office of Public Information, 1964).

At Providence Hospital nurses and physicians set up a triage system in the emergency department. Admissions personnel registered 108 people the first night, but only a few were critically injured. In the operating suites flashlights and battery-operated lights were available in addition to the auxiliary power; but one doctor delivered a baby by flashlight early Saturday morning when all power briefly failed. Sterilizers were not operational because there was no steam, and nurses washed instruments and sterilized them with Bunsen burners. They had to improvise in other ways, with one using snow as a substitute for hypothermia for a patient undergoing a craniotomy. Others heated water for infant formulas in the doctors' coffee urn, and they used distilled water for drinking purposes (Langston, 1964; Sister Phileas, 1964).

Public health nurses' roles in this disaster included investigating home-based cases, seeking out dislocated families, distributing food and clothing, performing health screenings, and helping survivors find shelter. The morning after the quake hit, public health nurses first went to Providence Hospital to see if they were needed. When told that the hospital had sufficient personnel, they went to the state's Civil Defense Headquarters where they assisted in evacuations (Haas, 1964). Nurses also opened clinics in outlying areas where they provided immunizations. Nurses, including volunteers from Juneau and Fairbanks, aided Anchorage school nurses, as did many retired nurses. One opined, "This was a very exciting experience of community cooperation" (Beltz, 1964). Other school nurses who were able to leave their families responded over the next 2 weeks, caring for more than 300 evacuated Aleuts from Old Harbor and Kaguyak where a tidal wave had destroyed their villages. Making formula for babies became a full-time job, and eventually Aleut midwives took over the responsibility from the local school nurses (Scott, 1964). Other nursing care required taking vital signs, dispensing medications, and listening to survivors' problems.

Farther away, a public health nurse from the Prince William Sound area was summoned to Anchorage from her post deep in the interior of the state. The village of Chenega was totally destroyed, 23 people died, and all the survivors were forced to move. This nurse and a team of physicians and sanitation engineers visited potential evacuation sites to evaluate available housing and water supplies for Chenega's residents (Bonehill, 1964).

Red Cross nurses were on the front lines to care for survivors in emergency shelter. Some nurses worked in typhoid immunization clinics and in shelters such as one that housed 166 Aleuts evacuated from Kodiak Island, which had suffered immense structural damage (Office of Public Information, 1964). It was 350 air miles from Anchorage, and it listed 19 dead or missing. This was the area to which Hazel Heywood, then Director of Nursing services for the Red Cross chapter in Milwaukee, Wisconsin, was assigned. Because communications had been knocked out, nurses' only contact with Red Cross headquarters was through the Alaska Communications System, with nurses and others manning the calls as they came through. The disaster teams supplemented the agencies already at the scene. To this end her first job was to relieve the fatigued nurse at a schoolhouse shelter where 600 to 700 people had congregated. Babies needed formulas and clean diapers, and someone was able to bring a washing machine into the schoolhouse. The Red Cross set up headquarters in a local church in Kodiak and provided nursing coverage for the schoolhouse shelter until April 7. It dispensed groceries and clothes to the needy, helped with housing, and fed evacuees waiting for stateside naval flights. Nurses checked for survivors, a monumental job because there were no transportation facilities, telephones, newspapers, or roads to reach outlying villages on the island (Farley, 1964).

American Red Cross volunteers went to other badly damaged areas. The greatest death toll was in Valdez, where 32 men, women, and children were killed when huge sections of land slid into the sea. A Red Cross representative from San Antonio, Texas, helped care for hospitalized and sheltered survivors there. Fairbanks experienced only a momentary swaying of buildings, and at St. Joseph's Hospital the local Red Cross nursing chairwoman helped screen evacuees from Valdez for communicable diseases and other needs for medical and nursing care (Benson, 1964).

Most of the nurses in Seward, which had been severely damaged, were on duty somewhere (Blue, 1964, p. 1),

> [H]erding children, gathering families together, setting up first aid stations. . . . The nurses did everything, scrubbed, cooked, set up trays, washed dishes, answered lights, comforted the hundreds who swarmed about the Hospital that first night and all the next day.

A Red Cross nurse from Oregon dealt with disrupted health and sanitation facilities and the dangers of communicable diseases.

Red Cross survey teams made daily trips into the remote, mountainous Alaskan countryside. To obtain information about distant villages, U.S. Public Health Service physicians and Division of Public Health nurses and sanitary engineers also visited sites in Prince William Sound and Kodiak Island. They provided medical and nursing care, preventive measures, health teaching, and further assessments of sanitary conditions. They worked in an advisory role with agencies responsible for the care of refugees, and as they returned to the areas badly damaged or destroyed, they helped in arranging temporary facilities (Office of Public Information, 1964).

CONCLUSION

Public health nurses' disaster work has a long history. The exemplars presented in this chapter are illustrative of the growing focus on expert practice, and they serve as windows for viewing changes in nursing practices. In the late 19th and early 20th centuries, nurses provided care, comfort measures, as well as fluid and nutrition. In fact, during the yellow fever epidemic and the 1918 flu pandemic, nursing care was usually the only treatment for the illness. As the 20th century progressed, nurses began participating in emergency first aid at the scene. They took vital signs, cared for physical and emotional wounds, administered plasma, and gave medications. Nurses, along with others, worked around the clock, often too busy to eat. Although many carried out traditional tasks of easing fears, they also worked with intravenous infusions, surgery, infection control, and pain relief. They possessed the knowledge and discipline needed for emergencies and did the skilled work they were educated to do. In the end, disasters created opportunities for nurses to expand their practice, blurring the disciplinary boundaries between medicine and nursing as they did so. Disasters also blurred the boundaries of race and class, as nurses and other responders worked to meet the needs of all people affected by the emergency situation.

After disasters such as 9-11 and Hurricane Katrina, public health nurses looked to lessons learned from the past. Disasters such as these demonstrate the need for qualified nursing, a task that nurses described in this chapter willingly assumed. For example, nurses in these disasters took charge, worked together, worked it out, and participated in case finding. As in the past, public health nurses today take charge of clinics and coordinate activities for vaccinations and the prevention of disease. They establish significant collaborative relationships with the American Red Cross and numerous other state agencies and organizations. They also reduce the impact of the disaster on the community's health and decrease morbidity and mortality from communicable diseases through case finding. Just as in Galveston in 1900 and Anchorage in 1964, today's disasters witness large numbers of individuals in hospitals and shelters. Nurses have to work without electricity and sustain adequate communication at all times. After September 11, 2001, for example, New York hospitals treated many patients with no electricity, gas, phone connections, or computers (Gaskill, 2006). Yet nurses learned, as in the past, that practicing in a disaster was something they could do, and do well.

References

American National Red Cross. (1947). *A preliminary report on the Texas City explosions.* Texas City file. Rosenberg Library, Galveston, Texas. St. Louis, MO: American National Red Cross, Midwestern Area.

Barry, J. (2005). *The great influenza: The epic story of the deadliest plague in history.* East Rutherford, NJ: Viking Press.

Bartholf, M. (1947). Co-operation. *American Journal of Nursing, 47*(8), 558.

Barton, C. (1900). To the people of the United States. 1900 Storm online manuscript exhibit, Red Cross Records, MSS # 05-0007. Retrieved July 5, 2006, from http://www.gthcenter.org/exhibits/storms/1900/Manuscripts/RecCross_7/index.html

Barton, C. (1904; reprinted 2005). *The Red Cross in peace and war.* Washington, DC: American Historical Press.

Beltz, A. (1964). Greater Anchorage health district. *Alaska Nurse, XIII*(4), 8.

Benson, R. (1964). Fairbanks reports. *Alaska Nurse, XIII*(4), 11.

Bixel, P. B., & Turner, E. H. (2000). *Galveston and the 1900 storm.* Austin: University of Texas Press.

Blagden, J. D. (2000). Letter to family, September 10, 1900. In C. E. Greene & S. H. Kelly (Eds.), *Through a night of horrors: Voices from the 1900 Galveston storm.* College Station, TX: Texas A&M University Press.

Blocker, V., & Blocker, T. G. (1949). The Texas City disaster: A survey of 3,000 casualties. *American Journal of Surgery, LXXVII*(5), 756–771.

Blue, E. (1964). Seward General Hospital. *Alaska Nurse, XIII*(4), 1.

Bonehill, B. A. (1964). Prince William Sound area as seen by a PHN after Alaska's disaster. *Alaska Nurse, XIII*(4), 10.

Boyle, H. (1947). Monsanto explosion offers foretaste of atom bomb. *The Houston Chronicle,* April 18, n.p.

Byerly, C. (2005) *Fever of war: The influenza epidemic in the U. S. Army during World War I.* New York: New York University Press.

Chronicles of the Sisters of Providence. (1964). Seattle, WA: Sisters of Providence Archives.

Crosby, A. (2003). *America's forgotten pandemic: Influenza 1918* (2nd ed.). Boston: Cambridge University Press.

D'Antonio, J., & Whelan, J. (2004). Moments when time stood still: A look at the history of nursing during disasters. *American Journal of Nursing, 104*(11), 66–72.

Dock, L., & Pickett, S. (1922). *History of the American Red Cross.* New York: The MacMillian Company.

Doty, P. M. (1919). A retrospect of the influenza epidemic. *Public Health Nurse, 11*(12), 949–957.

Farley, J. M. (1964). Alaskan earthquake jolts nurse's schedule. *The Milwaukee Journal*, April 26, n.p.

Fayling, L. R. D. (2000). Fear influenza outbreak among sailors may spread. In C. E. Greene & S. H. Kelly (Eds.), *Through a night of horrors: Voices from the 1900 Galveston storm.* College Station, TX: Texas A&M University Press.

Fieser, J. (1941). Report to Mr. Atkinson, January 15, 1941 re: Influenza Epidemic of 1918. NARA CP Records of the Red Cross, Box 557, 500.2 Influenza.

Fortier, E. J. (1964). Observations for Sister Philias on Providence Hospital and earthquake. Seattle, WA: Sisters of Providence Archives.

Gaskill, M. (2006). On their toes. *Nursing Spectrum.* Retrieved March 14, 2009, from http://include .nurse.com/apps/pbcs.dll/article?AID=20066 08280312

Geister, J. (1957). The flu epidemic of 1918. *Nursing Outlook, 5*(10), 582–584.

Girardeau, G. (1947). *Annual report*, July 1, 1946 to July 1, 1947. Galveston County Chapter. St. Louis, MO: American National Red Cross.

Givin, L. P. (1948). Memoir, Texas City disaster. University of Texas Medical Branch Library.

Haas, J. E. (1964). Some preliminary observations on the responses of community organizations involved in the emergency period of the Alaskan earthquake. Disaster Research Center Working Paper #2. Newark, DE: Disaster Research Center, University of Delaware.

Hilleman, M. R. (2002). Realities and enigmas of human viral influenza: pathogenesis, epidemiology and control. *Vaccine, 20*, 3068–3087.

Houston Chronicle. (April 21, 1947). Retrieved November 6, 2008, from http://www.redcross.org/ services/nursing/0,1082,0_389_,00.html# develope

Informer. (April 19, 1947). Many Negroes killed, scores injured in Texas City blast, p. 1. Employee of Texas City café tells of his escape, p. 10.

Johnson, N., & Mueller, J. (2002). Updating the accounts: Global mortality of the 1918–1920 "Spanish" influenza pandemic. *Bulletin of the History of Medicine, 76*, 105–115.

Johnston, M. E. (1947). Relatives claim dead at morgue. *Houston Post*, April 18, p. 20.

Kernodle, P. B. (1949). *The Red Cross nurse in action, 1882–1948.* New York: Harper and Brothers, Publisher.

Kilpatrick, E. (1919). Report of the Northwest ARC Division, 1919, in National Archives Records Administration, College Park (NARACP), 803.11 epidemics, Box 689, folder 1.

Kreps, G. A. (1990). The Federal Emergency Management System in the United States: past and present. *International Journal of Mass Emergencies and Disasters, 8*(3), 281.

Langston, D. V. (1964, July 27). Report of a hospital in a disaster area. *Journal of the American Medical Association*, 306–307.

Leake, C. D. (October, 1947). Copy of military medical principles applied to a civilian disaster. University of Texas Medical Branch Library.

Markel, H., Lipman, H., Navarro, J., Sloan, A., Michalsen, J., Stern, A., et al. (2007). Nonpharmaceutical interventions implemented by U.S. cities during the 1918–1919 influenza pandemic. *Journal of the American Medical Association, 298*(6), 644–653.

McLeod, T. (1948). When disaster strikes. *Hospital Progress, 408*, 411.

Minutaglio, B. (2003). *City on fire: The explosion that devastated a Texas town and ignited a historic legal battle.* New York: HarperCollins.

Molsbee, A. F. (1947). Students give disaster service in Galveston. *American Journal of Nursing, 47*(6), 414.

Moorehead, C. (1998). *Dunant's dream: War, Switzerland and the history of the Red Cross.* London: HarperCollins.

National Park Service, U.S. Department of Interior. (2006). Johnstown flood. Retrieved November, 14, 2008, from http://www.nps.gov/jofl/ faqs.htm

Noyes, C. (1918, September 25). Memo to all division directors. National Archives Record Administration (NARA). Memo found in CP Box 689 of the Influenza Epidemic records of 1918, Record Group 803.11.

Office of Public Information, Western Area, American Red Cross. (1964). Nurses answer call quickly for Alaskan disaster duty. American Red Cross Office, Anchorage, Alaska. n.p.

Rafferty, J. (1974). *Mercy Hospital, 1947–1972: An historical review.* Pittsburgh: Mercy Hospital.

Rubin, C. B. (Ed.). (2007). *Emergency management: The American experience, 1900–2005.* Fairfax, VA: Public Entity Risk Institute.

Scott, E. (1964). School nurses—Anchorage. *Alaska Nurse, XIII*(4), 6.

Sister Philias. (1964). Three c's for an operating room in disaster. Seattle, WA: Sisters of Providence Archives, PMCA, Box 32.

Special Report. (1964). Hospitals and the Alaskan earthquake. *Journal of the American Hospital Association, 38,* 23–24A.

Stephens, H. W. (1993). The Texas City disaster: A re-examination. *Industrial and Environmental Crisis Quarterly, 7*(3), 189–190.

Stephens, H. W. (1997). *The Texas City disaster, 1947.* Austin, TX: University of Texas Press.

1200 Feared dead in Texas blasts. (1947, April 17). *New York Times,* n.p.

Veenema, T. G. (2007). *Disaster nursing and emergency preparedness for chemical, biological and radiological terrorism and other hazards* (2nd ed.). New York: Springer.

Visiting Nurse Society. (1918) Newspaper clipping from scrapbook. VNS Collection, UPenn CSHN, Barbara Bates Center of the History of Nursing.

Wall, B. M. (2008). Healing after disasters in early 20th-century Texas. *Advances in Nursing Science, 31*(3), 211–224. Excerpts reprinted with permission.

Wheaton, E. L. (1948). *Texas City remembers.* San Antonio, TX: The Naylor Co.

PUBLIC HEALTH: COSTS, CHALLENGES, AND CONSIDERATIONS

MARY ALICE HIGGINS DONIUS

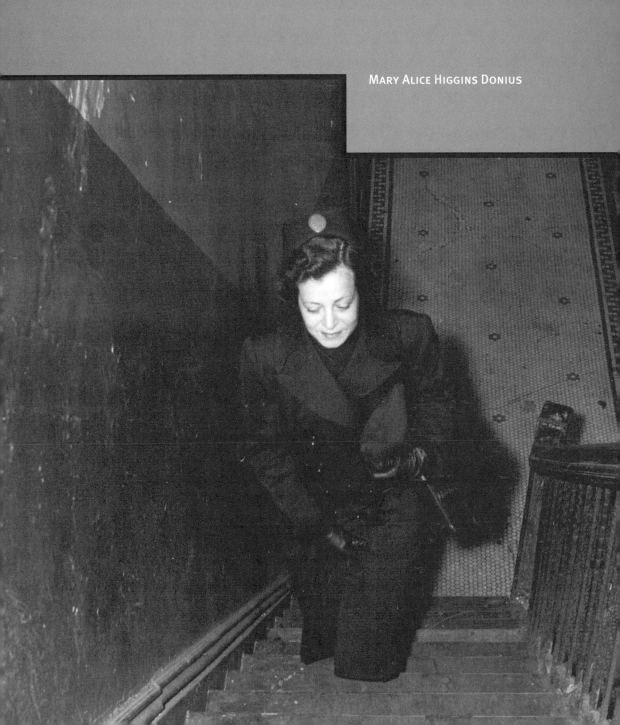

A comparison of the cost of treating tuberculosis patients in their homes and in hospitals is interesting and exceedingly important from an economic point of view. It costs no less than one dollar per day to care for one patient in a hospital. In most good hospitals the cost per day is from one dollar and fifty cents to two dollars and over. The sum so spent in caring for one patient for one year would be from four hundred to six hundred dollars. This sum is almost enough to supply a visiting nurse, who in one year, as has been shown, could and does visit from four to five hundred patients (Nutting, 1904, p. 501).

LEARNING OBJECTIVES

At the completion of this chapter, the reader will be able to

- Discuss the present state of the U.S. healthcare system with regard to cost and care.
- List the principal stakeholder participants in the U.S. healthcare system.

- Explore the competing interests of the "the 5 P's."
- Examine the various ways to reconsider healthcare delivery from a public health perspective.

KEY TERMS

- Gross domestic product
- "The 5 P's" principal participants
  - Payer
  - Policymaker
  - Population
  - Provider
  - Purchaser

The healthcare delivery system in the United States is complex, confusing, and often characterized by fragmentation. Part of the reason for this is the very existence of the multiple players within the system, all of whom have varying interest in direct contrast to one another. Many of these interests are directly rooted in economics. These conditions lead to unequal access for individuals, families, populations, and communities seeking care, often resulting in negative outcomes pertaining to health. The purpose of this chapter is to present to the reader a discussion pertaining to the cost of care, the challenges we face to ensure the health of the public, and considerations for the future.

COST AND CHALLENGES

The current financial state of healthcare delivery has evolved most significantly since the mid-20th century. Multiple factors influence the economics of and equality in, access to, and quality of health care. The Henry J. Kaiser Family Foundation (2009, para 5) spoke to the issue of the driving cost of health care and identified the following as major factors:

- Intensity of services
- Prescription drugs and technology
- Aging of the population
- Administrative costs

As this list illustrates, there are multiple forces that continue to drive the escalation of the healthcare expense. The overall population growth is a contributing factor, particularly if one considers the cohort representing individuals 65 years of age and older. Because of the advancing age of the largest cohort, the baby boomers, study projections published by the Center for Health Workforce Studies, School of Public Health at University of Albany in New York, suggest that between 2000 and 2020 the U.S. population will add 19 million older adults (Moore et al., 2005). This increase is expected to add to the strain on the healthcare system with the higher volume of healthcare services being projected. In addition, services required by this ever-expanding population have changed in the recent past decades. Despite the trend toward health promotion and disease prevention, chronic illness is still present along with the demands these long-term illnesses present on the healthcare system (Tyler-Evans, 2008).

Technological advances in the recent decades have facilitated the development of highly specialized and expensive equipment. Scientific research and evidence-based practice further increase specialization of knowledge. Ultimately, every hospital and medical center wishes to purchase this high-priced technology and provide the specialized services related to technology. Along with this increase in technology and research comes increasing specialization that requires education and training, all at considerable cost.

Advancements in pharmaceuticals are also noted. The Henry J. Kaiser Family Foundation (2009, para 1) identified that advances in pharmaceuticals in past decades for prevention, management, and cure of disease have sparked increases in spending: "In 2002, spending on prescription drugs in the U.S. grew 15 percent compared to a 9 percent increase for health care overall." The increase in spending associated with newly developed pharmaceuticals can also be traced to increased competition among the existing drug companies through increases in marketing and advertising costs that did not exist a decade ago.

Public policy is another influential factor in rising healthcare cost. Some view government-enacted mandates such as the Health Insurance Portability and Accountability Act as contributing to increased cost. Well-intended public policy mandates add complexity to an already overburdened system of healthcare delivery. In addition, legislative initiatives designed to increase access to care for vulnerable populations such as the elderly, disabled, poor, women, and children require the development of regulatory agencies necessary to monitor and enforce quality standards of care, thus enhancing administrative costs (Henry Kaiser Family Foundation, 2009).

Although these are noble initiatives, the cost to administer and monitor these initiatives adds to the rising costs of health care in the United States as evidenced by the increase in the **gross domestic product** (GDP).

GDP and Health Care

As the healthcare delivery system becomes more complex, the percentage of the GDP spent on health care increases. GDP is defined as the "overall measure of a nation's economic standing in terms of the market value of the total output of goods and services produced in that nation for a given period of time" (Pride & Ferrell, 2003, p. G-6). In 1960, for example, 5.2% of the GDP was spent on health care. There was a 2% rise in 1970 to 7.2% and again in 1980 to 9.1%. By 1990, however, the GDP for health care was 12.3%, and in 2000 the healthcare GDP was 13.8% (Shi & Singh, 2010). "In 2006, U.S. healthcare spending was $7,026 per resident and accounted for 16% of the nation's GDP" (Henry Kaiser Family Foundation, 2009, para. 1). The Centers for Medicare & Medicaid Services, National Health Statistics Group (2007, paras 1–2) also presents these staggering numbers and projected the following:

- National health spending increased from $2.2 billion in 2007 to $2.4 billion in 2008.
- National health spending will reach $4.4 trillion by 2018.
- National health spending will comprise over one-fifth (20.3%) of the GDP by 2018.

Where was all of this money allocated? The Centers for Medicare & Medicaid Services, National Health Statistics Group (2007) also addressed this question with the following information:

- Hospital care, 31%
- Physician/clinical services, 21%
- Other spending ,25%
- Nursing home, 6%
- Prescription drugs, 10%
- Program administration and net costs, 7%

Overview of the Financing of Health Care

The U.S. healthcare system is confusing, complex, and fragmented, partly because of the involvement of multiple players. According to the Henry J. Kaiser Family Foundation (2009):

> In the U.S., healthcare providers, insurers, employers, and the government are all unofficial partners in a complicated and loosely defined healthcare "system." In contrast to most other nations where the government finances health care for the majority of its residents, most Americans have some form of private health insurance sponsored by employers. A sizable share have government-sponsored insurance, with those over 65 years of age covered by a federal program (Medicare) and some poor children and their families eligible for a state-federal program (Medicaid). (para. 1)

The financing of individual health care, therefore, is generally provided by obtaining coverage through employers, individual coverage, or government programs (Shi & Singh, 2010). The way our healthcare system is set up facilitates an economically driven rather than socially driven system. In other words, this system and the processes that drive the system has made access to health care a social privilege and not considered a right of all individuals.

Principal Participants in the Healthcare Delivery System

The various interests of the stakeholders involved in the delivery and financing of health care often find their interests not just competing but in direct conflict. For example, free market competition creates a rivalry between the sellers of comparable goods and services for customers. The assumption is customers choose goods and services of equal quality on the basis of price, thus keeping the prices down. This applies only when all product attributes are standardized and the individual receiving the goods and services has the opportunity to choose the goods and services directly (Shi & Singh, 2001). For most Americans choice of health care as goods and services is decided by a third party, for example, their employers. Shi and Singh (2010) looked at the U.S. healthcare system and considered the multiple players:

> The key players in the system have been physicians, administrators of health service institutions, insurance companies, large employers, and the government. Big business, labor, insurance companies, physicians, and hospitals make up the powerful and politically active special interest groups represented before law-makers by high-priced lobbyists. Each player has a different economic interest to protect. The problem is that the self-interests of each player are often at odds. (p. 15)

In relation to Shi and Singh's work, this author has termed the stakeholders as key participants belonging to one of five groups known as "the 5 P's." Examining the 5 P's informs the reader about access, cost, quality, and choice of goods and services in relation to the health of the population.

"The 5 P's"

The five principal participants in the healthcare delivery system are purchasers, payers, providers, patients or populations, and policymakers. Each participant group has specific goals that influence its decision making and respective agendas and drive its individual initiatives for influencing the financing and delivery of health care in the United States. **Figure 15-1** provides a visual depiction of the 5 P's model.

PURCHASERS

Although individuals access medical care directly, most Americans rely on the health insurance benefits provided by their employers to cover the expenses of their care. Since the middle of the last century, employment benefits included health insurance. In fact, health insurance was an important part of bargaining between unions and employers (Shi & Singh, 2010). In recent years the increase in percentage of the GDP for healthcare delivery and the percentage of corporate profits required to meet the demands of the healthcare coverage for the employee prompted employers to consider ways to reduce their expenditures. According to the U.S. Census Bureau (2008):

> Both the percentage and the number of people without health insurance decreased in 2007. The percentage without health insurance was 15.3 percent in 2007, down from 15.8% in 2006, and the number of uninsured was 45.7 million

FIGURE **15-1**   **Visual depiction of "The 5 P's."**

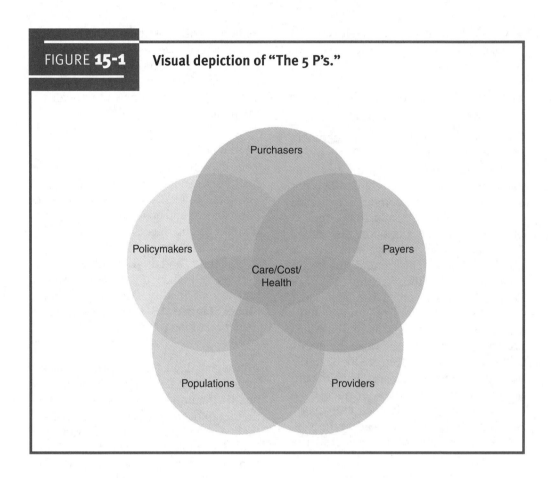

down from 47.million. . . . The number of people with health insurance increased to 253.4 million in 2007 (up from 249.8 million in 2006). The number of people covered by private insurance (202.0 million) in 2007 was not statistically different from 2006, while the number of people covered by government health insurance increased to 83.0 million up from 80.3 million in 2006. . . . The percentage of people covered by private insurance was 67.5 percent, down from 67.9 percent in 2006. The percent of people covered by employment-based health insurance decreased to 59.3 in 2007 from 59.7 percent in 2006. . . . (p. 19)

PAYERS

Third parties responsible for providing reimbursement dollars for the costs of health care are referred to as **payers**. These payers include for-profit insurance companies such as Oxford and Health Net, who are competing for business. In addition, payers include self-insured organizations that assume responsibility for the risks and the costs to minimize healthcare expenses as well as agencies responsible for public insurance such as Medicare and Medicaid and State Children's Health Insurance Program concerned with efficient, cost-effective access to and distribution of care (Shi & Singh, 2010).

Payers are interested in shifting costs and sharing risks associated with care provided. As payers negotiate with the purchasers for a compromise in sharing costs, they negotiate also the sharing of the risk associated with care. The three levels of risk related to costs are those incurred for episodic, chronic, or catastrophic care. Usually, episodic care for healthy individuals is the least costly type of care, and payers try to increase the numbers of enrollees in this category. An example of episodic care may be a visit to a primary care practitioner for acute otitis media. Chronic care requires ongoing treatment and follow-up, which becomes more costly as the chronic condition progresses. An example of this may be the ongoing care that is connected to diabetes. Catastrophic care is the unexpected and devastating disease or condition from which there is no full recovery and maintenance of life functions requires high cost technology and treatment. The payer prefers to assume the lowest level (Shi & Singh, 2001; Shi, 2010).

PROVIDERS

The **providers'** definition of cost of health care reflects the dollars required to provide the services to individuals and populations with a margin of profit. In today's healthcare environment providers have sought different ways to maximize their profits while still providing quality care. For example, group practices have replaced solo practitioners and hospitals have sought multispecialty practices to enhance their access to clients, thus increasing payments received. In addition, healthcare organizations such as acute care hospitals, outpatient clinics, long-term care facilities, and home care organizations also have joined together as an integrated system in an attempt to control cost and utilization (Shi & Singh, 2010).

The rise in the uninsured along with the decrease in employer-sponsored health insurance has spurred providers and policymakers to identify ways to address the healthcare financing issues. The nursing profession has been a major participant in this endeavor, especially the advanced practice nurse. Robinson and Smith (2008) noted that

> This new path is not one of paying physicians, hospitals, and drug manufacturers less to do what they have been doing; their overhead structures and income expectations require more of the same, not less. What is needed is the development of new and different products and processes. . . . (p. 1353)

These same authors go on to explain that a part of this process is the use of other professionals such as nurse practitioners in the provision of health care. Coddington and Sands (2008) carried out an evidence-based review regarding the cost of providing care and the quality of care that is provided in nurse-managed clinics. The outcomes of this review were as follows:

- Nurse-managed clinics facilitate the delivery of care to the poor and underinsured by prompting improved access and acceptability of service.

- This care improves the use of health promotion, preventive services, and compliance of treatments and enhanced patient satisfaction.
- Nurse-managed clinics have the potential to be cost effective in the provision of care.

The advanced nursing practice role and the potential positive outcomes have sparked what some view as a global trend. Sheer and Kam Yuet Wong (2008) spoke to this trend as the "impetus for members of the International Council of Nurses to launch an International Nurse Practitioner/Advanced Practice Nursing Network in 2000 to facilitate communication among nurses who share the same interest globally" (p. 204). The emphasis of this initiative is for the facilitation of better access to care and better cost containment in the global arena. There may be times, however, when providers are in conflict with each other as they vie for healthcare dollars.

POPULATIONS

Although individuals and **populations** are the ultimate recipients of health care, they are often the stakeholder with the least influence. Individuals who have access to health care by virtue of private or public insurance incur the costs according to the criteria negotiated between the purchasers, payers, and providers. Purchasers of healthcare benefits may offer different benefit plans to employees. Employees may have options; however, availability and accessibility to providers is governed by the financial contribution of the employee. Typically, the more directed the plan, the least costly to the employer and the employee. Plans with fewer utilization restrictions pass the

costs to the employee by increasing deductibles and copay requirements.

The growing numbers of uninsured and underinsured represent individuals from some of the most vulnerable populations in the United States, such as the unemployed, homeless, undocumented residents, elderly, women and children, and those with chronic diseases and mental illnesses. For example, according to the U.S. Census Bureau (2008):

> The proportion of people not covered by health insurance is lower among people with higher income. In 2007, 24.5 percent of people in households with annual incomes of less than $25,000 had no health insurance coverage. Uninsured rates decreased for each consecutive household income group to 21.1 percent for households with incomes of $25,000 to $49,999, 14.5 percent for households with incomes of $50,000 to $74,999, and 7.8 percent for households with incomes of $75,000 or more. (p. 23)

The consequence of not providing for these and other vulnerable populations continues to have significant financial impact on the providers of care.

POLICYMAKERS

Public policy is defined by Longest (1996) as "authoritative decisions made in the legislative, executive, or judicial branches of government" (p. 28). Harrington and Estes (2008) define health policy as "the art and science of making public policy decisions about financial organizations and delivery systems for healthcare services" (p. 437). Health policies are frequently a result of social policies and are developed by **policymakers** at the federal, state, and local levels of government. Legislation creates the statutes and laws to enact health

Case Study

Eliminating Cost Barriers for Patients and NP Practices
Stephen A. Ferrara, MSN, RN, FNP-BC, and Eileen T. O'Grady, PhD, RN, NP

Nurse practitioner practice was formally authorized in the New York State Nurse Practice Act in 1988. The original bill contained language consistent with independent nurse practitioner (NP) practice; however, in the final days of the legislative session an expensive compromise was made to change NP practice from "independent" to "collaborative."

Physician organizations believed that independent NPs posed an economic threat and pressured the legislature to limit NP practice and required one of their own to "collaborate" with NPs. This decades-old requirement, to collaborate with a discipline outside of nursing, has no evidence base and contributes to the cost of care because NPs must hire a "collaborating" physician to satisfy regulatory requirements and perform a retrospective review of an unspecified number of patient charts (this is to be decided between the NP and physician in New York State).

This health policy directly impacts the larger economic picture of rural communities. There are numerous instances where thriving rural practices in New York have nearly or temporarily closed down because the NP cannot locate a collaborating physician and therefore cannot legally practice. For example, NP Patricia Donnelly, co-owner of Donnelly & Oot, FNP, LLC in Syracuse, New York, spent 2 years networking locally to find a collaborating physician before opening their practice. The process of finding a collaborating physician is difficult because physicians are not obligated in any way to collaborate with NPs and there is no net gain to the physician. Perverse economic and resource barriers eclipse the cost savings patients would get from seeing an NP. For example, the collaborating physician must be credentialed for each insurance company with which the NP practice contracts; otherwise, the practice will not be reimbursed. The collaborating physician hired by Donnelly and Oot was paid a monthly consulting fee to review five charts per NP practitioner per quarter. After 8 years as an established practice, they nearly had to close their doors when the collaborating physician retired. A new collaborating physician was found after a 6-month search. Today, this practice serves over 2,500 patients, all of which hinge on the arbitrary regulation requiring a physician's willingness to serve as a collaborator.

Through a consensus process, the advanced practice nursing community developed standards that call for eliminating statutory collaboration because it serves no clinical purpose, contributes to rising healthcare costs, does not enhance healthcare quality, takes physicians away from important clinical duties, such as seeing patients, and creates access barriers for patients. When state legislatures allow politics to trump sound, evidence-based health policy, perverse consequences result. At a time when states are trying to expand access to care and reduce costs, New York has a law on its books that requires qualified professionals to hire an expensive collaborating physician because of the economic threat of one discipline. There are enormous workforce distribution imbalances in New York, and many rural areas cannot secure a healthcare provider for their community. Requiring a collaborative agreement costs practice time and money in hiring a physician, cosigning charts, which is not a good use of physician time and has no evidence to support enhanced quality in any way. As we work toward modernizing the nation's nurse practice acts, state legislators must consider the broader economic impact of their decisions.

policy and executive decisions and establish and support the programs related to health policy and the judiciary rules on the reasonableness of the laws. Though the branches of government are the arbiters of health policy, there are many interest groups that influence the government's policy agenda (Leavitt, 2008).

Each of the principal participants in health care have lobbying groups who try to influence health policy initiatives that reflect their perspectives, needs, and goals. For example, purchasers of healthcare benefits are concerned with policies that will reduce their direct costs of health care and contain the overall costs of health care delivered. Payers want health policies that minimize the risk of bearing the costs and maximize opportunities to share the costs associated with reimbursing health care to maintain profitability. For providers who are practitioners, maintaining income and professional autonomy are important policy issues. For provider organizations, policies to support profitability and ability to provide cost-effective and efficient quality care are key. Individuals and populations are interested in policies that ensure access to quality low cost care that meets their needs as well as those of their families and communities.

The model of the 5 P's illustrates the pull and tug that may take place between and among the players within the healthcare system. The pull and tug, however, may also be viewed as an essential dance as the players attempt to find their place within the ever-changing system in relation to cost, care, and their own interests.

The lived experience frequently provides the best teaching exemplars. The preceding case study is a lived experience of the authors. It is an example of the pull and tug that takes place between and

---

BOX **15-1** Field Exercise 1

- Who are the lobby groups in this case study?
- What major constituency do they represent?
- What is the major interest being protected?
- What role does policy serve?
- Which of "the 5 P's" are involved in this pull and tug?
- How is the individual's access to care hindered?
- How may this situation be changed or how may policy and law be altered?

---

among the 5 P's. Read the case study and take time to reflect on the field exercise questions in **Box 15-1**.

Role of Federal Dollars in Public Health

A discussion on the financing of health care cannot take place without a brief look at the federal government and its role in the financing of care pertaining to the population's health. An issue report, *Shortchanging America's Health,* by the Robert Wood Johnson Foundation (2009), opens with the following statement: "Every American should have the opportunity to be as healthy as he or she can be. Every community should be safe from threats to its health. Protecting the health and safety of Americans should be a top responsibility of our nation's leaders" (p. 1). Chapter 1 of this text addresses the

10 essential services of public health. If these 10 essential services are to be assured at the local level, then adequate and appropriate funding must be maintained. According to the Institute of Medicine (2003):

> State and local governments traditionally have had financial responsibility for basic governmental public health services, such as workforce training, the development of information system and the organizational capacity to conduct disease surveillance and prevention programs, the management of public health laboratories, the implementation of population-based prevention and health education programs, and other protections such as water and air quality management, waste disposal, and pest control. Yet the federal government also has a financial responsibility for assuring the capacity of the public health infrastructure at the state and local levels. (p. 147)

Programs for the public's health and protection are funded through a combination of federal, state, and local dollars. The U.S. Department of Health and Human Services (DHHS) is the principal government agency for protecting the public's health. The work of the DHHS is conducted by the Office of the Secretary and 11 agencies. **Box 15-2** illustrates these 11 agencies.

The role of the government is not limited to the federal level but is inclusive of state- and local-level agencies. For example, local public health agencies may receive their funding from three sources: federal, state, and local (Bernet, 2007). Each state department of health is responsible for identifying the priorities of their own state and setting the health agenda as well as identifying how to deliver ser-

---

BOX **15-2** Eleven U.S. Department of Health and Human Services Agencies

1. ACF—Administration for Children & Families
2. AOA—Administration on Aging
3. AHRQ—Agency for Healthcare Research and Quality
4. ATSDR—Agency for Toxic Substances & Disease Registry
5. CDC—Centers for Disease Control and Prevention
6. CMS—Centers for Medicare & Medicaid Services
7. FDA—Food and Drug Administration
8. HRSA—Health Resources and Services Administration
9. IHS—Indian Health Service
10. NIH—National Institutes of Health
11. SAMHSA—Substance Abuse & Mental Health Services Administration

Source: Adapted from U.S. Department of Health and Human Services (n.d.).

---

vices to the people of that state, whereas the local departments of health, such as county health departments, assures the following (Scutchfield & Keck, 1997):

> [T]he implementation of statures and regulations enacted and developed by federal, state, and local governments to protect the public's health. Traditionally, this has involved collecting and analyzing vital statistics, controlling communicable diseases, diminishing environmental risks to health, and providing maternal and child

Case Study

Margaret Macali, MS, RN, CS, Director of Public Health Nursing Service, Clinical Specialist, Public/Community Health Nursing

Cancer and the cancer education and early detection (CEED) programs are a result of continued passive surveillance and analysis of data that prompt policy development and grant funding at a federal and state level. One of the objectives of Healthy People 2010 is the overall reduction of cancer death rates. At a federal level the U.S. DHHS influences and supports states in providing healthcare services to specific populations by offering federal funding in the form of grants. At a state level, local counties are influenced and supported in providing these healthcare services to special populations by offering state funding in the form of grants to lead agencies within each county. These monies are then used in the development, implementation, and evaluation of programs that specifically focus on cancer prevention and early identification. In this way the process of case finding, screening, outreach, surveillance, and disease intervention regarding cancer slowly progresses from a federal to state to local public health intervention level.

Public health nursing is a population-based practice; therefore incorporation of cancer education and early detection is an essential aspect of their work—the doing of public health nursing. The CEED process starts with the defined target population and works down to the individual client. Outreach and education precede screening. The screening process provides case finding, disease and health event investigation includes case management, and that process provides follow-up of positives, referral for treatment, and ultimately data entry into the surveillance data system.

A northern New Jersey County Department of Health applied for and received grant funding to be a county lead agency for a CEED program. The goal was to reach targeted populations within the county that included older, uninsured, underinsured minorities experiencing income inequity who were at risk for specific cancers. Within this county, projected demographics indicated that by 2010 the European White community would be a smaller majority and the minority population would be primarily Asian, with the largest subset being Korean followed by Hispanic, then Black/African American, and then Native American and Other. Within the county's minority population, most will be foreign born with English as a second language. The population of Black/African American and Native American, who do speak English, present with a challenge because historically many are wary and resistant to participating in any health program. All the public health nurses and health educators at the time of the CEED program were White and none was bilingual. Outreach in this particular situation was a challenge, and the public health nurse workforce had to ask critical questions, the first of which was how to reach out to these communities in a culturally sensitive way that will demonstrate congruence with the identified targeted population(s) ideas, values, and beliefs.

The public health nurses in this Northern New Jersey County realized the importance of finding an answer to this very important question. Many members of this county's target population(s) considered breast, cervical, prostate, and colorectal cancer a health problem. The health department's problem was to find a method of outreach and provide clear, understandable, and accurate information in a culturally sensitive and congruent way, as noted above. Given the changing demographics of the county, planning for education and outreach meant engaging bilingual community members to work with the health educators and public health nurses in this outreach. Ultimately, the agency was successful in recruiting Korean bilingual female and male outreach interpreters, Hispanic bilingual female outreach interpreters, Polish bilingual female interpreters, and one Black/African American male outreach worker.

Service provider hospitals were identified and service agreements were developed using requirements of the grant. Public and private partnerships were formed, thus including even more stakeholders within the community. Partner/coalition members included local chapters of the American Cancer Society, Susan G. Komen affiliates, nurse practitioners from provider hospitals, and other local health departments.

Londrigan and Macali (2006) addressed the need of a lead agency to develop partnerships and coalition building to have a successful outreach, education, and screening program. They listed potential members of these coalitions as being key stakeholders living in the community, social service organizations, health and/or voluntary agencies, hospitals, community centers, houses of worship, volunteer organizations, and transportation agencies.

So how successful was the program in outreaching the target communities? Initially, the program had fairly "good" success in its outreach to the Polish, Korean, and Hispanic female target communities. The Black/African American community, however, both male and female, participated initially in very small numbers despite the public health nurses' best efforts.

A senior public health nurse in charge of the CEED program initiated the involvement of a retired Black/African American football player. In finding out about the CEED program, this former player offered to help with the outreach process. As this effort gained momentum, the senior pastor from a local community church whose members were predominantly Black/African American joined this outreach team. The results were dramatic. As the athlete and the pastor donated their time at educational and screening events, many more men within the targeted population participated in the program. Ultimately, an educational DVD on prostate cancer and the screening program was developed and shared throughout the state. The two men were responsible for opening the door to the Black/African American population by donating their time. An additional grant award funded the process. Although the work and the process of the work are critical here, what is of equal importance is noticing the origins of the funding and the stream of the funding. Without the monies the question would be would this program and the positive results ever been realized?

---

health services, adult personal health services, health education, and other services required by their particular community. (p. 87)

An example of funding initiated at the federal level but enacted at the local level is presented in the preceding case study. Read the case study and take time to reflect upon the field exercise questions in **Box 15-3**.

The importance of this discussion in relation to health financing is critical, especially considering the concerns of some when it comes to whether financing of public health initiatives has been sustained in past years. The Robert Wood Johnson Foundation (2009) addressed a shortfall of funds that involved state, local, and federal government funding of public health programs. Specifically, the Foundation noted ". . . federal funding (through CDC) for public health varies, often significantly, with a per capita low of $12.74 to a per capita high of $52.78. . . . The median state spending on public health is $33.71 per person, with a range of $3.37

BOX **15-3** Field Exercise 2

- What is the major public health issue identified in this case study?
- Who is the population being served?
- What Minnesota Department of Health Population-Based Public Health Nursing Practice Intervention Wheel Strategies are enacted in this case study?
- Where did the initial funding begin for this initiative?
- Who were the major players in the partnership at the local level?
- In what way was cultural competence and culturally congruent care addressed at the local level?
- What other strategies might you have initiated to improve the delivery of culturally congruent care?
- How successful was this initiative?

---

per person in Nevada to $172.21 per person in Hawaii" (p. 1). Furthermore, Bassett (2009) stated "The United States spends under 2% of its health dollars on population health, proportionally less than any other wealthy nation" (p. 587). A comparison of these numbers in relation to what is spent on other health costs is a cause of concern.

The purpose of presenting this information is not to cause alarm but to bring home again the need to reconsider how we do business in health care. Farley (2009) asked the following question: "How important is medical care taken as a whole, to health?" (p. 588). This question requires contemplation especially if one considers the amount of money allocated to our medical healthcare system compared with the public healthcare system.

FUTURE CONSIDERATIONS

The first part of this chapter presented the 5 P's. These 5 P's spoke about providers of care and the need to permit these professionals to practice more effectively so that access to care by the population would result. In addition to this, the focus of health promotion and disease prevention is critical now more than ever. The Robert Wood Johnson Foundation (2009) considers a focus on prevention outside the "doctor's office" as well as prevention "inside the doctor's office." Factors outside are community-driven programs that help people to make healthy choices easier choices:

- Keeping schools open after hours for play
- Providing access to fresh produce via farmers markets
- Evidenced-based interventions for those trying to quit smoking

Factors inside the healthcare provider's office include

- Immunizations
- Weight management support and counseling
- Screening for cancers and chronic illnesses

Each of these services has the potential to save in healthcare costs and enhance quality of life for the citizens of the United States.

CONCLUSION

The pull and tug of the competing interests within our healthcare system and the factors that have influenced the cost of health care in the past must be reconsidered with a new "eye" to reconfigure how the delivery of health care will take place today as well as in the future. A medically driven healthcare system that values scientific research and medical technology with an emphasis on specialization may not necessarily facilitate a healthcare system that is less fragmented with positive health outcomes. According to Farley (2009):

> One could conclude from this that the only problem with our healthcare system is a shortage of primary care and an excess of specialty care. It certainly seems likely that more-accessible, higher-quality primary care could prolong life in people with the chronic conditions that are so common and so inadequately treated today, such as hypertension and diabetes. . . . If so, then medical care reform could contribute to closing the mortality gap between the United States and other developed countries. But there is reason to believe that wider population-based approaches would contribute far more. (pp. 588–589)

The goal of healthcare reform will continue to be a national priority. Challenging questions that will stimulate discussion are as follows:

- Should the medical model centered on treatment and cure of illness and disease be the dominant model for the delivery of health care?
- Should a public health population–based healthcare system model centered on health promotion and disease prevention be the dominant model of delivery?
- Is there a need for both models given the United States' own historical and cultural heritage?
- Is there a model yet to be discovered?

Deliberation of questions from the perspectives of the 5 P's must be a part of the conversation on health care and on the delivery of that care to the population. The fragmentation of the nonsystem may continue if the competing interests of the participants as well as the competing goals are not considered simultaneously, finding the balance necessary and reflecting the interests of all the participants.

References

Bassett, M. (2009). Bold steps for the health of Americans: Yes we can. *American Journal of Public Health, 99*(4), 587.

Bernet, P. M. (2007). Local public health agency funding: Money begets money. *Journal of Public Health Management Practice, 13*(2), 188–193.

Centers for Medicare & Medicaid Services, National Health Statistics Group. (2007). Where it went. Retrieved March 8, 2009, from http://cms.hhs.gov/NationalHealthExpendData/downloads/PieChartSourcesExpenditures2007.pdf

Coddington, J. A., & Sands, L. P. (2008). Cost of health care and quality outcomes of patients at nurse-managed clinics. *Nurse Economic$, 26*(2), 75–83.

Farley, T. (2009). Reforming health care or reforming health? *American Journal of Public Health, 99*(4), 588–590.

Harrington, C., & Estes, C. L. (2008). *Health policy: Crisis and reform in the U.S. health care delivery system* (5th ed.). Sudbury, MA: Jones and Bartlett.

Henry Kaiser Family Foundation. (2009). Issues modules: U.S. health care costs. Retrieved March 5, 2009, from http://www.kaiseredu.org

Institute of Medicine. (2003). *The future of the public's health in the 21st century.* Washington, DC: National Academy of Sciences.

Leavitt, J. (2008). Getting involved: Public policy and the decision-making process. In S. B. Lewenson & M. Truglio-Londrigan (Eds.), *Decision-making in nursing: Thoughtful approaches for practice* (pp. 179–191). Sudbury, MA: Jones and Bartlett.

Londrigan, M. T., & Macali, M. K. (2006). Screening. In C. L. Edelman & C. L. Mandle (Eds.), *Health promotion throughout the lifespan* (6th ed., pp. 202–203). St. Louis, MO: Mosby Elsevier.

Longest, B. B. (1996). *Seeking strategic advantage through health policy analysis.* Chicago: Health Administration Press.

Moore, J., Salsberg, E., Wing, P., Dill, M., McGinnis, S., Stapf, C., et al. (2005). *The impact of the aging population on the health workforce in the United States.* Albany, NY: University of Albany, Center for Health Workforce Studies, School of Public Health.

Nutting, M. A. (1904). Visiting nurses in the homes of tuberculosis patients. *American Journal of Nursing, 4*(7), 500–506.

Pride, W., & Ferrell, O. C. (2003). *Marketing: Concepts and strategies* (12th ed.). New York: Houghton Mifflin.

Robert Wood Johnson Foundation. (2009). Short-changing America's health. A state-by-state look at how federal public health dollars are spent and key state indicators. Retrieved February 20, 2009, from http://www.healthyamericans.org

Robinson, J. C., & Smith, M. D. (2008). Cost-reducing innovation in health care. *Perspective: Innovation, 27*(5), 1353–1356.

Scutchfield, F. D., & Keck, C. W. (1997). *Principles of public health practice.* New York: Delmar.

Sheer, B., & Kam Yuet Wong, F. (2008). The development of advanced nursing practice globally. *Journal of Nursing Scholarship, 40*(3), 204–211.

Shi, L., & Singh, D. (2001). *Delivering health care in America: A systems approach* (2nd ed.). Gaithersburg, MD: Aspen.

Shi, L., & Singh, D. A. (2010). *Essentials of the US health care system* (2nd ed.). Sudbury, MA: Jones and Bartlett.

Tyler-Evans, M. (2008). Right on the money: Economics and decision-making. In S. B. Lewenson & M. Truglio-Londrigan (Eds.), *Decision-making in nursing: Thoughtful approaches for practice* (pp. 159–177). Sudbury, MA: Jones and Bartlett.

U.S. Census Bureau. (2008). Income, poverty, and health insurance coverage in the United States: 2007. Washington, DC: U.S. Government Printing Office. Retrieved March 30, 2009, from http://www.census.gov/prod/2008pubs/p60

U.S. Department of Health and Human Services [DHHS]. (n.d.). U. S. Department of Health and Human Services Organizational Chart. Retrieved March 14, 2009, from http://www.hhs.gov/about/orgchart/index.htm

NURSING EDUCATION AND PUBLIC HEALTH NURSING

CATHLEEN M. SHULTZ
KAREN KELLEY

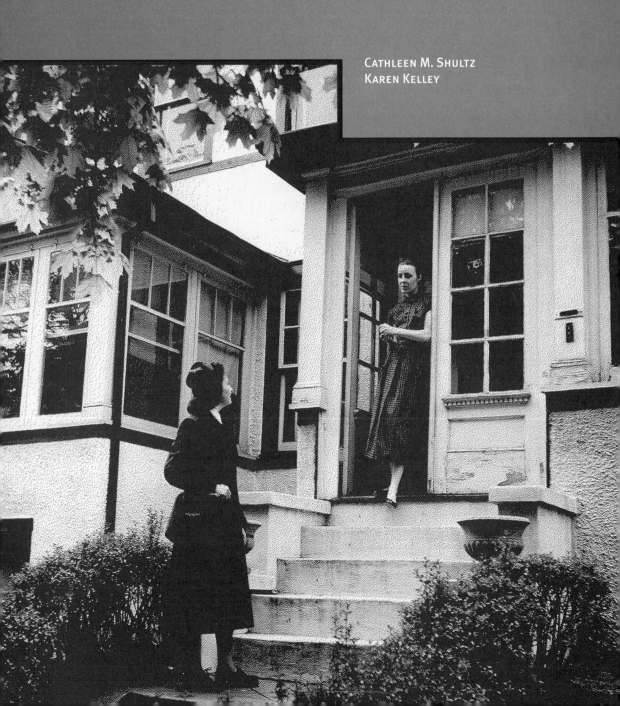

. . . by 1950, more than 17 years would have been added to the average span of American life. . . . It could not have been accomplished without skilled nursing for the sick; the participation of nurses in immunization and case-finding programs; persuasive teaching of health principles by nurses in homes, schools, hospitals, industries, clinics, and health centers; and the public information for groups of community leaders (Roberts, 1954, p. 4).

LEARNING OBJECTIVES

At the completion of this chapter, the reader will be able to

- Identify three challenges related to public health and nursing education.
- List two of the public health clinical experiences described in this chapter.

- Describe the intervention wheel strategies applied in at least one of the public health clinical experiences identified above.
- Explore additional creative public health clinical experiences.

KEY TERMS

- *Essentials of Baccalaureate Nursing Education for Entry Level Community/ Public Health Nurses*
- Healthy People 2020
- Institute of Medicine reports for nursing education

- Population-focused care
- Service learning
- Social justice
- Teaching–learning strategies

N ursing is in an ideal position to respond to numerous challenges facing the healthcare system today. The list of challenges related to the health needs of our nation and our global neighbors is nearly endless: skyrocketing costs of health care and the resultant need for a renewed emphasis on prevention and health promotion measures, healthcare inequalities and disparities, the epidemic of childhood obesity, immigration, the increasing complexity of care for those with chronic illness, anticipated pandemics, emerging and reemerging infectious diseases, threats of bioterrorism, the burden of disease, the enormous expansion of technology, the HIV/AIDS epidemic, unemployment, homelessness, violence, increasing globalization, and increasing evidence of the major impact that the economic and social environments have on health, to name some of these challenges. As the nation responds to the healthcare system crises, public health has regained attention as a viable response to meet many of these challenges. Nurses are a large workforce with a lengthy history of practicing in public health settings. Many nurses practice in positions that place them in people's homes, schools, workplaces, houses of worship, public clinics, and other settings where public health expertise is needed.

Although barriers exist to specializing in public health nursing, it is imperative that nursing education programs prepare graduates who are skilled in use of public health practices, able to work as a member of multidisciplinary public health teams, are knowledgeable of the determinants of health affecting populations, and know how to integrate this knowledge into interventions that positively impact the health of individuals, families, and communities. This chapter explores the educational mandates for nursing students as related to public health, educational challenges, and practical learning exemplars that integrate these into learning experiences that can develop public health skills, knowledge, and aptitudes in nursing students—in other words, "applying and doing" in nursing education. Graduates must be prepared as professionals ready to meet rapidly changing healthcare system demands.

CHALLENGES TO NURSE EDUCATORS

Nursing and nursing education have come full circle. History seems to repeat itself, but the context changes. From the early days of the colonies to the present, the United States has struggled with its nursing numbers, the preparation of its nursing workforce, and containment and conquering of its infectious diseases and other major causes of maiming and death. Recently, our states and federal governments coasted through the last five decades and reduced resources that were needed to build a strong public health workforce and infrastructure, which are now costly to reconstruct and repair. There is a pressing need to graduate nurses capable of understanding and meaningfully contributing to the public's health. As mentioned elsewhere in this book, leaders such as Florence Nightingale, Lillian Wald, and Clara Barton pressed to create, implement, and sustain public health initiatives that changed health and disease practices for decades after their deaths. They modeled perseverance and courage and met the challenges of their times. They were among the first nurse systems thinkers.

Historically, public health nurses were valued by society and functioned autonomously. They practiced in settings and with populations that were of minimal interest to other healthcare disciplines. Traditionally, public health nursing care encompassed the unempowered and the invisible—women, children, poor, immigrants, and other disenfranchised groups. Gradually, practice shifted from personal healthcare services, such as home care, to public health issues and activities. It is beyond the scope of this chapter to comprehensively explore major discoveries and movements that altered public health needs and practices. Dramatically, the cataclysmic events that redirected the nation's public health policies, urgencies, and attention were the terrorist attacks on the World Trade Center and the Pentagon and the brave passengers of a hijacked airliner that crashed outside Pittsburgh, Pennsylvania, on September 11, 2001. Thousands were murdered and even more were injured and sustained chronic conditions due to their part in that day's activities. Shortly thereafter, the anthrax exposures of thousands in New York, Florida, and Washington, DC, forced a reexamination of the weakened public health infrastructure and ultimately the preparation of nurses for a timely response to population needs.

The Institute of Medicine (IOM, 2003) developed seven public health priorities, which are summarized in **Box 16-1**. Nursing education programs are addressing these priority needs as well as other

---

BOX 16-1 Institute of Medicine's Seven Public Health Priorities

1. Understand and emphasize broad determinants of health
2. Create a policy focus on population health
3. Strengthen the public health infrastructure
4. Build partnerships
5. Develop systems of accountability
6. Emphasize evidence-based practice
7. Enhance communication

Source: IOM (2003).

Following a tornado, these lone steps mark a reminder of the homes that were present hours before. Inhabitants are at a local shelter receiving health care and aid from nursing students and relief organizations. *Source:* Courtesy of Cathleen Shultz.

initiatives such as disaster preparedness. Public health issues are competing with bioterrorism activities for resources. The worldwide economic depression remains unresolved, and its full effects are yet to be seen. Regardless of the pressures felt by nurse educators and nursing students, preparation for effective public health needs is central to developing and sustaining a prepared nursing workforce and a healthy population.

RESPONDING TO THE PUBLIC HEALTH NEEDS

Teaching of IOM: Implications of the Institute of Medicine Reports for Nursing Education, based on the series of **IOM reports for nursing education** aimed at improving the safety and overall quality of healthcare in the United States, addresses areas of interest to nurse educators in preparing students in public health (Finkelman & Kenner, 2007). The IOM (2003) reports view education of health professionals as a "bridge to quality care" (p. 9) and state that education must change to meet the needs of current and future healthcare systems. The authors provide understanding that adding content is nearly impossible in already overfilled curriculums but offer that threads such as cultural competence and informatics (Shultz, 2009b) can be woven into other public health learning activities, allowing the student to gain the knowledge and experience its application. Suggestions also involve students from different health-related professions located in the academic institution to have joint educational opportunities.

In addition to legislative expectations such as a state's nurse practice acts, nursing program approval standards and health laws, and other requirements such as clinical agency expectations, numerous organizations, such as accrediting bodies, affect nursing education in the United States. National initiatives that push for increased competence in gerontology, women's health, safety, healthy work environments, and end-of-life practices add to the challenges facing nursing students and educators. Currently, programs' lengths and types are defined by law and graduates enter practice after passing the National Council Licensure Examination that tests practice expectations within 6 months of graduation. Faculty must create learning activities that quickly involve students in increasingly complex case situations to graduate competent, dedicated, lifelong learners.

Students at all educational levels need exposure to relevant definitions of nursing, public health, and public health nursing and understanding of public health nursing as a specialty (**Table 16-1**). Beyond basic understandings, faculty program decisions involve collectively selecting methods to incorporate learning public health concepts and nursing roles (**Table 16-2**). Faculty may choose a public health total curriculum, a multicourse focus, or a single-course focus. Complex learning, such as public health nursing, most often takes time to learn. An early curriculum introduction to the concepts and roles fosters deeper understanding before graduation. The greater the lack of experienced public health nursing clinicians, the more faculty will need to creatively develop relationship-based clinical experiences.

Table 16-1 Relevant Nursing Public Health Definitions

Term	Definition
Nursing	The protection, promotion, and optimization of health and abilities, prevention of illness and injury, alleviation of suffering through the diagnosis and treatment of human response, and advocacy in the care of individuals, families, communities, and populations (American Nurses Association, 2003, p. 6; 2004, p. 7)
Public health	Science and art of preventing disease, prolonging life, and promoting health and efficiency through organized community effort (Winslow, 1920, as cited in Turnock, 1997, p. 9)
Public health practice	What we as a society do collectively to ensure the conditions in which people can be healthy (IOM, 1988, p. 1; 2003, p. 28)
Public health nursing	The practice of promoting and protecting the health of populations using knowledge from nursing, social, and public health sciences (American Public Health Association, 1996, p. 1)
	A specialty practice of nursing defined by scope of practice and not by practice setting (Council on Linkages Between Academia and Public Health Practice, 2001; Quad Council of Public Health Nursing Organizations, 1999)
Public health nursing specialty	Contains 8 core foundation principles of public health nursing identified and discussed in the *Public Health Nursing; Scope and Standards of Practice* (American Nurses Association, 2007; Association of Community Health Nursing Educators, 2003)

INTEGRATING LEARNER KNOWLEDGE, SKILLS, AND APTITUDES TO DEVELOP PUBLIC HEALTH–FOCUSED NURSING CARE

Because of the limited time for educational experiences (both didactic and clinical) there is a need to create learning experiences that meet multiple outcome objectives. Carter, Kaiser, O'Hare, and Callister (2006) urged **teaching–learning strategies** based on public health nursing practice (Quad Council of Public Health Nursing Organizations (1999), public health nursing competencies (Quad Council, 2004), and *Essentials of Bac-*

Table 16-2 Select Examples of Public Health Concepts and Public Health Nursing Roles

Public Health Concepts	Public Health Nursing Roles
Population-focused care	Advocate
Disaster planning and response	Collect, monitor, and analyze data
Public health surveillance	Case manager
Outbreak investigation	Health policy and legislation involvement
Community and population assessment	Referral resource
Use of evidence-based interventions	Literacy assessor
Infectious disease prevention, recognition and care	Educator
Vulnerable populations	Identify community needs
Partnerships	Create and implement educational activities
Health agency roles (federal, state, local)	Direct primary caregiver
Epidemiology—the scientific core	Organize public health services
Service learning	
Social justice	
Violence	
Cultural competency	

calaureate *Nursing Education for Entry Level Community/ Public Health Nurses* (Association of Community Health Nursing Educators, 2000). Program, course, and class decisions affecting learning rest with faculty. Exemplar teaching and learning examples are provided in the narrative that follows. They are modifiable depending on learner expectations and placement of the learning strategies in the nursing program.

Where possible, faculty align clinical assignments directly to theory application. For situations where finding appropriate clinical experiences is difficult, either clinical experiences or simulations are created. Theory and application are at the individual, family, and community levels. Many class activities are discussed at the national and global levels, with some students participating in international experiences. Application of national and global issues to the local situation is made. Nurse educators, from novice to expert, build real-world learning activities that use cognitive, affective, and psychomotor skills. Evidence-based teaching, learning, and evaluation methods are increasing in numbers and scope as the science of nursing education is pursued (Shultz, 2009a). Many of these are applicable to teaching public health nursing that faculty are urged to use and further research.

In the beginning of the public health–focused nursing course, students are introduced to the learning outcomes. For most students, viewing the community as the client is difficult to grasp, as is the idea of **population-focused care**. As the semester's content outline, clinical rotations, and learning assignments are reviewed, the students begin the journey of combining concepts that seem to be unrelated, such as healthcare financing and epidemiology, into what they will come to know as public health nursing. As each content area is covered, the learning links between them are explained and experienced. By the end of the semester, bridges between those links are stronger and the students view the interrelated concepts of public health more clearly.

An example of an assignment that encourages these connections involves the students locating and presenting a current event article in class. They prepare the public health news item for display on the classroom's bulletin board after the in-class verbal presentation. Connections to the various concepts in public health are made during the classroom discussion. The assignment increases student awareness of media interpretation of health-related news items and their relevance to nurses. An example is the media events announcing the severe acute respiratory syndrome, caused by a virus that led to illness and death in many in 2003. From China the disease spread rapidly to other countries by airline passengers traveling internationally. In this situation the media coverage lasted several months and was timely for class discussions. News items that involve health promotion and prevention studies are especially useful for class discussions because of the nature of these studies and the amount of rapidly conflicting information that often appears simultaneously.

Early in the semester, healthcare financing, healthcare systems, health policy, and political issues are taught. Emphasis is on their interconnectedness and the dramatic influences they bear on health status and needs. Extensive discussion regarding effects on vulnerable populations and concern for social justice dominate learning. At this section's conclusion students produce an in-class debate on the pros and cons of universal health care. It is typically a lively debate. Preparation requires knowledge of public health concepts and assigned readings. In a reflective summative evaluation of the activity, students report a broader view of the issue and additional insight into how populations and the healthcare system are affected.

PUBLIC HEALTH CLINICAL EXPERIENCES

Clinical experiences involve nursing in schools, local health departments, rural health clinics, home health settings, screenings (hearing, vision, scoliosis, body mass index, laboratory and wellness focused), area agency on aging, and disaster management simulation (Bambini, Washburn, & Perkins, 2009). Students use clinical experience guidelines for each separate experience (see example in **Figure 16-1**). Each requires a student self-assessment (establishes goals and monitors progress toward them), which is a technique that enhances self-directedness (Nicol & Macfarlane-Dick, 2006). Fitzpatrick (2006) determined that self-assessment positively influences students' development, particularly their sense of

FIGURE **16-1**   **Sample clinical experience journal template.**

Clinical Experience Journal

Clinical Experience in: Local Health Department

Date:_____   **Setting:** <insert name of agency>   **Location:** <insert town or city>   .

This clinical experience is guided by your clinical teacher and supervised by agency personnel. The clinical teacher will visit the site during the experience and is available during the experience by phone or text at <insert number> or <insert email address>.

You are expected to complete preparatory materials prior to the experience, participate in nursing care at the agency, and meet this experience's learning objectives. Following the experience, complete a reflective self-assessment evaluation of your experiences. Evaluation is comprehensive and is also completed by agency personnel and the clinical teacher.

Purposes of the Experience:
- To participate in public health nursing at a local health department
- To determine services offered at a local and state health department

Preparation:
Review the State Department of Health (SDH) website. What programs are offered by the SDH? What is the structure of the organization? How is the SDH funded?

Objectives:
1. Describe the major health promotion and disease preventing programs delivered at the HD (family planning, WIC - Women, Infants and Children, Immunization, Communicable Disease, TB, STD, Breast Care). List the requirements for participation in each program, how is it funded, the cost to the participant, what specifically is provided, and describe what occurs during a visit for each of these major programs. What is the protocol if someone is/has a positive TB test? Is HIV positive? Tests positive for syphilis? What immunizations are required? Offered?
2. Describe the cultural diversity of the health unit's target population. How is this diversity being addressed? (Review population statistics for the county.)
3. Use the nursing process to assess, plan, implement and evaluate public health care given to members of the community during your experience. Identify public health nursing roles observed and examples of each.
4. Discuss what referrals are most often needed by patients. How are they made?
5. Describe the process used for reportable diseases. How is the information gathered and reported?
6. What skills did you perform? Describe how you maintain safe nursing practice? Specifically, be prepared to do venipunctures, injections, urine pregnancy tests, fingersticks, assist with pelvic exams, etc.
7. Describe the computer charting and database for record keeping, including vaccination records. Accurately document any findings. Discuss how charting is related to reimbursement for the health unit.
8. Demonstrate professional and ethical standards. Discuss specific issues encountered and their method of resolution.
9. Incorporate teaching/learning principles to provide education to patients and family members. Give examples of education offered at the health department. Also discuss education programs implemented at the community level from the local HD and from the state health department. Select a written health education tool and determine its reading level.
10. Give examples of primary, secondary, and tertiary prevention measures offered at the HD.

Self-assessment evaluation of clinical experience: <Insert Clinical Judgment Rubric>

Arrival Time: _____   Departure Time: _____

autonomy and thinking skills (Maclellan & Soden, 2006). When shared, faculty members gain insight into students' thinking (Davies, 2002), and it becomes a mechanism for personalized feedback (Cato, Lasater, & Peeples, 2009).

The goal of each experience is to develop clinical judgment (Tanner, 2006), which facilitates students thinking like a public health nurse. The reflective self-assessment activity incorporates the four phases of Tanner's clinical judgment model (2006) (noticing, interpreting, responding, and reflecting) with students describing their responses to clinical situations using behavioral descriptors. The learning strategy fosters clinical judgment (Craft, 2005; Lasater, 2007a, b; Lasater & Nielsen, 2009; Nielsen, Stragnell, & Jester, 2007)

Creating Clinical Experiences: Wellness Screening

With the increasing emphasis in the United States on controlling healthcare costs, a growing interest in prevention is occurring in all sectors of health care. Both governmental and private stakeholders are urgently implementing ways to control costs. Public health professionals have long advocated prevention as a way to meet that goal. Students in the community health nursing course learn a variety of skills and concepts that consider both risk factors and interventions at the primary, secondary, and tertiary levels of prevention.

Each semester the community health nursing students conduct a wellness screening for faculty, staff, and students at the university. The screening involves two interactions between students and participants. The first interaction involves actual screening assessments. Partici-

pants choose from a selection of laboratory tests including lipid panels, high sensitivity C-reactive protein, complete blood counts, glucose, hemoglobin A1c, complete metabolic panels, prostate-specific antigens, testosterone levels, arthritis profiles, vitamin D levels, thyroid screens, and HIV. Body fat analysis and health risk appraisals are also offered. In clinical conferences the students learn which screenings, such as lipid panels, are recommended for the general population and which are targeted screenings based on risk factors. This provides an excellent application of screening theory. The students then learn to analyze results and provide written counseling to each participant. With guidance they recommend additional screenings such as mammography or colonoscopy based on the age and sex of the participant. Students ensure that all screenings are returned from the laboratory and organize and package the results. From this experience students learn many skills and abilities needed to manage a screening program. These skills include clinic set-up, managing traffic flow, involvement with forms that order and report results, and dismantling the clinic. The following week, students are available for participants to receive results, be counseled regarding needed lifestyle changes, and refer to local health providers as needed.

The nursing program partnered with a local wellness company affiliated with a certified laboratory to provide the wellness clinic on campus. Approximately 200 people participate each semester. The nursing program works with the campus human resources department, and the cost to those on the university's insurance plan may be reimbursed through an employee wellness benefit. Students experience an example of

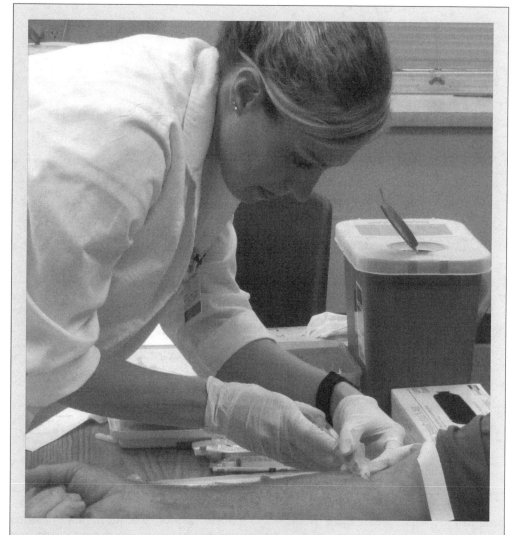

Nursing student participant in a campus wellness screening clinic. *Source:* Courtesy of Cathleen Shultz.

healthcare financing previously discussed in class and the cost-saving benefits that would appeal to a company that chooses to implement wellness programs. The students learn basic phlebotomy skills and draw blood samples. The experience emphasizes prevention and health pro-

motion and how lifestyle affects biophysical indicators of health.

Before the wellness screenings, students prepare an educational poster that addresses at least one Healthy People 2010 objective that is applicable to the target audience for the screening

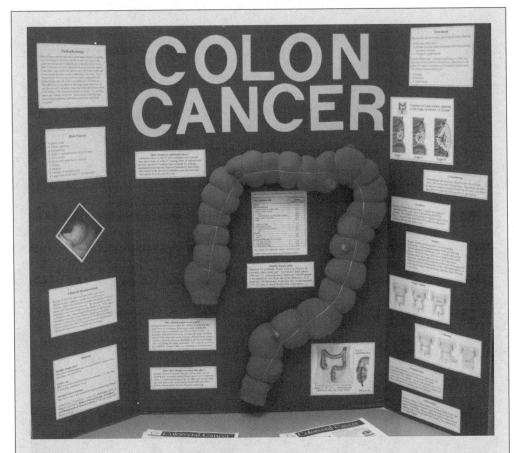

Wellness screening clinic poster created by students. The 3D colon model is constructed from fabric with marbles mimicking locations of tumors. *Source:* Courtesy of Cathleen Shultz.

program. Students search for Healthy People objectives, currently 2010 and soon **Healthy People 2020**, consider the audience attending the wellness screening, obtain educational material to supplement the poster, and develop a distributable fact sheet to expand the poster's information. They search the Internet to find reliable sources to order educational materials. They must consider relevance to their poster topic, the cost, time for delivery, and any copyright issues with use. When screening partici-

pants wait for appointments, consume donated breakfast foods and drink, and exit the screenings, they visit the displayed posters. Campus wellness screenings were started by the nursing faculty over two decades ago. There exists a loyal, repeat clientele who depend on these cost-saving services.

Simulation Experiences

DISASTER DRILL

Veenema (2006) reinforces that as the largest sector of the healthcare workforce

A damaged church building remains in a neighborhood devastated by Hurricane Katrina in Louisiana. *Source:* Courtesy of Cathleen Shultz.

in the United States, nurses must be prepared in all aspects of disaster management. Although this article explores formal certificate and degree programs to train nurses in various aspects of disaster management, it also notes the overall importance of preparing nurses to effectively communicate with the wide variety of disciplines represented in disaster management teams. The skills to collaborate, assess, plan, problem solve, and make decisions are noted as essential for nurses being fully prepared to respond to disasters. Landry and Stockton (2008) describe adding disaster management content to undergraduate nursing education and emphasize the importance of both inclusion in theory content and hands-on simulated practice.

Disaster Drill/FEMA Course Online

Almost two decades ago, the nursing program initiated simulated disaster drills for student learning in the community health nursing course and another senior clinical course. Over time, and especially after 2001, the drill has morphed into a university–community partnership experience with win–win results. Hundreds of students, community agencies, and personnel now participate and the event is described in the following narrative.

Each spring semester the university conducts a disaster drill where nursing students and other community agencies respond to simulated events such as tornadoes and fires affecting a dorm or other campus buildings. Initiated by the College of Nursing as part of the community health nursing course, the drill has merged into a university- and community-wide event. The merging began as a conversation between nursing and theater faculty. Both disciplines realized the learning value potential of the experience for students. The first interdisciplinary drill was planned

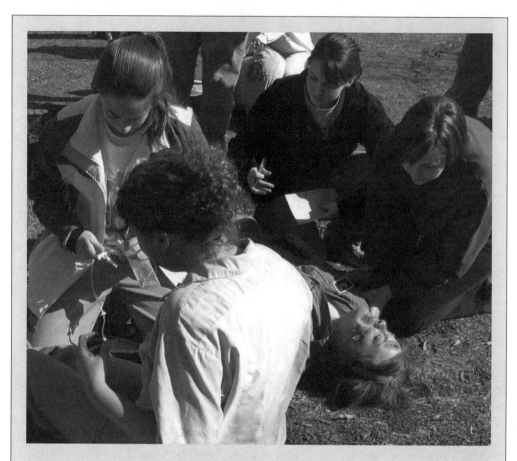

Interdisciplinary students triage those injured in a simulated community disaster drill that meets community emergency management requirements. *Source:* Courtesy of Cathleen Shultz.

in the fall of 2001, and, due to the timing related to the events of September 11, interest and participation grew rapidly. Community agencies now participating are the local police, fire, emergency medical services, and hospital. Fire trucks, police cars, and ambulances and the uniformed responders add to the authenticity of the experience. These community agencies use the drill as training for their personnel, which provides increased community preparedness for actual events as well. The Public Safety Office coordinates university participation, and nursing faculty coordinate the participation of health-related academic areas. The local hospital receives "victims" and uses these victims to have a mass casualty drill for the emergency department. Senior nursing students in the community health nursing course plan the injuries and evaluate the response. Senior nursing students in an advanced medical-surgical nursing course respond to triage and treat victims. They bandage wounds, simulate starting intravenous fluids, and perform other emergency care at the scene. They provide information as to the number of victims and conditions to the medical officer in charge of the scene and observe the communication within the Incident Command System.

The theater students add an essential element of realism to the drill by accurate portrayal of victims and application of stage makeup to create very realistic injuries. The community health nursing students also learn the details of how the injury will appear and what signs and symptoms would be expected so they can portray the injuries appropriately and advise the theater students. The physician assistant and pharmacy students on campus are also victims and responders. Working with interdisciplinary teams is practiced under simulated but intense situations. Journalism and public relations students participate and the health-related students practice relating to the media. A first aid course is completed during a clinical day before the drill. Students view first hand the Incident Command System operationalized on a local level, which they cover in class before the drill. They also complete the Introduction to the Incident Command System online Federal Emergency Management Agency (FEMA) course certification (www.fema.gov/emergency/nims/IncidentCommandSystem.shtm) as part of the preparatory work for the clinical experience.

The disaster drill is a simulated experience that provides opportunity to meet a variety of objectives. The most obvious is the clinical application of disaster management theory. Critical thinking is nec-essary to appropriately triage and treat victims. The students, through clinical conference discussion, also are aware of the positive influences that the drills have on preparedness for the university and the community. One of the first results was creation of an Emergency Management Committee for the university. A nursing faculty is on this committee that has members, both academic and administrative, from many areas of the university. During one drill, which simulated a dorm fire, the fire department had difficulty with master key access to all rooms during the search and rescue phase of the drill. This resulted in their recommendation to install Knox boxes, which allow the fire department access to entire buildings during an emergency. After installation on campus buildings, the fire department then discussed the key difficulty with other community businesses and industries; many had them installed as well. Each time the drill is conducted on campus, ways to increase safety are found and most are implemented. The drill enables the community to meet FEMA standards and the university to obtain excellent disaster management standards. Debriefing follows the drill to evaluate the response. University-involved academic areas and departments, as well as community agencies, participate to create an excellent way to maximize the learning experience.

Immunization Clinic

Students participate in the local health department's annual influenza immunization clinic. This clinic is also used by the department of health as a mass vaccination drill to prepare for a bioterrorism event. The dual purpose event provides an effective immunization learning opportunity. Many community members receive flu vaccine free of charge and the health department prepares for a disaster. Students work directly with the nurses at the local health department for this event. The students complete screening forms, educate patients, and administer the immunizations. They learn both concepts and skills related to mass vaccination and immunization status of populations.

Service Learning

Lawler (2008) explored the development of professional nursing values through service-learning experiences. She noted the importance of reflection to the process of **service learning** and that guided reflection and discussion facilitated by faculty are crucial to students developing a deeper and broader understanding of the complex social issues commonly found in those utilizing services such as those found in public health nursing. Her findings supported the development of professional values, including **social justice** (Lawler, 2008). Describing a clinical experience that placed nursing students in a setting where they would be in direct and personal contact with those who are poor, DeLashmutt and Rankin (2005) noted that novice students' understanding "about poverty's impact on physical, mental and spiritual well-being is usually inadequate and undeveloped" (p. 143). At the conclusion of the experience, nursing students demonstrated a much better understanding of the complex nature of poverty and the effective interventions to assist those who are poor.

Students must develop an understanding of poverty to effectively work with the poor who frequently engage public health

services. *In Bridges Out of Poverty*, Payne, DeVol, and Smith (2001) outlined typical resources, such as financial, but focused on additional resources, such as emotional, mental, spiritual, coping strategies, knowledge of hidden rules of the social classes, and support systems, that those experiencing poverty frequently lack. The book provides practical ways professionals can assist individuals in acquiring missing resources so that students can effectively engage those in poverty in their health care and assist those in poverty to interact with and hopefully transition into a middle class work environment.

Faith-Based Clinic

A decade of planning that involved nursing faculty resulted in the opening of a free-standing clinic, staffed by various healthcare and other volunteers, within a mile of the university. Clinical experiences at the faith-based clinic for uninsured, low-income individuals provide opportunities for students to meet impoverished individuals who are the faces of the statistics and issues discussed in class. Many clients are homeless, experiencing intimate partner violence, or addicted to substances. Immigrant populations also attend this clinic, allowing opportunity to develop skills in cultural competence. As the semester progresses, examples of poverty and related issues are from the students' clinical experiences. Connections are made between the determinants of health and poor health status. Students compare the health status of this population with the wellness screening clinic participants. The differences are dramatic, making meaningful learning experiences.

Faith-based clinic that provides interdisciplinary services to low-income, uninsured individuals.
Source: Courtesy of Cathleen Shultz.

School Health Screenings

The students spend 1 or more clinical days assisting school nurses in the community area with the state-required screenings of hearing, vision, scoliosis, and body mass index. The students quickly realize the value of this service to the school nurses, the students at the school, and the community-at-large. They appreciate the difficulty of school nurses providing multiple required screenings in underfunded settings without assistance. The experience allows meeting multiple objectives. An interesting related clinical conference focuses on the discrepancy between laws that are passed to mandate screenings and the frequent nonallocation of funding for adequate personnel to conduct the screenings. Outcomes data on the effectiveness of each type of screening program are researched and discussed during conference so that the student can evaluate whether the screening is necessary based on those findings. The political process to make any needed future change is explored to further model the public health nursing role of advocacy. In this rural setting, over three decades of nursing students' active involvement in school health have dramatically increased school children's overall health while meeting nursing student learning needs.

PARADIGM SHIFT FROM "LOCAL WORLD" TO "GLOBAL WORLD VIEW"

Nurses practicing in future settings will be required to change their thinking paradigm from a local to a global world view. Recognizing this need, faculty members have identified concepts and learning experiences to prepare graduates for the changing world. The umbrella concepts are social justice, healthcare missions, culture of poverty, global learning, and systems thinking.

Social Justice

A recent study on developing competencies in social justice, equity, and the social determinants of health explored how nursing education programs developed knowledge and skills in these three areas (Cohen & Gregory, 2009a, b). Findings supported that content should be included in theory; further, these concepts also need to be embedded throughout the curriculum and exposed to areas in clinical experience where these factors can be explored. These are included in most clinical experiences in the community health nursing course. Elective courses are offered that strengthen this content.

Boutain (2008) describes the education of nursing students for social justice as "an urgent, yet complex undertaking" (p. 2). She describes student learning experiences about social justice in three stages: "1) social justice knowledge development, 2) social justice knowledge integration and issue identification, and 3) social justice action" (p. 3). Stages are described as built into the curriculum, and by the end of the senior community health nursing course, students were expected to take action on a social justice concern. A method of evaluation is described. "Without the action component, social justice teaching cannot be viewed as transformative" (Boutain, 2008, p. 1). In developing a model of faculty scholarship, Boyer (1990) suggested that academia explore ways to respond to social needs. He stated that the reality of the many social crises cause academicians to ask if all the resources of higher education could be of greater service to the nation and to the world.

The goal of educating nursing students about issues of social justice is that the knowledge they gain and experiences they have will be transformative, becoming part of their lifelong practice. Like past leaders, nurses who actively work to promote social justice are needed to address the many social ills of today (Boutain, 2005). With nurses on the front lines in public health agencies in communities across the nation and the world, they are ideally placed for service. Having skill sets not just to care about the issues but to address them effectively is critical. Skills in community assessment and building community partnerships provide the groundwork for intervention, whereas skills in advocacy and engaging in the political process can be used to bring change to systems. Skills to work with those who are vulnerable enable nurses to develop interventions with individuals, families, and communities most at risk.

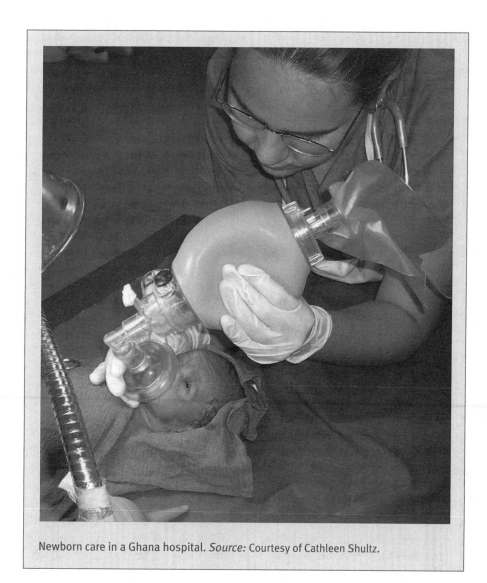

Newborn care in a Ghana hospital. *Source:* Courtesy of Cathleen Shultz.

Healthcare Missions

Since the mid-1970s, when the nursing program began, students and faculty have participated in domestic and international health mission experiences. The program now co-offers an interdisciplinary health missions minor and numerous courses that can be taken by majors from other disciplines. Some of the courses also meet global literacy degree requirements. One of these elective courses is "Healthcare Missions," which many students choose to take. This course is taught by nursing faculty experienced in providing health care in the developing world and is cotaught by a missions faculty member who has experience in development work in these countries. The class includes content on global health issues such as tuberculosis, AIDS, and malaria, emphasizing their devastating impact on developing countries. Learning activities such as how to make the World Health Organization's oral rehydration solution, treat parasites, and use of culturally appropriate skits to provide health teaching that might not be taught in traditional nursing courses in the United States are explored. As part of the course, students complete a weekend immersion experience a few miles from campus at the university's global village, where they practice bartering skills; cook with very limited ingredients and facilities; live in authentic housing such as an African hut, a Mexican barrio, or an Appalachian shack; and learn development strategies while working through cultural barriers.

Culture of Poverty

This elective course provides in-depth insight into understanding poverty and the world view of those who are poor and the skills needed to effectively engage with those who are poor. Emphasis is on the culture of generational poverty, but situational poverty is also explored. Poverty, from U.S. and global perspectives, is analyzed for impact. Practical methods to understand and develop interventions to work with those who are poor are explored in depth with strategies such as the use of microdevelopment loans. An excerpt from the introduction

of one course textbook states the urgency of community problems and why education in sustainable, effective solutions is necessary:

> The economic insecurity of low-wage and the middle class threatens the viability of our communities. When members of the middle class flee the cities, taking the tax base and spending power with them . . . when Main Street empties of viable businesses and refills with pawn shops, used clothing stores, social service storefronts, and payday lenders . . . when people can't afford to stay in the community to raise their children because of the lack of well-paying jobs . . . and when the free and reduced-price lunch rate at the schools hits 50%, our communities are becoming unsustainable. (Payne, DeVol, & Smith, 2001, p. 5)

Emphasis is on the connection between poverty and health status.

Global Learning

The College of Nursing offers three annual international experiences in which students can participate. One is a spring break trip to Haiti where the students participate in community primary care clinics. The College of Nursing partners with a larger group from several area churches for this experience. Nursing faculty accompany the students as well as a variety of other professionals. During the spring semester the students also have an opportunity to go with a faith-based group on a medical mission trip to Guatemala. The group has an established hospital and clinics and coordinates multiple healthcare mission trips during the year. The recent focus of the students' experiences was gynecological surgery and plastic surgery for children with cleft lip and palates. The students work with nurses and provide around-the-clock postoperative care for those undergoing surgeries. One memorable story and photograph captured students and patients who were recovering from gynecological surgeries forming a "conga line," led by the volunteer nurses and nursing students, to provide postoperative ambulation.

In the summer the College of Nursing selects a site in Africa, and students go with a faculty member with advanced practice credentials who has long-term experience working as a nurse in Africa. In this immersion experience the students work in clinics and a mission hospital while gaining experience in pediatrics and labor and delivery. They also obtain first-hand experience with global health issues such as poverty, HIV/AIDS, tuberculosis, malaria, and parasites. Students see death in those who are young and wrestle as never before with why the inequalities exist. Some of these sites have been managed for one to two decades, and long-term health improvements have been realized. Students receive ongoing

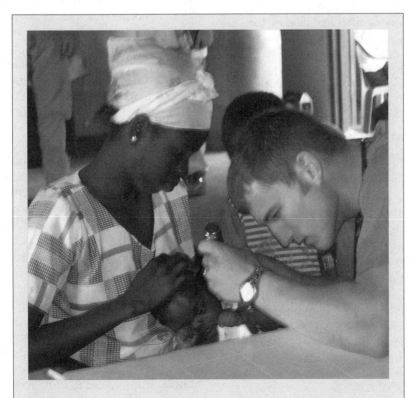

Assessing a sick child's ears in a Tanzania clinic. *Source:* Courtesy of Cathleen Shultz.

preparation for months before entering another culture and are debriefed to assist with acculturation upon return.

These trips are all voluntary, but many students do choose to go and bring back those experiences they then share with other students, thus enriching the classes on global health issues. The programs aid all students in experiencing the ties to our global neighbors. Over 80% of the nursing majors voluntarily participate in healthcare missions and global learning, both of which develop their public health nursing knowledge, abilities, and aptitudes.

Systems Thinking

As the semester progresses, linking the information together and guiding the student to make the connections is an educational objective. By the end of the course, the student is expected to make the connections between the determinants of health and health status. The clinical project that ties all these concepts together is the community assessment. The students, through collaborative learning strategies, work on this all semester in groups of four to five. They divide the assessment data to be gathered and then, during the semester, have meetings with faculty who guide them in connecting theory to their findings, evaluating the strengths and weaknesses of the community, and establishing priority health-related problems. Goal setting at the population level is a complex process usually requiring faculty guidance. During this process students become able to develop interventions and population-focused plans of care.

Debriefing

Debriefing after public health nursing experiences occurs during clinical con-

ferences. Debriefing, and evidence-based teaching and learning strategy, has historically been used in nursing education as a method to focus on learning outcomes and intended objectives of experiences (Jeffries & Rogers, 2007). The practice of debriefing varies by teacher. When debriefing involves reflection, students analyze accomplishments and events and think about enhancing and creating more skillful nursing practice. The process involves active engagement and maturing as a learner who evaluates self and others.

Dreifuerst (2009) identifies the attitudes of debriefing as reflection, emotion, reception, and integration and assimilation. Reflection involves reexamining the experience. Exploring and releasing emotions related to learning enhance experiences, but they can also inhibit learning if distraction from active engagement takes place. Teachers facilitate emotional expressions to promote reflective learning. Reception, as openness to feedback, addresses knowledge, skills, and aptitudes. This is a meaningful time to coach students to be open to receive feedback. Using formative feedback for critique and correction makes affective learning more visible (Kuiper, Heinrich, Matthias, Graham, & Bell-Kotwell, 2008). Integration of the experience may be the most difficult because it urges the learner to frame (i.e., attributes of meaning to a set of facts [Pesut, 2004]) learning, usually for clinical settings, into the nursing process of the public health nurse. This sets the stage for accommodation and assimilation, the transfer of learning and experiences from one situation to the next. Anticipation, asking "what if" as a process of accommodation, represents higher order clinical judgment and reasoning based on metacognition (Benner,

Stannard, & Hooper, 1996; Pesut, 2004; Tanner, 2006). "What if" questions that change the details and nursing process frame encourage students to think beyond the boundary of the experience and anticipate the next question. All defining attributes work in tandem during debriefing and optimize the clinical experiences. Omitting, minimizing, or discounting debriefing attributes may be harmful to student learning and future development within a program.

NURSE EDUCATORS: EMBRACING PUBLIC HEALTH IN TEACHING, LEARNING, AND EVALUATION

Much of the clinical faculty responsibility is creating learning situations that facilitate public health learning outcomes. Clinical experiences can be developed in an educational culture that encourages partnerships with resources and support. Creating positive relationships with agency staff is an essential faculty skill. Because of the nature of clinical experiences related to public health, many of the experiences are mentored. For students to have positive experiences and therefore develop an interest in public health, they must have meaningful, engaging learning experiences. The importance of positive learning environments cannot be overstated. Because of the rural locations or nature of the public health experiences, students may be without peers or faculty present in the agency. If students do not feel welcomed by staff who convey that they want them there, and are willing to help them learn, they will have a less than optimal learning experience. Positive relationships with clinical agency

staff assist nurse educators in planning learning and receiving student performance evaluations.

Created and simulated learning experiences require a great deal of time and coordination between academic and administrative departments at the university and community agencies. Faculty who teach these types of clinical experiences must be flexible, have excellent organizational abilities, and be able to make adjustments quickly. When such a large number and variety of people and agencies are involved with learning, rescheduling or changing plans is almost a certainty. So that students are not overwhelmed, the faculty ensures that all plans and changes are clearly communicated to students and that expectations are clear. Being actively engaged in university committees that are involved in the wellness program and emergency management are crucial to planning the wellness screenings and the disaster drill. Much work done by these committees has positively impacted the university and created excellent learning opportunities for the students that continue to improve.

Faculty, fully engaged in the faculty role, continue to develop while teaching. In addition to competence attainment for specialty practice, faculty members can use evidence-based teaching, learning, and evaluation practices. Although the latter task may seem daunting, attempting and refining select teaching practices through the annual review process builds one's expertise. The authors of this chapter have summarized essential teaching resources to strengthen development of learning and evaluating public health nursing content and experiences. Clearly these are fostered in a civil, healthy work environment.

CONCLUSION

Critical to developing a future public health nursing workforce is the response of nursing education programs to public health needs. While acknowledging barriers to preparing fully specialized public health nurses, nursing faculty are encouraged to address the basic elements in all nursing programs. Through a review of major national documents used as a public health approach framework, evidence-based teaching and learning strategies are shared. Most have been developed over decades with seasoned faculty and willing students.

An overview of faculty and curriculum activities includes decisions to be made at the program, course, and learning experiences levels. Specific learning strategies such as the clinical self-assessment journal, simulation, and clinical experiences that foster clinical reasoning and judgment while incorporating public health concepts and nursing roles are discussed. Student knowledge, skills, and aptitudes development as public health nurses are encouraged in each learning experience.

A major goal of teaching public health nursing is shifting the learner's thinking paradigm from a local to a global world view. Equally important is relating that global world view back to the local level. In other words, the world is now local. Strategies are discussed using these concepts: healthcare missions, culture of poverty, global learning, systems thinking, and debriefing. By using a variety of community agencies and experiences, students see the network of agencies, organizations, professionals, and others in the communities that comprise the local public health system.

In Boyer's (1990) work on models of scholarship, he describes the scholarship of integration that illuminates the faculty role in teaching public health nursing, "making connections across the disciplines, placing the specialties in larger context, illuminating data in a revealing way . . . what we mean is serious, disciplined work that seeks to interpret, draw together, and bring new insight to bear on original research" (pp. 18–19).

> The connectedness of things is what the educator contemplates to the limit of his capacity. No human capacity is great enough to permit a vision of the world as simple, but if the educator does not aim at the vision no one else will, and the consequences are dire when no one does. (Mark Van Doren, in Boyer, 1990, p. 19)

Public health and nursing are both complex disciplines. Integration of the knowledge of both is necessary for the nurse educator teaching public health nursing. Nurses need the skills to look at entire systems and see how they affect populations and individuals.

References

American Nurses Association. (2003). *Nursing's social policy statement* (2nd ed.). Silver Spring, MD: Author.

American Nurses Association. (2007). *Public health nursing: Scope and standards of practice*. Silver Spring, MD: Author.

American Public Health Association. (1996). *The definition and role of public health nursing: A statement of the APHA public health nursing section, March 1996 update*. Washington, DC: Author.

Association of Community Health Nursing Educators. (2000). *Essentials of baccalaureate nursing education for entry level community/public health nurses*. Pensacola, FL: Author.

Association of Community Health Nursing Educators. (2003). *Essentials of master's level nursing education for advanced community/public health nursing practice*. Lathrop, NY: Author.

Bambini, D., Washburn, J., & Perkins, R. (2009). Outcomes of clinical simulation for novice nursing students: Communication, confidence, clinical judgment. *Nursing Education Perspectives*, *30*(2), 79–82.

Benner, P., Stannard, D., & Hooper, P. L. (1996). A "thinking-in-action" approach to teaching clinical judgment: A classroom innovation for acute care advanced practice nurses. *Advanced Practice Nursing Quarterly*, *1*(4), 70–77.

Boutain, D. M. (2005). Social justice as a framework for professional nursing. *Journal of Nursing Education*, *44*(9), 405–408.

Boutain, D. M. (2008). Social justice as a framework for undergraduate community health clinical experiences in the United States. *International Journal of Nursing Education Scholarship*, *5*(1), 1–12.

Boyer, E. L. (1990). Scholarship reconsidered: Priorities of the professoriate. San Francisco: Jossey-Bass.

Carter, K. F., Kaiser, K. L., O'Hare, P. A., & Callister, L. C. (2006). Use of PHN competencies and ACHNE essentials to develop teaching–learning strategies for generalist C/PHN curricula. *Public Health Nursing*, *23*(2), 146–160.

Cato, M. L., Lasater, K., & Peeples, I. (2009). Nursing students' self-assessment of their simulation experiences. *Nursing Education Perspectives*, *30*(2), 105–108.

Cohen, B. E., & Gregory, D. (2009a). Community health clinical education in Canada. Part 1. "State of the art." *International Journal of Nursing Education Scholarship*, *6*(1), 1–17.

Cohen, B. E., & Gregory, D. (2009b). Community health clinical education in Canada. Part 2. Developing competencies to address social justice, equity, and the social determinants of health. *International Journal of Nursing Education Scholarship*, *6*(1), 1–15.

Community-Campus Partnerships for Health. (1998). *Principles of good community-campus partnerships*. Retrieved April 19, 2009, from http://depts.Washington.edu/ccph/principles.html#principles

Council on Linkages Between Academia and Public Health Practice. (2001). *Core competencies for public health professionals*. Washington, DC: Public Health Foundation.

Craft, M. (2005). Reflective writing and nursing education. *Journal of Nursing Education*, *44*(2), 53–57.

Davies, P. (2002). Using student reflective self-assessment for awarding degree classifications. *Innovations in Education and Teaching International*, *39*(4), 307–319.

DeLashmutt, M. B., & Rankin, E. A. (2005). A different kind of clinical experience: Poverty up close and personal. *Nurse Educator*, *30*(4), 143–149.

Dreifuerst, K. T. (2009). The essentials of debriefing in simulation learning: A concept analysis. *Nursing Education Perspectives*, *30*(2), 109–114.

Finkelman, A., & Kenner, C. (2007). *Teaching IOM: Implications of the Institute of Medicine reports for nursing education*. Silver Spring, MD: American Nurses Association.

Fitzpatrick, J. (2006). An evaluative case study of the dilemmas experienced in designing a self-assessment strategy for community nursing students. *Assessment & Evaluation in Higher Education*, *31*(1), 37–53.

Institute of Medicine [IOM]. (1988). *The future of public health*. Washington, DC: National Academies Press.

Institute of Medicine [IOM]. (2003). *The future of public health in the 21st century*. Washington, DC: National Academies Press.

Jeffries, P. R., & Rogers, K. J. (2007). Theoretical framework for simulation design. In P. R. Jeffries (Ed.), *Simulation in nursing: From conceptualization to evaluation* (pp. 21–33). New York: National League for Nursing.

Kuiper, R., Heinrich, C., Matthias, A., Graham, M. J., & Bell-Kotwell, L. (2008). Debriefing with the OPT model of clinical reasoning during high fidelity patient simulation. *International Journal of Nursing Education Scholarship*, 5(1), Article 17.

Landry, L. G., & Stockton, A. (2008). Evaluation of a collaborative project in disaster preparedness. *Nurse Educator*, 33(6), 254–258.

Lasater, K. (2007a). Clinical judgment development: Using simulation to create an assessment rubric. *Journal of Nursing Education*, 46(11), 496–503.

Lasater, K. (2007b). High-fidelity simulation and the development of clinical judgment: Students' experiences. *Journal of Nursing Education*, 46(6), 269–276.

Lasater, K., & Nielsen, A. (2009). Reflective journaling for clinical judgment development. *Journal of Nursing Education*, 48(1), 40–44.

Lawler, K. B. (2008). *Service-learning and the development of professional nursing values in adult undergraduate students*. Retrieved April 18, 2009, from http://proquest.umi.com/pqdweb?index=null&did=1609700001&SrchMode=5&Fmt=2&re

Maclellan, E., & Soden, R. (2006). Facilitating self-regulation in higher education through self-report. *Learning Environments Research*, 9, 95–110.

Nicol, D. J., & Macfarlane-Dick, D. (2006). Formative assessment and self-regulated learning: A model and seven principles of good feedback practice. *Studies in Higher Education*, 31(2), 199–218.

Nielsen, A., Stragnell, S., & Jester, P. (2007). Guide for reflection using the clinical judgment model. *Journal of Nursing Education*, 46(11), 513–516.

Payne, R. K., DeVol, P. E., & Smith, T. D. (2001). *Bridges out of poverty: Strategies for professionals and communities*. Highlands: AHA Process, Inc.

Pesut, D. J. (2004). Reflective clinical reasoning. In L. Hayes, H. Butcher, & T. Boese (Eds.), *Nursing in contemporary society* (pp. 146–162). Upper Saddle River, NJ: Pearson-Prentice Hall.

Roberts, M. M. (1954). *American nursing: History and interpretation*. New York: Macmillan.

Quad Council of Public Health Nursing Organizations. (1999). *Scope and standards of public health nursing practice*. Washington, DC: American Nurses Association.

Quad Council of Public Health Nursing Organizations. (2004). Public health nursing competencies. *Public Health Nursing*, 21(5), 443–452.

Shultz, C. M. (Ed.). (2009a). *Building a science of nursing education: Foundation for evidence based teaching-learning*. New York: National League for Nursing.

Shultz, C. M. (2009b, April/May). Preparing to work in an informatics-based world. *Imprint*, 36–39.

Tanner, C.A. (2006). Thinking like a nurse: A research-based model of clinical judgment. *Journal of Nursing Education*, 45(6), 204–211.

Turnock, B. J. (1997). *Public health: What it is and how it works*. Gaithersburg, MD: Aspen.

Veenema, T. G. (2006). Expanding educational opportunities in disaster response and emergency preparedness for nurses. *Nursing Education Perspectives*, 27(2), 93–99.

GLOSSARY

A

advocacy: Acting on someone's behalf with the intention to ultimately build the capacity of the individual, family, community, or system so that they may ultimately support their own cause.

agent: That which causes or contributes to a health problem or condition. The agent may be infectious, chemical, or physical, and is one of the parts of the epidemiological triangle.

age-specific rate: Provides information about a disease for a particular age group.

American Red Cross: The lead emergency response agency in United States, founded by Clara Barton in 1881.

analytic epidemiology: Illustrates the causal relationship between a risk factor and a specific disease or health condition. It seeks to answer the questions how and why with regard to the cause of a disease and the effects.

assessment: The process of gathering data from a wide variety of sources and critically analyzing that data to identify strengths and weaknesses and to prioritize the weaknesses.

assurance: Requires that public health agencies provide needed services and that the services are guaranteed for those unable to afford them.

attack rate: The incidence of a disease in a particular population over a period of time. This is important for the study of a single disease outbreak or epidemic during a short time period.

B

Black Death: The second recorded pandemic of the disease known as the *bubonic plague* swept across Europe from Central Asia in the fourteenth century, causing millions of deaths and devastating entire villages.

C

case finding: Actions and activities that help the healthcare professional locate individuals and families with identified risk factors and/or active disease and connect them with resources.

case management: Activities and actions that facilitate the seamlessness of a system's operation, thereby enhancing the capacity of the system. A system functioning at maximum capacity enhances the coordination and provision of services that optimize self-care of an individual and family.

chain of infection: Description of how an infectious disease results from the interaction between and among the agent, host, and environment. Transmission, direct or indirect, of an infectious agent takes place after the agent leaves its *reservoir* (host) by a *portal of exit*, such as the mouth when coughing. The agent then enters the *susceptible host* via a *portal of entry*, such as a skin wound, to infect the susceptible host.

coalition building: Promotes and develops partnerships among agencies and organizations for a common purpose. The coalition, via the partnership, serves to bring about change as all members work together toward the common vision and solve problems or enhance an already existing healthcare initiative.

collaboration: The working together of two or more individuals or organizations to achieve a common goal.

community health nurse: Any nurse who works in the community setting and focuses on the health of the community.

community organizing: Activities that bring together various community groups with a common goal and mobilize resources in the identified community to develop, implement, and evaluate the outcome of their initiative as they work collectively.

consultation: Interactive problem solving with a community, system, family, or individual that generates optimal and optional solutions to issues.

core functions of public health: Assessment, policy development, and assurance. Each of the functions requires a specific set of skills to ensure that the ten essential services that fall under the three core functions are accomplished.

counseling: An interpersonal relationship between a health professional and a community, system, family, or individual with the intention to increase self-care and coping.

crude rates: Measure of the experience of an entire population in a specific area with the certain disease or condition being investigated.

culturally competent care: A healthcare provider's set of attitudes and behaviors that takes into account a client's or population's cultural beliefs, values, health practices, and ways of behaving in social interactions, which may differ widely from the expectations of the healthcare provider.

culture: The lifeways, folkways, rituals, taboos, and practices of a group of people who share symbols, values, and patterns of behavior.

D

data: Discrete elements or entities that are objective and that have not been interpreted.

database: A system or structure that allows for data to be stored in an organized way so that it may be easily accessed.

data mining: Discerning patterns and relationships from large aggregate data sources.

delegation: Direct care tasks a registered professional nurse carries out under the authority of another healthcare practitioner as permitted by law. Delegation also includes any direct care tasks a registered professional nurse entrusts to other appropriate personnel to perform while still being responsible for that task.

descriptive epidemiology: The extent of an outbreak in terms of *who* gets the disease, *where* the disease occurs, and *when* the disease occurred. It is concerned with the acquisition of information about the occurrence of states of health, such as characteristics of person, place, and time. Descriptive epidemiology is essential for the description of the characteristics of disease occurrence and in the development of a hypothesis.

disaster: A sudden, devastating occurrence within a community that demands a nursing and medical response.

discrimination: The process by which people are treated differently because they are members of a particular group. Particular -*isms* such as racism (bias against racial and ethnic groups), sexism (bias against women), ageism (bias against elders), heterosexism (bias against gays and lesbians), ableism (bias against disabled), and classism (bias against class) are forms of discrimination.

disease and health event investigation: The systematic collection and analysis of data about a threat to a population that ascertains the source of the threat, identifies cases and others at risk, determines strategic measures for action, and evaluates outcomes.

district nurse: A mid-nineteenth century English term that refers to a nurse whose main focus was caring for the sick poor in their homes.

E

emergency preparedness: Completion of the steps and actions to prepare for unexpected emergency situations and to be able to deal with the emergency as it is taking place as well as in its aftermath.

environment: A factor that is considered extrinsic, which has an effect on the agent and the opportunity for exposure. It is one of the parts of the epidemiologic triangle.

epidemiology: The scientific discipline that studies the distribution and determinants of diseases and injuries in human populations.

epidemiological triad: The traditional model of infectious disease causation. The triad has thee components: the agent, the host, and the environment.

Essentials of Baccalaureate Nursing Education: A publication that identifies the framework for designing and assessing professional practice nursing education programs.

essentials of public health: The 10 essential public health services includes responsibilities of local public health systems as well as strategies necessary for building a healthy, integrated public health system capable of facilitating the health of the public.

ethnocentrism: The interpretation of the world according to the norms of one's own culture.

evidence-based medicine: The application of research evidence as the best evidence to guide decision-making. The term was first developed and used by medical professionals and was noted to be the new way of medical practice.

evidence-based practice: A systematic framework for decision-making that uses the best available evidence in conjunction with the professional's expertise and the client's values and preferences to guide problem solving about how to best approach a situation.

G

gross domestic product: The overall measure of a nation's economic standing in terms of the market value of the total output of goods and services produced in that nation for a given period of time.

H

health disparities: Gaps in health care related to the existence and the quality of health care for individuals, families, populations, communities, and systems.

health literacy: The degree to which individuals have the capacity to obtain, process, and understand basic health information and services needed to make appropriate health decisions.

health promotion: A primary level of prevention that includes strategies and behaviors that an individual engages in to enhance health. These strategies are not focused on any one particular disease, but rather focus on the individual, family, or population's overall health and optimal level of wellness.

health teaching: The communication of knowledge, facts, ideas, and skills that change competencies, attitudes, values, beliefs, behaviors, and practices of individuals, families, communities, and systems.

Healthy People 2010: A comprehensive, nationwide health promotion and disease prevention agenda that serves as a roadmap for improving the health of all people in the United States.

Healthy People 2020: A collaborative process that will build from the goals and objectives set forth in Healthy People 2010.

home care nurse: A nurse who provides care to individuals and families across the health continuum within their homes.

host: Individual affected by intrinsic factors and environmental exposure, susceptibility, and/or response to a causative agent. It is one part of the epidemiologic triangle.

I

incidence rates: The number of new cases of a specified disease reported during a given time interval.

income inequity: Describes where wealth is concentrated and who controls the wealth in society. Income inequality measures the degree of income variation in a population.

information: Data that is interpreted, organized, and structured.

information technology: The study, development, and implementation of computer-based technology that the healthcare professional can use to access information; identify information for best practice; and apply technology in educational initiatives, communication, and in the support of research.

Institute of Medicine Reports for Nursing Education: Publication based on the series of IOM reports aimed at improving the safety and overall quality of health care in the United States that addresses areas of interest to nurse educators in preparing students in public health.

K

knowledge: Information that is synthesized so that relationships are identified and formalized.

L

life-course model: A model that suggests that the socioeconomic position of the family during childhood affects the child's health status, educational choices, and occupational choices in the future.

M

maintaining health: Engagement in activities that sustain an individual's present level of health.

morbidity rate: The rate of illness, injury, or disability in a population (i.e., the number of people ill during a time period divided by the number of people in the total population).

mortality: A measure of the frequency of occurrence of death in a defined population during a specified interval.

multilevel analysis: An analysis necessary to understand all of the factors that contribute to disease. In a multilevel analysis, all factors are examined on an individual level and on an environmental level, such as a neighborhood, community, city, state, and so forth.

N

nursing informatics: The integration of nursing science, computer science, and information science to manage and communicate data, information, knowledge, and wisdom in nursing practice.

O

outreach: The process of locating individuals, families, and/or populations of interest for the purpose of information dissemination and/or provision of service.

P

participant observation: A technique in which the nurse makes careful observations of specific processes, actions, or communications while providing care as a participant in the activity.

payer: Third-party responsible for providing reimbursement dollars for the costs of health care.

policy development and enforcement: Actions and activities that place health issues on decision makers' agendas, acquire a plan of resolution, and determine needed resources. Policy development results in laws, rules, regulations, ordinances, and policies. Policy enforcement compels others to comply with the laws, rules, regulations, ordinances, and policies created in conjunction with policy development.

policymaker: Individual involved in decision making in the legislative, executive, or judicial branches of government.

population: A group of individuals who share specific characteristics such as social, physical, cultural, economic, or environmental characteristics.

population-focused care: Application of intervention wheel strategies that will access and provide care to a specific population.

population perspective: Viewpoint that suggests that an individual's risk for health problems cannot be isolated from the community in which he or she resides or from the population or society in which he or she belongs.

prevalence rate: A measure of the number of people in a given population who have a specific existing condition at a given point in time.

primary prevention: Actions taken to prevent disease and/or injury and require strategies including health promotion and specific protection.

provider: One who delivers services to individuals and populations with a margin of profit.

public health: Both a science and an art that assures the public's health by engaging in interventions that promote health and prevent disease, prolonging life through organized community efforts.

public health informatics: The systematic application of information, computer science, and technology to public health practice and learning.

public health nurse: A term coined by Lillian Wald in the early twentieth century that describes the work of the visiting nurse who cares for the sick at home and provides health promotion and disease prevention measures in the community. The work of the public health nurse is population focused and takes place on three practice levels: individual/family, community, and system.

purchaser: An individual, group, or organization that purchases health insurance benefits.

Q

quarantine: The isolation of a contagious individual from the remainder of the population.

R

rate: The primary measurement used to describe the occurrence of a health problem. It is a measure of the frequency of a health-related event in a specific population within a given period of time. A rate consists of a numerator and a denominator and calculated by dividing the number of conditions or events of time, and multiplying by a base multiple of 10.

referral and follow-up: Actions and activities that serve to assist individuals, families, and/or populations by connecting them to needed services for possible treatments and other resources, including follow-up to identify outcomes.

risk: The probability that an event will occur within a specific time period.

risk reduction: Completion of specific strategies designed to reduce risk or the probability that an event will occur.

ritual: An act often associated with key life events. It may enhance joy, as in the case of celebratory traditions such as weddings and holidays; provide a sense of comfort, as in the case of death and dying; or promote a gracious lifestyle, as exemplified by table manners and the offering of food to guests.

S

screening: A strategy of the Intervention Wheel that serves to identify individuals with disease who are asymptomatic or those individuals with health risk factors.

secondary prevention: Strategies that facilitate early detection of disease, thus resulting in early diagnosis, early treatment, and prevention of spread to others as well and long-term disability. An example of secondary prevention would be screening.

service learning: A hands-on approach to education where community service, instruction, and reflection serve as a meaningful learning experience.

social capital: Social resources such as parks, medical facilities, schools, and economic investments that are needed to ensure that communities have the resources to maintain health.

social context: A guiding concept of social epidemiology. The social context of behavior addresses individual behavioral risk factors such as smoking and drinking and examines these behaviors in a larger social context, or examines the social influences or conditions that contribute to specific behaviors.

social epidemiology: The study of epidemiology that deals with social distribution and social determinants of health and disease. Social epidemiology makes the case that social determinants of health, which con-

sist of socioeconomic status (income, occupation, and education), socioeconomic position, and discrimination, can influence health outcomes.

social justice: Justice as it is considered and applied to every aspect of society and to every member of society.

social marketing: Actions and activities that operationalize social marketing principles and the application of appropriate technology for program design with the expressed purpose of influencing the knowledge, attitudes, values, beliefs, behaviors, and practices of a population of interest.

socioeconomic position: Determined by an individual's socioeconomic status. How much money an individual has, his or her educational attainment, and his or her occupation have a bearing on and reflect the individual's socioeconomic position, or standing in society.

socioeconomic status: Consists of family income, educational level, and occupation.

Spanish Influenza: An epidemic of 1918–1919 (caused by the virus H1N1) that developed towards the end of World War I and was estimated to have caused a global mortality of between 50 and 100 million.

specific protection: Considered in the primary level of prevention, it focuses on a particular disease and/or injury and the prevention of those situations before they take form by stopping the causal event. Examples of these actions include immunizations, environmental sanitation, and nutrition.

state-sanctioned control measures: Government-implemented measures to control the spread of a disease. During the Black Death, Italian city states were at particular risk. These states were the first to introduce systematic measures to protect their populations from plague.

surveillance: The monitoring of health events and the facilitation of the ongoing systematic collection, analysis, interpretation, and evaluation of data for the purpose of planning, implementing, and evaluating public health initiatives.

T

teaching–learning strategy: Method of education to meet the needs of and enhance the learning of a specific individual, family, community, population, or system.

tertiary prevention: Strategies that stop a disease from progressing and prevent further disability. An example of tertiary prevention is rehabilitation and education on maximum use of an individual's capabilities, thus supporting their human capital.

the 5 A's: A framework for the healthcare practitioner to use when working with populations at the individual/family, community, and systems levels of practice to assess how well the population can gain entry into needed resources and use those resources with ultimate positive outcomes.

the 5 P's principal participants: The various interests of the stakeholders involved in the delivery and financing of health care as well as the competition between and among the stakeholders.

V

visiting nurse: A term used interchangeably with district nursing in the United States, this term refers to the trained nurse who provided care for the sick public in their homes.

vulnerable populations: A group of individuals who are at greater risk than other populations and who also share specific characteristics such as social, physical, cultural, economic, or environmental characteristics.

X

xenophobia: The conscious fear of foreigners.

CHAPTER OPENER PHOTO CREDITS

Chapter 1: Courtesy of the Visiting Nurse Service of New York.

Chapter 2: Courtesy of the Visiting Nurse Service of New York.

Chapter 3: Photograph Collection, Center for the Study of Nursing Historical Inquiry, University of Virginia School of Nursing.

Chapter 3 Appendix: U.S. Department of Health and Human Services, 2000.

Chapter 4: Courtesy of the Visiting Nurse Service of New York.

Chapter 5: Courtesy of the Visiting Nurse Service of New York.

Chapter 6: Courtesy of the Visiting Nurse Service of New York.

Chapter 7: Courtesy of the Visiting Nurse Service of New York.

Chapter 8: Charlottesville-Albemarle Public Health Nursing, Imogene Bunn Collection: University of Virginia.

Chapter 9: Courtesy of the Visiting Nurse Service of New York.

Chapter 10: Courtesy of the Visiting Nurse Service of New York.

Chapter 11: Courtesy of the Visiting Nurse Service of New York.

Chapter 12: Courtesy of the Visiting Nurse Service of New York.

Chapter 13: U.S. National Library of Medicine, Images from the History of Medicine.

Chapter 14: © National Library of Medicine.

Chapter 15: Courtesy of the Visiting Nurse Service of New York.

Chapter 16: Courtesy of the Visiting Nurse Service of New York.

INDEX

Italicized page locators indicate a figure; tables are noted with a *t*.

A

Absolute income inequality, 110
Abuse
  of frail elderly, 241
  women, gender-appropriate
    behavior and, 168
Acceptability, access and, 61, 81*t*
Access, to technology,
  150–152
Access to care
  assessing, 257
  PHNAT tables and assess the
    seven A's, 81*t*
Action research, 170
Active surveillance, TB
  control and, 208
Actors, in public health
  system, 6, 7
Acute diseases, incidence rate
  and, 98*t*
Acute pulmonary
  tuberculosis, 207
Adaptability, technology and,
  150–152
Addiction, 250
Adequacy, access and, 61, 81*t*
Adolescence, regular physical
  activity during, 291
Adolescent juvenile offenders,
  intervention programs
  for, 176

Adolescents, overweight, 287
Adolescent smokers, quit
  attempts among, 128
Adults
  body mass index-defined
    categories for, 287
  obesity among, 287
Advanced practice nursing
  community, standards
  developed by, 351
Advanced practice public
  health nurse, 49
Advocacy, 286, 287, 293, 301
Advocacy case management,
  294 (box 12–2)
Advocacy interventions, 224
Affordability, access and,
  61, 81*t*
African American
  adolescents, culture, drug
    abuse, and sexually risky
    behaviors among, 176
African American nurses,
  marginalization of, 29–30
African Americans
  cancer rates among, 143
  physical inactivity issues
    and, 273
  rural domestic violence
    project and, 179
  Texas City ship explosion,
    1947 and, 335
African American women,
  participant observation in
  study about cocaine use
  by, 170–171

Age, in analytical
  epidemiology, 100
Ageism, 111
Agency for Healthcare
  Research and Quality, 126,
  142 (box 6–1), 196
Agent, 204
  in epidemiological triad,
    101, *101*
Age-specific rates,
  96, 98*t*
Aging, biological
  determinants of health
  and, 253
AHRQ. *See* Agency for
  Healthcare Research and
  Quality
AIDS, 95, 118, 169, 173, 307,
  320, 360, 379
  awareness campaigns on,
    318–319, 320
  in contemporary Britain,
    316–319, 320
  prevention of, 317
  transmission of, 317
Air pollution, 148
Alaska earthquake of 1964,
  336–339
Alcoholics Anonymous, 169
Altice, F., 189
Altman, D., 4
American Academy of
  Nursing, 172
American Association
  of Colleges of
  Nursing, 50